KETTLEBELL
AND CH...

Kettlebell wor...
Beginner to advance... ...natives.

With links to videos

40+ WORKOUTS WODS

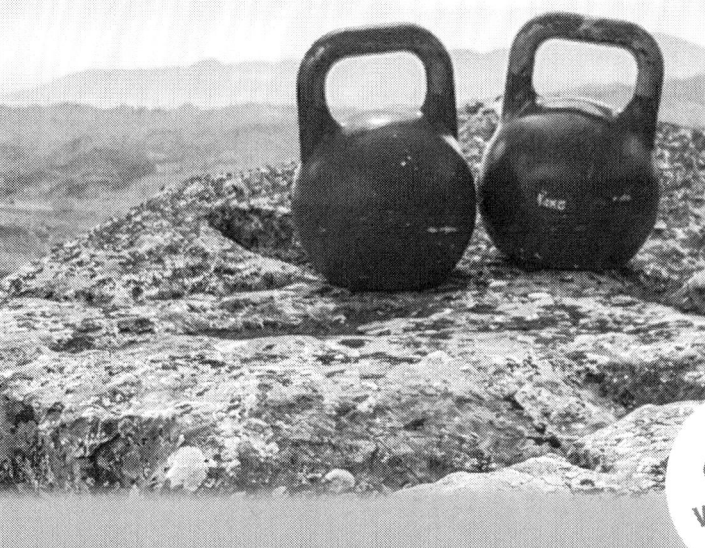

By Taco Fleur
Cavemantraining.com

Cardio. Strength. Endurance. Flexibility...

Kettlebell Workouts and Challenges 2.0
Designed and written by the owner of Cavemantraining

Workouts that have a story. Workouts that motivate. Workouts that can be adjusted.

In this book I provide an adventure, a story, motivation, education, the best workouts, all combined. I include photos of my own adventures to give you the sense to want to explore, to make you feel like you were there. All photos are real there is no photoshop or tricks, if you see me on a 3,500 meter high mountain with a kettlebell, I lugged it there, if you see me under a waterfall with a kettlebell, I climbed down and in the process might have unintentionally hurt a kettlebell or two.

This book is targeted to **at-home kettlebell enthusiasts**, **MMA** and **BJJ** fighters, and **crossfitters** that use their open box time for kettlebell WODs. This book is even for budding trainers who want to know more about the *Cavemantraining* programs, and learn the basics on how to run them.

40+ serious kettlebell workouts and several kettlebell challenges, many paired with very detailed videos.

- Beginners to advanced workouts.
- How to score AMRAP workouts.
- Finer details on many of the exercises.
- Quality emphasis on warming-up and mobility.
- Full details of the popular *Thorax Workout* included in this book.
- Additional ideas on how to make your WODs even more popular and exciting.
- Additional little tips and information for personal trainers.

Each workout is either 100% kettlebells, combined with bodyweight, or other equipment. Most workouts will have alternatives and progressions.

40+ kettlebell workouts designed with passion, for beginners and hardcore kettlebellers. Workouts that will make you feel good, look good, stronger, more flexible, fitter, or simply make you want to cry.

"These are not shoddy quick workouts put together for a book. I've performed each and every workout listed in this book, and so have hundreds of others."
—*Taco Fleur*

I highly recommend to just read the whole book first, even if you're at beginner level, and then pick a workout. After reading all of the information the workouts will make more sense to you. Remember, I'm always available for questions.

The title is prefixed with 2.0 as we'll be putting out plenty more books with new workouts. If you are a beginner I recommend one of the following resources to help you get a better understanding of the kettlebell and train with ease:

- *Kettlebell Guide for Beginners* (available on Amazon https://amzn.to/2WLEFwf)
- *Kettlebell Training Fundamentals* (Amazon https://amzn.to/2WygRvA)
- *21-Days to Kettlebell Training for Beginners DVD* (Amazon https://amzn.to/2WzkIsa)
- *21-Days to Kettlebell Training for Beginners Online Course* (Udemy http://bit.ly/udemy-kb-beginners)
- *21-Days to Kettlebell Training for Beginners Android App* (Google http://bit.ly/kb-beginners-app)

If you're interested in any of the above kettlebell resources, I've listed discount codes for 50% off toward the end of the book.

BONUS:

1. Information for trainers on how to run your own *Caveman Circuit,* and *Boot Camp*.
2. Downloadable workout PDF that can be printed and taken to the gym.
3. Downloadable kettlebell grip PDF that will improve your kettlebell training instantly.
4. Downloadable PDF that will improve your racking for resting and endurance.
5. Free kettlebell workouts mobile app for Android.

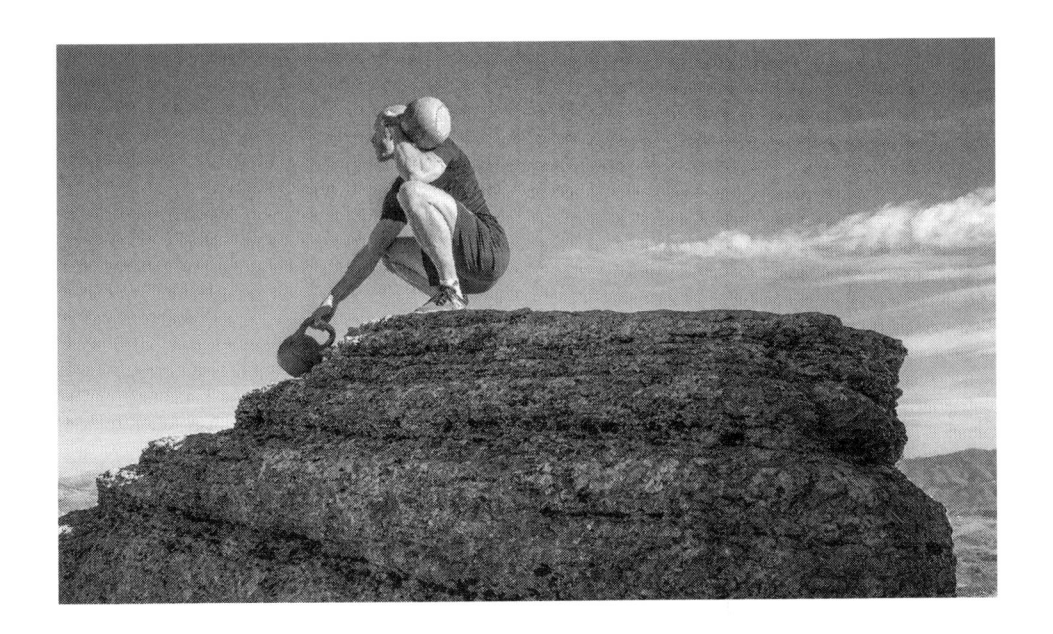

Nothing's ever perfect. Neither is this book. The great thing is, you can get answers by posting in one of our discussion groups. Not only will you get the answer you're looking for, you'll also be helping us improve the book. Since this book is electronically maintained, it allows us to update it frequently, which we do. You can see which revision the book is below. If our revision is more up to date, you can get a free copy of the new version. Simply email us your proof of purchase with a request for an updated copy of the book.

go.cavemantraining.com/kbwc-link20

Last updated: 4/12/19
Revision: 17

Flaws. Allow me to point out some flaws to you right off the bat. I've been writing and creating kettlebell books for a while, and as I progress I do take feedback onboard. In my earlier books I left photos out as the description for the exercises were there, it also had a video, and it's a workout book not a kettlebell exercise book, however, this time I added some screenshots from the videos to quickly give an idea of the movements. The screenshots are not of high quality but I know if you follow instructions in this book and read all workouts, you'll find that there is more than enough to get the details across. I previous books I had complex links that could not be typed easily, I'm now using easier links to type but they are case sensitive, so make sure you type them lower-case.

Free gift if you point out two grammar/spelling mistakes. Email me@tacofleur.com

Who/what is Cavemantraining?

Cavemantraining is a team of fitness experts, specializing in the field of kettlebells, who provide online education/certifications, weekly workouts, customized programming, and much more unconventional training resources worldwide. Cavemantraining runs a website with an enormous amount of free information, articles, interviews, mobile apps like KB workouts, KB exercises, and advanced variable workout timer, online courses, and also runs a highly popular *YouTube* channel. On social media you'll see Cavemantraining just about anywhere there is a kettlebell, or talk of unconventional training.

Some of Cavemantraining's most famous online programs and courses include:

- **Caveman Inner Circle**
  Private group of people who get a new workout each week and train with with me online
  http://bit.ly/online-kettlebell-workouts

- **Online Snatch Certification**
  Learn and get certified for the king of kettlebell exercises
  http://bit.ly/online-snatch-cert

- **Kettlebell Fundamentals Trainer L3.0**
  Online certification for kettlebell trainers that want to lay a foundation to become PRO
  http://bit.ly/online-certifications

- **Master The Kettlebell Clean**
  An online kettlebell course that teaches and certifies you for one of the most important kettlebell exercises
  http://bit.ly/online-clean-cert

- **From Zero To Kettlebell Superhero**
  An online kettlebell course for people at home who want to get started with kettlebells and learn how to avoid pains and aches
  www.cavemantraining.com/shop/online-training/zero-kettlebell-superhero-4-weeks/
  www.udemy.com/from-zero-to-kettlebell-superhero/

- **21-Days to Kettlebell Training for Beginners**
  An online kettlebell course to learn the ins and outs of kettlebell training
  www.udemy.com/kettlebell-training-for-beginners/

Popular social media channels:

- **Cavemantraining Magazine** Community
  www.facebook.com/Cavemantraining.Magazine/

- **Cavemantraining** Page
  www.facebook.com/Cavemantraining

- **Kettlebell Enthusiasts** Discussion group
  www.facebook.com/groups/kettlebell.enthusiasts/

- **Kettlebells For Complete Beginners** Discussion group
  www.facebook.com/groups/kettebells.for.beginners/

- **Kettlebell Workouts (new one each week)** Discussion group
  www.facebook.com/groups/kettlebell.workout/

- **Nothing but training matters—Cavemantraining** Discussion group
  www.facebook.com/groups/unconventional.training/

- **Fitness Motivational Quotes** Discussion group
  www.facebook.com/groups/fitness.motivational.quotes/

- **Kettlebell Swing** Discussion group
  www.facebook.com/groups/kettlebell.swing/

- **Kettlebell Training** Discussion group
  www.reddit.com/r/kettlebell_training

Thanks for buying the book *Kettlebell Workouts and Challenges*, I hope you'll achieve the same awesome results I've achieved from these workouts.

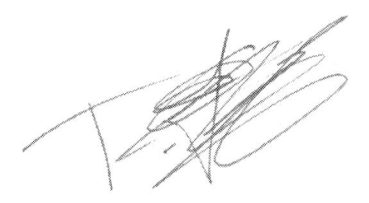

Printable Copy

Since this is a book, it's more detailed, has photos, links and much more. Hence, it's not suitable to print and take to the gym. So, I've created a plain PDF of just the workout info which you can download for free with the coupon code that's listed toward the end of the book.

Layout and structure of the book

After each workout or topic I end with a decorative line which looks as following, this allows you to recognize the end of one workout/topic, and the start of a new one.

About the Author

My name is Taco Fleur, and I'm an IKFF Certified Kettlebell Trainer, Russian Girevoy Sport Institute Kettlebell Coach, Kettlebell Level 1 + 2 Trainer, Kettlebell Science and Application, CrossFit Level 1 Trainer, MMA Conditioning Level 1, Kettlebell Sport IKMF Rank 2, MMA Fitness Level 1 + 2, Punchfit Trainer and Plyometrics Trainer Certified, with a purple belt in Brazilian Jiu-Jitsu. Featured in 4 issues of the Japanese Iron Man Magazine 2019. I have owned and set-up 3 functional kettlebell gyms in Australia and Vietnam, and lived in the Netherlands, Australia, Vietnam, and Thailand. I'm currently living in Spain.

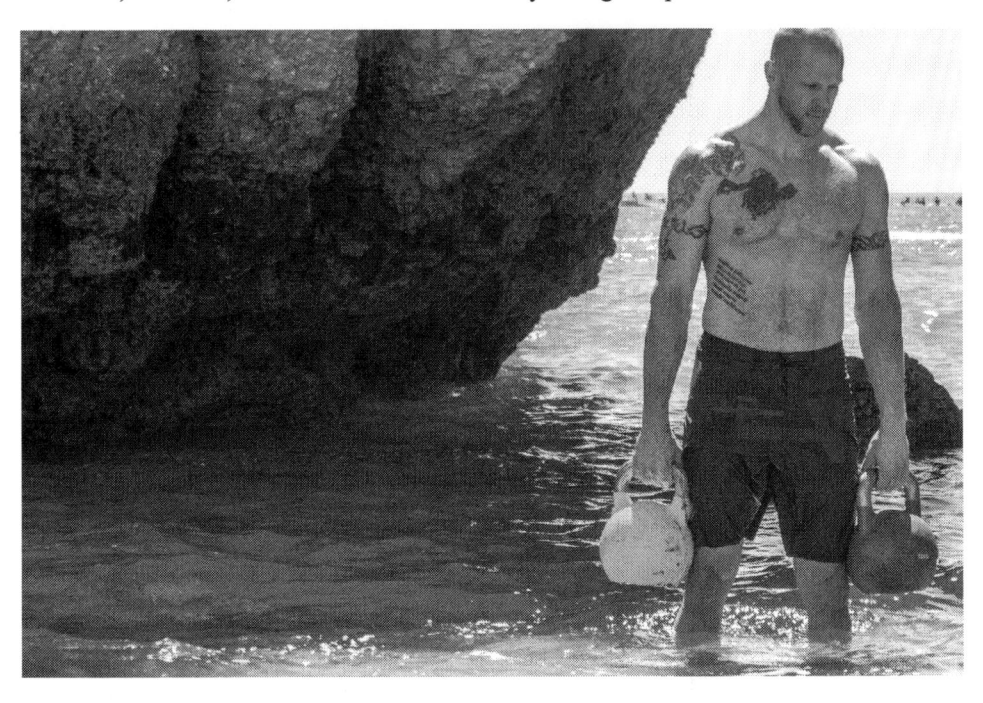

The first thing I'd like you to know about me is that I do **not** know everything, I don't pretend to know everything, and I never will. I'm on a path of life-long learning. I believe there is always something to learn from someone, no matter who they are. I've been physically active since the day I arrived on this earth in 1973. I got serious about training in 1999, touched a kettlebell for the first time in 2004, and got serious about kettlebell training in 2009. I'm here to do what I love most, and that is to share my knowledge with the world.

Some of my personal bests are 400 burpees performed in under one hour; 500 kettlebell snatches, 500 swings and 500 double-unders all completed in one session; 250 alternating dead clean and presses in one session with 20kg; 200 pull-ups in one session; 200 unbroken kettlebell swings with a 28kg; most kettlebell swings completed in one session with a 28kg (1,501); most total kettlebell swings done in 28 days with a 28kg (11,111); windmill with a 40kg kettlebell; lugged a kettlebell up a 1,184m mountain; 160kg dead lift; 250 alternating dead clean and presses in one session with 20kg; 100 snatches on sand with a 24kg kettlebell; 300 unbroken clean and jerk with 20kg/44lbs; 85kg Olympic Squat Snatch; Gold medalist with 30 minutes of unbroken 16kg half snatches for a total of 532 reps; and one of my favorites is lugging the first kettlebell up the highest mountain in mainland Spain 3,479m/11,414f with 16kg. I mention these PBs not to boast but to demonstrate that I have a good understanding of technique and movement across different areas. This demonstrates especially with the high reps, an area in which most commonly tearing of the hands occurs.

My own training and goals are geared around GPP (General Physical Preparedness) which involves kettlebell training, calisthenics, and CrossFit. I like high-volume reps but also like greasing the groove now and again. My main goals are to remains as agile as possible, remain mobile, train in as many planes of movements as possible, and learn as many different exercise combinations and movements as possible while having fun and enjoying Brazilian Jiu Jitsu. I'm no Arnold Schwarzenegger and never will be, but strength is not solely defined by physical appearance and huge bulging muscles.

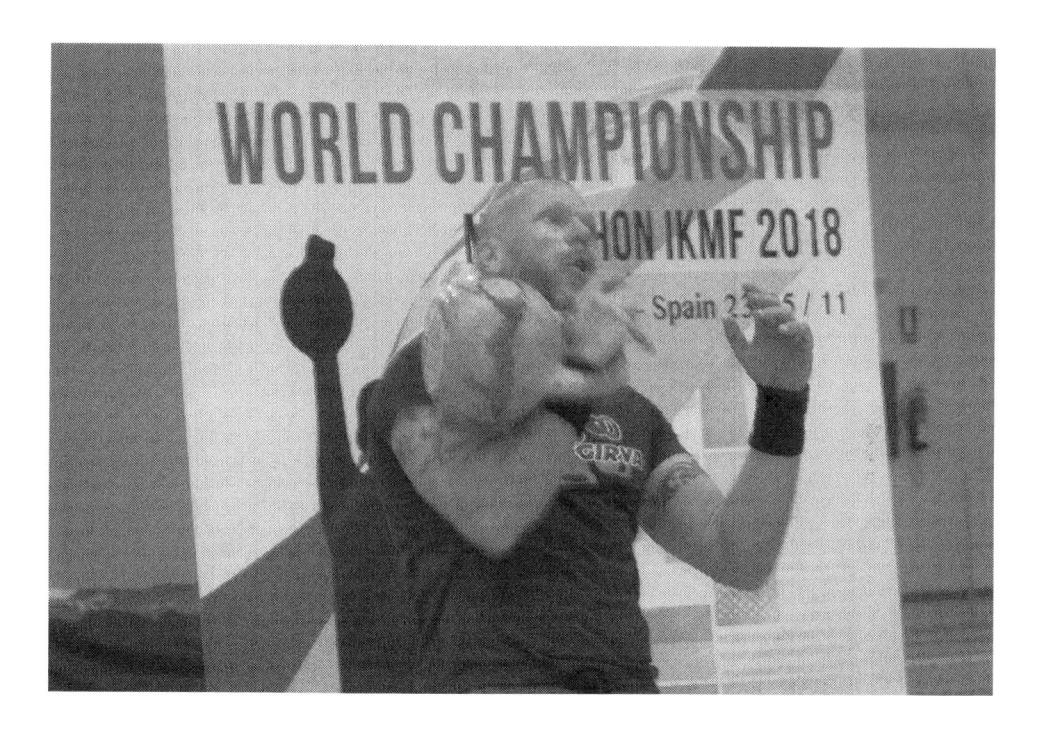

You can read more about my training, philosophy, and other ramblings on my website, www.cavemantraining.com, and on my YouTube channel, bit.ly/youtube-cavemantraining, which at the time of writing has over 35,000 subscribers and more than 6 million views.

SUBSCRIBE

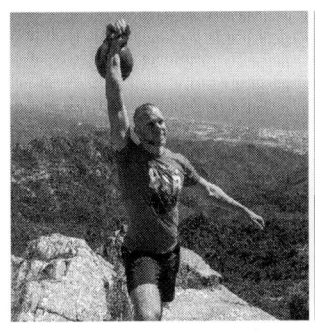

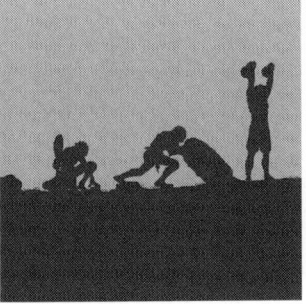

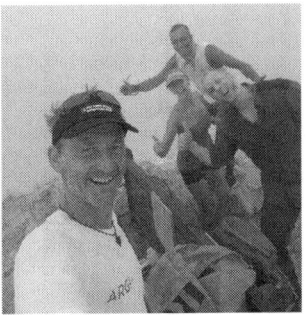

Add me: Facebook.com/taco.fleur or Facebook.com/coach.taco.fleur

Facebook.com/Cavemantraining or Facebook.com/Cavemantraining.Magazine
for up-to-date articles and news.

Please note that this material may not be reproduced or publicized elsewhere without the written consent of the author me@tacofleur.com.

If you bought this as a PDF/electronic copy, it is digitally signed and password protected with identifiable information.

All *Cavemantraining* owned images are copyrighted © Cavemantraining

Note: Most of the kettlebell stock images used in this book have literally been created with blood, sweat, and tears - I'm talking lugging kettlebells for hours up mountains, through canyons, running out of water, etc. Please respect the effort that has gone into producing the photos.

Photos are available for purchase or in some cases made available for educational purposes with appropriate credits/links in return.

Table of Contents

About the Author 8
Workout Index 14
WOD Terminology 25

- How to Score AMRAP Workouts ... 29
  - How to Structure a Caveman WOD ... 33
  - Caveman Buddy System ... 38
- Warm-up and Mobility ... 40
  - Bodyweight warm-up routine ... 40
  - Warm-up and Mobility Exercises ... 42
    - Generic warm-up ... 43
- Kettlebell Workouts ... 45
  - The Man of Steel Workout ... 47
  - FUSION4.5 ... 52
  - Simple 8-minute Kettlebell Workout ... 55
  - Quicksilver Kettlebell Workout ... 58
  - Kettlebell Workout Nova ... 60
  - Iron Man Kettlebell Workout ... 63
    - Military press ... 66
  - MORTUUS GEMINUS 50 ... 68
  - David Keohan Kettlebell Workout ... 72
  - Procerus Fortis 14 ... 76
  - Clean and snatch Workout ... 83
  - 10 Minute Kettlebell Workout ... 85
  - 4 in 1 Kettlebell Workout ... 87
  - Kettlebell Snatch Workout ... 93
  - RKC Monster Workout ... 96
  - The Grinding Warrior ... 99
  - Killer. Killa. Workout ... 104
  - This workout will bring you to your knees! ... 106
  - The Undaunted Warrior ... 110
  - SHORT, HEAVY, AND EXPLOSIVE. ... 112
  - Short, But Insane. ... 114
  - Gorilla Blackback Workout ... 118
  - Roses and Babies 96 ... 121
  - Kettlebell Drop Set Shoulder Workout ... 126
  - Magnus Dorsi ... 129
  - Raven 3×5 100 ... 131
  - Kronos Workout ... 135
  - A Kick-Ass Lower-body Kettlebell Workout ... 140
  - Simple Kettlebell Cardio Workout ... 142
  - Simple Kettlebell Workout #2 ... 145
  - Quick Kettlebell Cardio Workout ... 152
  - ZATANNA ... 157
  - Armory Workout ... 161
  - Caveman Kettlebells Silverback Workout ... 166
  - Workout Mulhacén ... 182
  - The Best Upper-body Workout ... 186
  - Fourforty WOD ... 190
  - BBKB10-4 ... 193
  - Thorax Mobility Workout ... 195
  - World Kettlebell Video Workouts ... 217
    - WKV1 ... 218
    - Beginner ... 219

  Intermediate 220
  Advanced 220
  WKV2..221
  Beginner..221
  Intermediate 221
  Advanced 222
  WKV3..223
  Beginner..223
  Intermediate 224
  Advanced 224
Kettlebell Challenges...226
 300 Clean and Jerk Challenge..227
 11-Day Sots Press Challenge by Cavemantraining.....................................231
  Sots Press Tutorial 234
  Double Kettlebell Alternating Sots Press Tutorial 245
 The HULK Test 252
  Kettlebell Half Snatch...259
Kettlebell Training Instructions (fundamentals) 268
 Day 1 Warming up and priming for kettlebell training................................269
 Day 2 Stretching and mobility for kettlebell training 284
 Day 3 Kettlebell anatomy and grip 297
 Day 4 Safely lifting the kettlebell with a squat...299
 Day 5 Safely lifting the kettlebell with a hip hinge 302
 Day 6 Assisted kettlebell clean 305
 Day 7 Kettlebell squat swing 312
 Day 8 Kettlebell hip hinge swing..316
 Day 9 Kettlebell pendulum swing 321
 Day 10 Double arm swing clean 325
 Day 11 Kettlebell dead clean 330
 Day 12 Kettlebell swing clean 338
 Day 13 Kettlebell racking 342
 Day 14 Kettlebell pressing 345
 Day 15 Kettlebell rowing 348
 Day 16 Kettlebell American swing 351
 Day 17 Double kettlebell dead swing clean 354
 Day 18 Recap and additional kettlebell tips...358
 Day 19 Kettlebell programming and goals 360
 Day 20 Kettlebell workout 362
 Day 21 Common kettlebell injuries and annoyances 365
  Got back pain?..366
How To Kettlebell Swing...372
 What Muscles Are Used With The Kettlebell Swing?.................................373
 Hip Hinge Swing..379
 How To Swing 380
  The Single Arm Kettlebell Swing 383
  Kettlebell Squat Style Swing..383
  Kettlebell Sport Style Swing AKA Fluid Style 386
 Kettlebell Swing Clean Fluid 391
 Clean and Jerk (push press) 394
 Gorilla Cleans AKA Alternating Hang Cleans 401

Double Kettlebell Half Snatch 404
Full Snatch Fluid 409
Kettlebell Snatch Hardstyle 414
Kettlebell Halo 418
Bonus Content 421
Bonus: How to Design and Administer a Caveman Circuit 421
Bonus: How To Run Caveman Boot Camp 429
Difference Between 'Workout' and 'Complex'? 434
Looking for adventure? Add an experience! 436
Inspiration 437
VOUCHER CODES 439

Workout Index

Following is an index to all the workouts. Due to the way page numbers change based on whether this is an electronic or printed version of the book I can't provide page number here, please use the main index above to find the page numbers for each one.

The Man of Steel Workout

Level: Intermediate

Weight: Heavy

Kettlebell(s): 🔔🔔 (or 1 if you just do the workout)

Type: Strength and mobility

Duration: 40 minutes

Other: Full-body, legs, shoulders, back, chest; slow

FUSION4.5

Level: Intermediate to advanced

Weight: Medium to heavy

Kettlebell(s): 🔔🔔

Type: Strength, endurance, cardio, mobility

Duration: 27 minutes

Other: Full-body with emphases on the legs

Simple 8-minute Kettlebell Workout

Level: Beginner

Weight: Light to medium

Kettlebell(s): 🔔
Type: Cardio
Duration: 8 minutes
Other: Full-body

Quicksilver Kettlebell Workout

Level: Beginner to intermediate
Weight: Medium
Kettlebell(s): 🔔
Type: Cardio, endurance
Duration: 25 minutes
Other: Full-body with focus on the trapezius and gluteus maximus; high volume; FOR TIME

Kettlebell Workout Nova

Level: Advanced
Weight: Medium
Kettlebell(s): 🔔🔔
Type: Cardio, endurance, strength
Duration: 25 minutes
Other: Full-body with focus on core, legs, shoulders, and back; buy-in; FOR TIME

Iron Man Kettlebell Workout

Level: Intermediate
Weight: Medium
Kettlebell(s): 🔔🔔
Type: Cardio, endurance, strength
Duration: 35 minutes
Other: Full-body with focus on shoulders, core, and legs; AMRAP; buy-in

MORTUUS GEMINUS 50

Level: Intermediate
Weight: Medium
Kettlebell(s): 🔔🔔

Type: Cardio, endurance, strength
Duration: 8 minutes
Other: Full-body with focus on the legs and back; interval

David Keohan Kettlebell Workout

Level: Intermediate to advanced
Weight: Medium
Kettlebell(s):
Type: Cardio, endurance, strength, flexibility
Duration: 25 to 30 minutes
Other: Full-body; FOR TIME; AMRAP

Procerus Fortis 14

Level: Intermediate to advanced
Weight: Medium
Kettlebell(s):
Type: Strength
Duration: 14 minutes
Other: Full-body with focus on triceps, shoulders, upper back, and legs; EMOM

Clean and snatch Workout

Level: Intermediate
Weight: Medium
Kettlebell(s):
Type: Cardio and strength
Duration: 15 minutes
Other: Full-body with focus on the lower-body; FOR TIME

10 Minute Kettlebell Workout

Level: Intermediate to advanced
Weight: Medium
Kettlebell(s):
Type: Cardio, strength, and flexibility

Duration: 10 minutes
Other: Full-body with focus on the lower and upper-body; FOR TIME

4 in 1 Kettlebell Workout

Level: Intermediate
Weight: Medium
Kettlebell(s):
Type: Cardio, strength, and flexibility
Duration: 30 minutes
Other: Full-body; training; EMOM; AMRAP

Kettlebell Snatch Workout

Level: Intermediate
Weight: Medium
Kettlebell(s):
Type: Cardio and strength
Duration: 35 to 40 minutes
Other: Full-body with a focus on legs and cardio; FOR TIME; AMRAP

RKC Monster Workout

Level: Intermediate
Weight: Medium to heavy
Kettlebell(s):
Type: Cardio, strength, and power
Duration: 25 to 30 minutes
Other: Full-body with a focus on the upper back and legs; FOR TIME; AMRAP

The Grinding Warrior

Level: Intermediate to advanced
Weight: Medium
Kettlebell(s):
Type: Strength and flexibility
Duration: 22 to 25 minutes

Other: Full-body, training, slow

Killer. Killa. Workout
Level: Intermediate
Weight: Medium to heavy
Kettlebell(s):
Type: Cardio and strength
Duration: 30 to 40 minutes
Other: Full-body; buy-in; FOR TIME

This workout will bring you to your knees!
Level: Intermediate
Weight: Medium
Kettlebell(s):
Type: Cardio and endurance
Duration: 20 to 40 minutes
Other: Full-body; high reps

The Undaunted Warrior
Level: Intermediate
Weight: Medium
Kettlebell(s):
Type: Cardio and endurance
Duration: 30 to 40 minutes
Other: Full-body; high reps; Concept2; chipper

SHORT, HEAVY, AND EXPLOSIVE.
Level: Intermediate
Weight: Heavy
Kettlebell(s):
Type: Cardio and endurance
Duration: 12 minutes
Other: Full-body; low reps; barbell; AMRAP

Short, But Insane.
Level: Intermediate
Weight: Heavy
Kettlebell(s):
Type: Strength and power
Duration: 20 to 25 minutes
Other: Full-body; short

Gorilla Blackback Workout
Level: Advanced
Weight: Medium
Kettlebell(s):
Type: Strength
Duration: 20 minutes
Other: Full-body; low reps; AMRAP

Roses and Babies 96
Level: Intermediate
Weight: Medium
Kettlebell(s):
Type: Cardio
Duration: 20 to 30 minutes
Other: Full-body; Concept2; partner workout; interval; FOR TIME

Kettlebell Drop Set Shoulder Workout
Level: Beginners
Weight: Heavy
Kettlebell(s):
Type: Strength
Duration: 24 to 30 minutes
Other: Shoulders and triceps; upper-body; slow

Magnus Dorsi

Level: Beginners
Weight: Heavy
Kettlebell(s):
Type: Strength
Duration: minutes
Other: Back; slow

Raven 3×5 100

Level: Intermediate
Weight: Medium
Kettlebell(s):
Type: Cardio, strength, and endurance
Duration: 25 to 30 minutes
Other: Full-body with focus on legs, chest, and shoulders; AMRAP; FOR TIME; unbroken

Kronos Workout

Level: Beginner to intermediate
Weight: Medium
Kettlebell(s):
Type: Strength, flexibility, and mobility
Duration: 30 to 45 minutes
Other: Full-body with focus on rotation, shoulders, core, and legs; slow

A Kick-Ass Lower-body Kettlebell Workout

Level: Intermediate
Weight: Light to medium
Kettlebell(s):
Type: Strength and endurance
Duration: 3 minutes
Other: Full-body with focus on the legs, shoulders, and triceps; stability; high reps

Simple Kettlebell Cardio Workout

Level: Beginner
Weight: Light to medium
Kettlebell(s):
Type: Cardio and strength
Duration: 30 to 35 minutes
Other: Full-body with focus on the core

Simple Kettlebell Workout #2

Level: Beginner
Weight: Medium
Kettlebell(s):
Type: Strength
Duration: 20 to 25 minutes
Other: Full-body with focus on the legs, shoulders, and biceps

Quick Kettlebell Cardio Workout

Level: Intermediate to advanced
Weight: Light to medium
Kettlebell(s):
Type: Cardio
Duration: 12 minutes
Other: Full-body; AMRAP

ZATANNA

Level: Beginner
Weight: Medium
Kettlebell(s):
Type: Strength and cardio
Duration: 12 to 15 minutes
Other: Full-body; FOR TIME; complex/flow

Armory Workout

Level: Intermediate

Weight: Medium

Kettlebell(s):

Type: Strength and cardio

Duration: 24 minutes

Other: Full-body; EMOM; interval

Caveman Kettlebells Silverback Workout

Level: Advanced

Weight: Medium

Kettlebell(s):

Type: Strength and light cardio

Duration: 20 minutes

Other: Full-body; short; low reps; AMRAP

Workout Mulhacén

Level: Intermediate

Weight: Medium to heavy

Kettlebell(s):

Type: Strength and cardio

Duration: 22 to 26 minutes

Other: Full-body; FOR TIME; low reps

The Best Upper-body Workout

Level: Intermediate

Weight: Heavy

Kettlebell(s):

Type: Strength

Duration: 60 minutes

Other: Upper-body and back; slow

Fourforty WOD

Level: Beginner to intermediate
Weight: Medium
Kettlebell(s):
Type: Strength and cardio
Duration: 26 to 30 minutes
Other: Full-body; AMRAP; FOR TIME

BBKB10-4

Level: Intermediate
Weight: Heavy
Kettlebell(s):
Type: Strength and cardio
Duration: 25 to 30 minutes
Other: Full-body; FOR TIME

Thorax Mobility Workout

Level: Beginner
Weight: Light
Kettlebell(s):
Type: Mobility and flexibility
Duration: 45 to 60 minutes
Other: Full-body but focus on the thoracic area, but not neglecting the hips, knees, and ankles

I like to stress again that although the workouts have been classified as beginner, intermediate, or advanced, this does not mean that some of the intermediate workouts can't be done by beginners. Some workouts will have alternatives or progressions. Some workouts can be adjusted by yourself with a bit of thinking, removing 1 kettlebell, reducing reps, reducing intensity, or breaking up the duration etc. If in doubt, post online and ask "How do I……?".

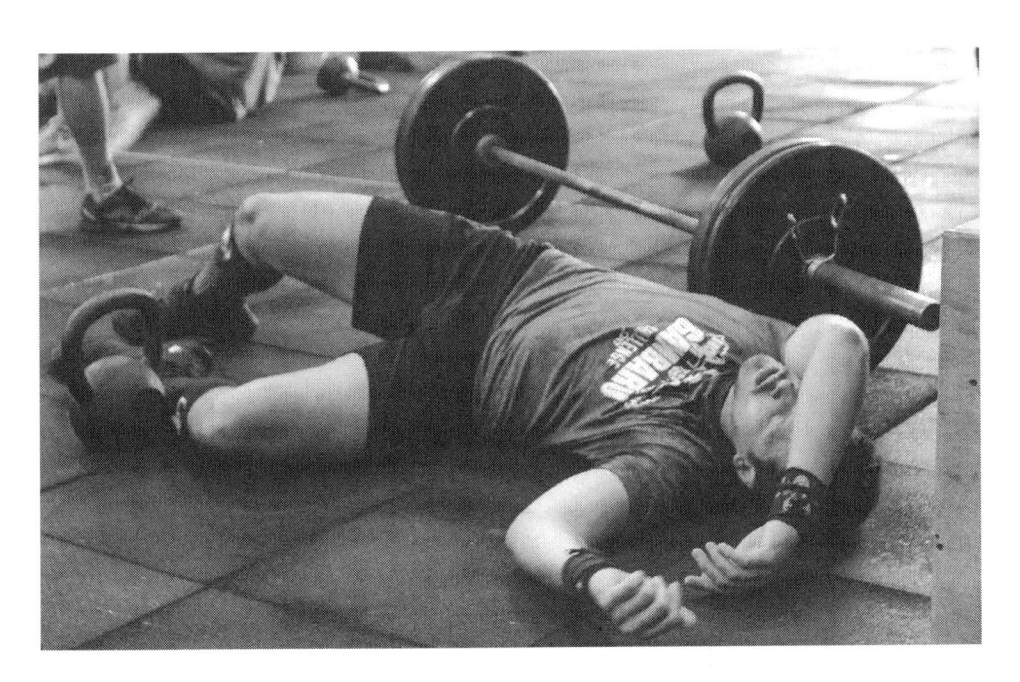

WOD Terminology

- **WOD**
  Workout Of the Day
  Usually something different every-time, but repeated over an x period of time to measure progress

- **Task**
  Part of your workout which can be any number of tasks to complete

- **AMRAP**
  As Many Rounds as Possible; or
  As Many Reps as Possible
  Complete a set task as many times as possible within the set time

- **FOR TIME**
  Complete a set task in the fastest time possible

- **Rx (R)**
  Prescribed or recommended weight to use as a benchmark

- **Scaled**
  Using a weight or exercise that's more suitable than what's prescribed

- **Buy in**
  Something you perform once before starting the task at hand

- **Buy out / check out**
  Something you perform once after finishing the task at hand

- **DNF**
  Did not finish

- **EMOM**
  Every minute on the minute

With the workouts I try to provide as much information as possible. I'm not categorizing workouts by level in order. I do this on purpose, as I hope you'll also learn to get creative, meaning the workout may be marked as advanced, but you'll be able to see that you can swap a snatch for a clean and press, a jerk for a push press, reduce total time worked, reduce number of reps, break the task into multiple parts, and so on. These workouts are so good you should experience each and everyone of them. **Justin did** go.cavemantraining.com/kbwc-link7

Bonus Downloads

This book would become very bulky if I included all of the following important kettlebell information, but I wanted to make it available to you, as each and every part of the information is truly going to make you so much better at kettlebell training and perform better in your workouts.

- **Kettlebell grips PDF**
  www.cavemantraining.com/shop/ebook/kettlebell-grip-ebook/
  Knowing correct grips is extremely important, especially for snatching and cleaning.

- **Kettlebell racking PDF**
  www.cavemantraining.com/shop/ebook/kettlebell-racking-pdf/
  Knowing how to rack properly is extremely important, especially for jerking, resting, and endurance.

Safety and Other Important Information

Safety first! Ego at the door. Use common sense. That's really all I need to say, but... this is not a personal training session, I'm not with you, I don't know your goals, I don't know your history, etc. This book is intended to be as generic as possible, providing information that will teach you to make your own decisions. You will need to do so rather than blindly taking what's written. We do have a team of pro's ready to help you online, so, if in doubt, or you want more customized training plans, just contact us.

If a workout is done with two kettlebells, and you only have two uneven kettlebells with not too much weight difference between them, let's say up to 8kg/17.6lbs max, use them. There is absolutely nothing wrong with using uneven weights, more difficult in most cases, yes, but bad, no. It does not create muscle imbalance either, in fact the opposite, assuming you don't do anything stupid like training for months with the lighter weight on your left side, and the heavier one on the right side. Swap weights after a round or two.

Use progression and regression wisely. If you see an awesome workout you want to do, it has snatches in it, and you're not ready for those yet, then use progression. Start with clean and press, progress to clean and push press, clean and jerk, half snatch, and finally you end up at full snatches over time. If you grab a nice heavy weight as prescribed, but your form sucks, you'll more than likely end up injured if you continue, regress, regress to a lower weight, regress to a previous progression of the exercise if you need to. Just because you were ready to snatch a few 24's yesterday, does not mean you can today. Safety and remaining injury free is priority numero uno.

Since this book contains information for personal trainers as well, you might want to skip over any information only applicable to trainers, I've marked it as such with an icon. I'm using the following icons to clearly mark other important parts of a workout.

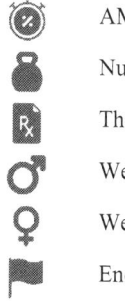

⏱	AMRAP or FOR TIME
🔔	Number of kettlebells used 1, 2, or more
℞	The prescribed weights
♂	Weight for males
♀	Weight for females
🚩	End of the workout
	Penalties apply
▶	A link to a YouTube video
	Rest time
🔄	Number of cycles or rounds

How to Score AMRAP Workouts

WODs—Scoring And Keeping Score

Scoring AMRAP workouts appropriately is super important in competitive exercise. Use the following formulas when calculating your score for AMRAP workouts published on Cavemantraining, or elsewhere.

I've been programming, running, and participating in WODs for over a decade now, I'm here to share my experience on how to score them.

For demonstration purposes, let's use the *Sneaky Anna WOD* (included in Kettlebell Workouts and Challenges 1.0), which consists of:

- 4 half snatches
- 4 burpees
- 4 squat deadlifts

20 minutes AMRAP

Scoring remains pretty simple. You just keep track of rounds, plus the rep you stopped at when the timer went off. If you completed one squat deadlift when the timer went, you would look at the number of rounds you did plus 9 (4 snatches + 4 burpees + 1 deadlift). If you did 24 rounds that would be 24.9 or 297 ((24 x 12) + 9) reps.

If you're programming short WOD cycles with rest, like this for example:

- 10 Russian kettlebell swings
- 2/2 dumbbell snatches
- 2 deadball over the shoulder

6 minutes AMRAP

2 minutes rest

⟳ 3 cycles

You count full rounds plus the number of reps, meaning, if you completed 8 full rounds, and then just finished 2 dumbbell snatches when the timer went off, you would have done 12 reps that round (10 swings + 2 snatches). Write down 8.12 for that round. At the end of your three cycles, if you have for example a score of:

Cycle 1 — 8.12

Cycle 2 — 8.2

Cycle 3 — 7.13

You would add the rounds (the number before the dot) up, as 8 + 8 + 7 = 23. You then add the reps that did not make a full round (those marked after the dot) as 12 + 2 + 13 = 25. We know that one full round equals 16 reps, 25 can only be divided once, equals, one round, leaving 9 reps, thus, your final score would be 24.9, 24 full rounds and 9 reps, or written as a total of 393 reps, which is 24 x 16, equals 384 plus the remainder of 9, is a total of 393.

If you want to score fairer, taking into consideration the amount of weight lifted, you'd use the following Contraindicating scoring formula. For demonstration purpose we'll use *The HULK Test* which is a WOD designed to test every inch of your being—you either smash HULK, or HULK smash you!

- 1 minute of strict presses with double kettlebells weighing approx. 70% of your 1RM
- 2 minutes of half snatch into squat with double kettlebells medium weight
- 5 minutes rest
  If you're working with a partner, it's 1 minute and then you're counting or no repping for them

⏱ **AMRAP**

⟳ 5 cycles

In this case we add the total weight used multiplied by the number of reps to get the final score. If you've programmed a WOD which uses the same weight throughout, but the athlete scaled back to lighter weight half-way through, then the lowest weight is used to calculate score for the whole workout.

Let's continue with *The HULK Test* as an example, I completed the test as follows:

- 22kg + 22kg for strict press equals 44kg (97lbs)
- 16kg + 16kg for snatches and squat equals 32kg (70lbs)
- Total of 76kg times 134 equals 10184
- Hence, my final score is 10184

As you can see, there are many different ways to score fairly. How you score and keep track depends on the type of workout you programmed. Make sure you subscribe to our mailing list for weekly WODs in your inbox. I'm not just talking the regular workouts you can get anywhere, I'm talking 100% original WODs, designed at *Cavemantraining*.

Subscribe www.cavemantraining.com/newsletter/

Experimenting

I've been experimenting with some of the approaches to scoring different ways, taking endurance into account, like for example issuing penalties when weights are put down during a set time frame, or a set is broken, partnering people up into teams and scoring as a team.

Keeping score

If you do not have someone to count for you, then keeping score is another task you need to get good at. After all, you don't want to be called out for cheating. Trust me, nothing worse than cheaters in a class. No one speaks about them in the open, but behind closed doors they're the topic of conversation. Everyone knows better though. They don't fool anyone but themselves, so, if you don't have any tools at your disposal to keep a good record of your score, and you lose count, take the approach of "Let's do one or two extra to be sure!"

Putting that aside, here are some tools to keep track of your score.

If you're completing a WOD with low reps and it's one that can easily be completed unbroken, then you don't want to be writing each round down. You can repeat the round number in your head, i.e. let's say the WOD is 2 push-ups, 2 squats, 2 pull-ups. You would simply repeat the round for each rep, i.e "one" for all six reps in round one, then "two" for all six reps in round two, "three" (push-up), "three"(push-up), "three" (squat), "three" (squat), "three" (pull-up), "three" (pull-up), and so on. This way you don't confuse round three with round four, or even worse, deduct one.

Shouting rounds out loud is also fun, but with lots of people in a class, it can become noisy. The great thing is that you're aware of where your competition is at, and that makes you work even harder. There's also less chance of cheating/mistakes, because for sure someone will pick you up on it.

Writing down your rounds or reps on a whiteboard is also an option, but this usually takes time to get to the board. If you lay the board on the ground, it will become a puddle of sweat mixed with ink. Great option if you want to program in a slight 3 to 5 second rest, however, you do need to make it clear that everyone needs to write down their round after completion, rather than some people writing them down, and others only writing them down after they've completed 5. This only works with long rounds though, for example rounds that take a minute or so to complete. If they're short, you can decide at which number they write it down, i.e. 5 rounds equals one marker. Whatever it is, be clear upfront, and write it on the board.

If you find a whiteboard marker becomes messy, you can write the names down, then next to each name draw a line or multiple, and simply have the athletes wipe away part of the line for each round. Be careful not to use two fingers, or wipe some else's line!

In my opinion, the fastest and most authentic way to keep score is with a piece of chalk, marking your rounds on the ground! Not every box seems to appreciate this, but a real gym is where people sweat puddles and throw chalk around (in moderation of course)!

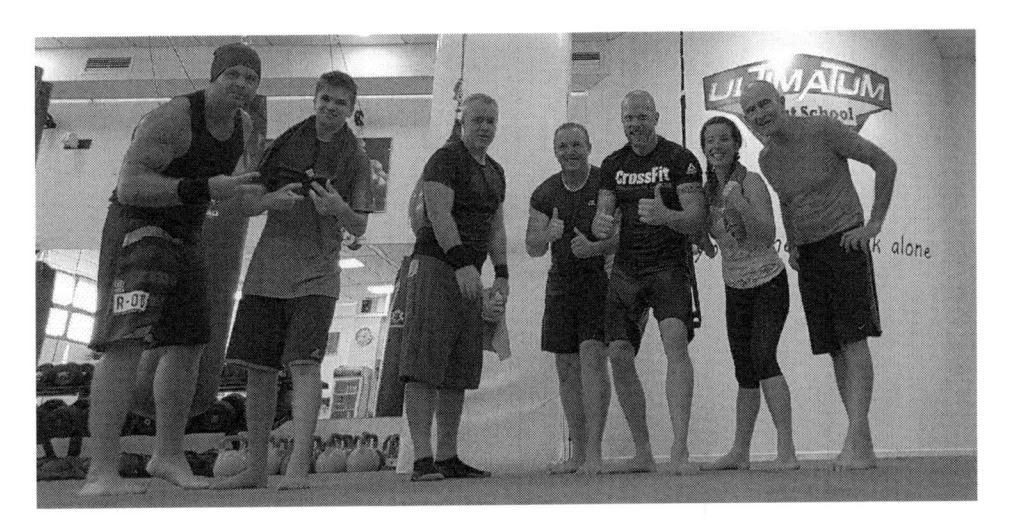

How to Structure a Caveman WOD

This topic is suitable for trainers. There are many ways to structure a workout of the day, but here's what we consider the most optimal structure for any type of workout, but especially WODs:

- Warm-up
- Work on mobility / strength
- Demo
- Training
- Demo
- Workout and monitor
- Cool down and stretch
- Provide feedback

Why warm-up?

We warm-up to achieve an increased heart rate, body temperature, get the blood pumping through the system, increase blood flow to the muscles and loosen the joints. Not only is a warm-up good physically, but also mentally. You warm-up with body or light weight, gently increasing intensity during the duration of the warm-up. The most important reason for a warm-up is to prevent injury like muscle strain etc. If after your warm-up you focus on mobility, and/or training, then you can reduce warm-up time to about 5 to 10 minutes. If you're using running as a warm-up, start with a light jog or high knees, then run, and finish with sprinting. Squats, burpees, jumping jacks, jump rope, and alternating reverse lunges are all good for warming-up. A warm-up should be full-body, but should focus more on the areas that are going to be worked.

Why mobility?

It's not necessarily a bad thing to focus on mobility before the warm-up, but a warm body means increased range of motion.

You focus on mobility, to increase range of motion, increase flexibility to achieve a better overhead lockout, to be able to hold the bar/kettlebell overhead during a squat without it impacting the lower-back, and so on.

Some of the areas to focus on are, but not limited to: thoracic spine, shoulders, ankles, hips. This can also be a good time to focus on mind-muscle connection, lat activation, core activation, glute activation, preventing excessive pelvic tilt etc. Some of the mobility drills can be, but not limited to: resistance band work, bodyweight windmills, even lunges are great, but should be performed in a slow controlled manner focusing on range. Add rotation to make it even better. Put your hands behind your head and you're also opening up the chest.

With mobility it's best you focus on the work to come. If you're going to do a lot of overhead stuff, focus on shoulders, chest, scapula, thoracic spine, lats, lower traps etc. The plank is great for lat activation, or just hang from a bar and activate the lats. Alternating superman or cobra are also great for the back, and throw in some rotational work as that's mostly overlooked.

Why work on strength separately from the workout? For optimal strength, control, focus, and removing the competitive quality of most WODs is required, hence the reason to separate strength.

Why demo?

You can talk and get lots of "Yesses" paired with blank stares, and you know they're too afraid to say, "I have no clue what you're talking about." A quick demonstration will prevent this. Pair it with some cues, and you're reinforcing technique through visualization and verbalization. A demo is different from training; there is no need to cover the complete exercise and every detail for regulars. Carefully pick the right cues, muscle groups to activate, and common mistakes made. Each time you demo, try and cover something new. You might even cover something specific you know someone in the group needs to know. This is a great way to cover things that might otherwise be awkward to discuss. For example, with the deadlift, you could talk about trap activation, glute activation, shaving the shins, full hip extension but not hyperextension and so on. If you're lost for ideas, then it's time to learn more about the exercises.

Why training?

Training is where you get the group to go through the exercises, correct the technique, assess, progress or regress, provide alternatives, keep an eye out for injured people—yes some people train when injured. You can pick up this and talk to them, tell them you recommend rest and recovery, or if they insist on training, tell them to go lighter or halve the reps. Maybe you can see that they're fatigued. You might know they're capable of easily smashing this WOD in a recovered state, but today you can see they need rest. Provide the guidance you're paid for. Break things down during training. If you're going to be jerking, then you would start with a push press, and work on the second dip without weight. If it's a push jerk then you want to work without bar as well, and work on the feet coming off the ground and outwards, stand up and reset. You might even work on the drop. Break things down, and work on the issues. Training is also a great time to work on strength and MMC, include static holds, like the plank or hang, which are all great for lat activation (MMC).

Why workout?

Working out is to push yourself further, compete against others, compete against your yesterdays self. Working out is not about training' it's about using what you've learned during training. It's about conditioning, repetition, improving muscle endurance, improving cardiovascular endurance, increasing reps; it's about learning how to pace yourself, listening to your body and above all, it's about increasing mental toughness. Read about the difference between training and working out.

Why monitor?

Monitoring is what you do while the participants are working out. There is a plethora of things to monitor for -- muscle activation, technique, pacing, effort and so on, but most importantly, monitor potential for injury. If someone is pressing with a hyper-extended back instead of jerking, it's time for rest, lower weight, and a scheduled technique session. If someone is squatting RX overhead and their heels are coming off the ground every-time, squat depth is minimal, then it's time to lower their weight for that exercise and make a note to have them work on flexibility. And my favorite, picking someone out of the crowd and monitoring their reps. Hey, everyone makes a mistake sometimes, for sure, but always 7 = 10 requires some group directed motivational talk about why you're working out, that coming in numero uno isn't your main objective, well, not at the cost of technique, reps, and potential for serious injury.

Why cool down and stretch?

The body is now in a perfect state for static stretching and foam rolling, well deserved time to thank and take care of the muscles for the performance they've given. Static stretches are great for increasing muscle length, which in turn helps prevent injury, and greater range of motion. It's also a good time to relax, and reflect on your performance. Let me tell you a secret, I don't always stretch, as I don't think it's a requirement to always stretch, but this depends entirely on what you do outside of the workouts and/or what was involved in the workout, for example a session which involved a lot of dynamic stretches and/or grinding moves that go to the edge of flexibility. But having said that, cooling down and stretching after a session is good for the mind.

Why provide feedback?

Time to talk about the notes you made during your monitoring. It can be a quick addressing of the whole group if the majority of the group made the same mistake. It can be pulling someone aside, and giving them some tips in private or even suggesting personal training, whether to increase technique, strength, flexibility or other.

We have always made feedback a big part of our service. We talk to people afterwards and if we don't get to talk to them afterwards, we make a mental note and take them aside next time if they're in early, and we have a few minutes to spare. It could even be things like improvements we've seen, it doesn't always need to be about learning more. It would even go as far as life tips, general health tips, little things like talking about smoking, excessive drinking, nutrition, rest and mental state.

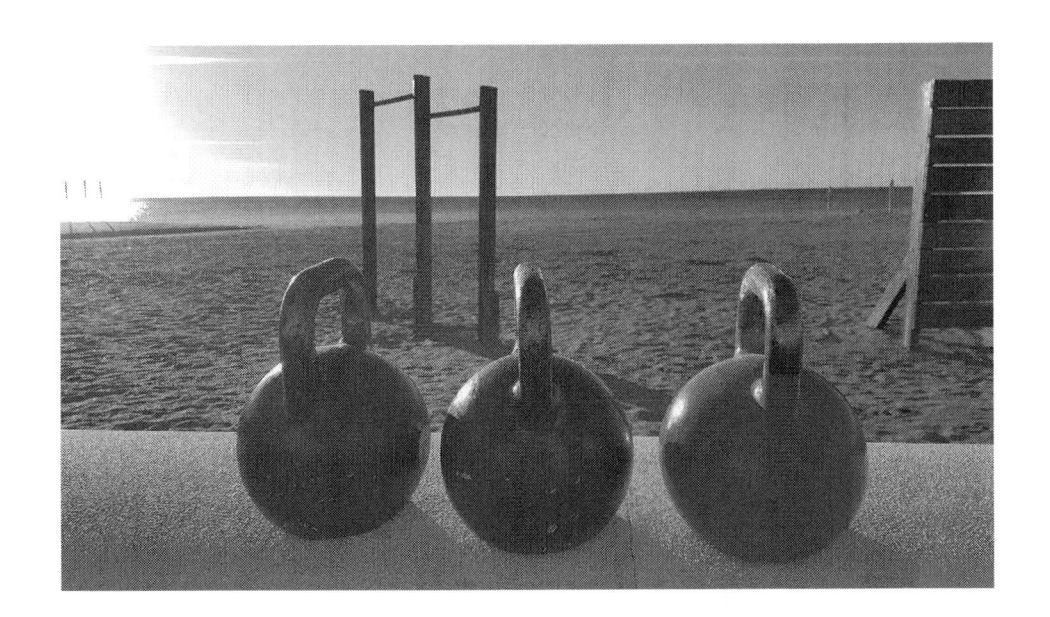

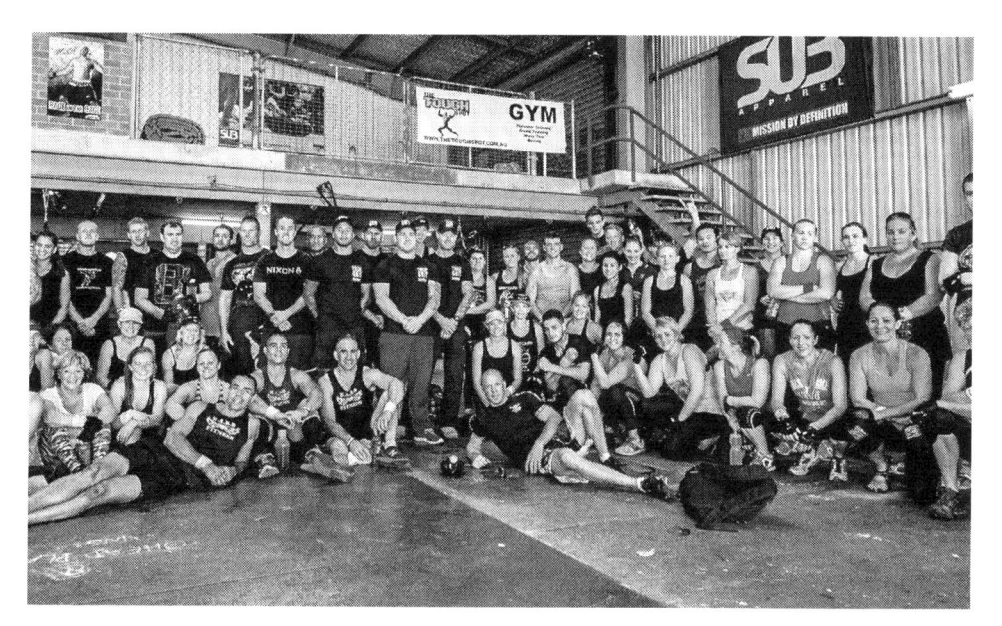

Caveman Buddy System

This topic is suitable for trainers but can also give a home user ideas. Many years ago we started something that we like to call the 'Caveman Buddy' system, and we've been implementing it in different formats of training, circuit training, boot camp, WODs and strength training. It's awesome, and if you're not doing it yet, you should!

We first started using this in our *Caveman Circuit Training* many years ago back in Australia. We then implemented it in our *Caveman Strength* sessions as well, and it's absolutely perfect. People love it. In *Caveman Strength* the coaches pair up people with similar ability so can they then work together for the whole session. In the WODs it's more about pairing so that all teams are equal.

In circuit training it's awesome because you get to use one station for two people, allowing you to take in more people for your session. Working with the 'Caveman Buddy' system is great for many reasons. Not only does it provide motivation to work harder than your buddy, it also allows you to ask questions and get support during the session, not just from the coach, but also from your buddy.

Where I personally love the whole 'Caveman Buddy' idea is in our Caveman Strength sessions. As a coach, your focus is on warming your clients up, explaining the exercises, explaining how to spot/assist their buddy and what they should be looking out for. Then you spend your time walking through the class doing what you normally do. The awesome thing with the 'Caveman Buddy' system is that people get their required rest in, which is especially important in strength classes.

We use the Caveman Buddy system in our Caveman Strength program, which is usually structured as follows:

- 60 to 90 minutes in duration
- Slow controlled movements
- Isometrics
- Negatives (eccentric phase)
- Caveman Buddy system
- 5 to 7 stations, duplicated if dealing with a larger class
- Functional exercises
- Preference for unilateral exercises
- Free weights (no machines used)
- 1 minute per station, sometimes 2 minutes depending on the program
- Aiming for 6 to 10 reps per station

Further more, we use the *Caveman Buddy* system in our *Caveman Circuits*, and even in *Caveman WODs*.

Some of the exercises we use in our Caveman Strength, but not limited to, are:

- Weighted pull-ups
- Weighted chin-ups
- Back squats
- Front squats
- Weighted push-ups
- Weighted tricep push-ups
- Barbell curls
- Tricep press
- Chest press
- Strict shoulder press
- Weighted pistol squat
- Weighted step-ups
- Flyes
- Squat dead lifts
- Sumo dead lifts
- Hip hinge dead lifts
- Heavy swings

The *Dead Renegade Farmers WOD*, and *Strength Workout Helios* discussed in the *Kettlebell Workouts and Challenges 1.0* book are great workouts that utilize the Caveman Buddy system.

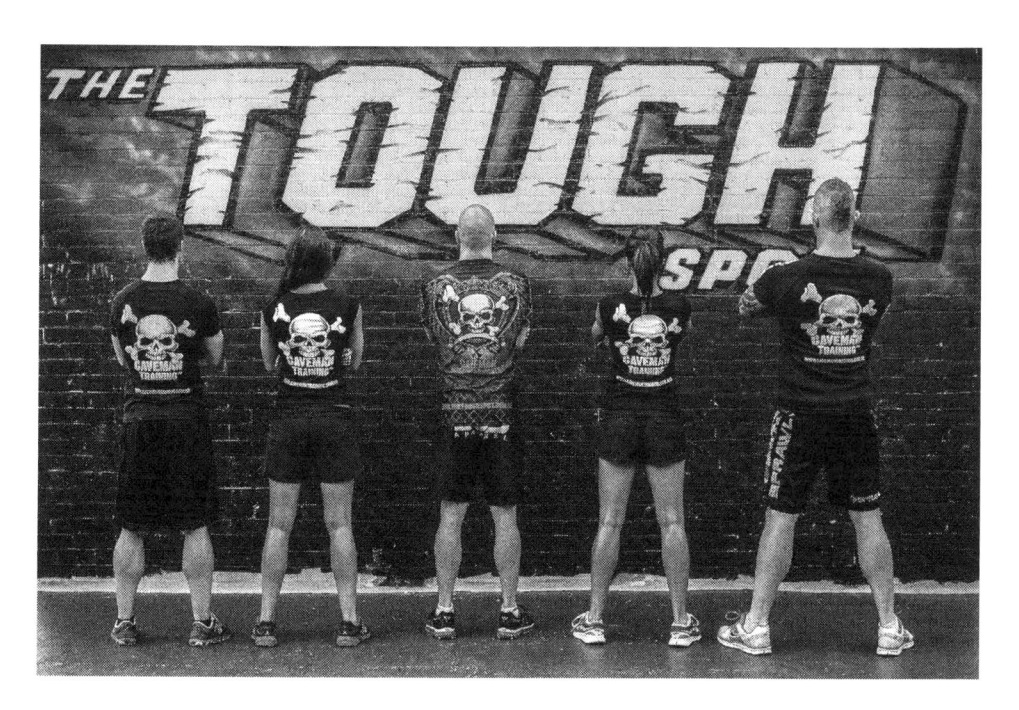

Warm-up and Mobility

This section is dedicated to warming up and mobility. Warming up prior to every workout is vital. Mobility is what keeps you injury free and performing better.

Bodyweight warm-up routine

If I walk to the gym and am already warm, I normally start this warm-up routine right away. If I did not walk, I would first do some star jumps (jumping jacks) to get the body warm. Depending on how cold my body is, I would also throw in some burpees.

I like to go top down, and usually start with:

- Arms in and out http://bit.ly/kb-wk-vid1
  Thoracic and scapula

- One arm up and one down http://bit.ly/kb-wk-vid2
  Shoulders and scapula

- Arm circles http://bit.ly/kb-wk-vid3
  Shoulders

- Shoulder circles http://bit.ly/kb-wk-vid4
  Shoulders and scapula

- Thoracic rotation (same as demonstrated but without the lunge) http://bit.ly/kb-wk-vid5
  Thoracic
- Hip hinge
  Hips, and knees
- Squat
  Hips, ankles and knees
- Reverse lunge and twist (first exercise demonstrated) http://bit.ly/kb-wk-vid5
  Hips, knees, ankles, and thoracic
- Reverse lunge and arm raise (second exercise demonstrated) http://bit.ly/kb-wk-vid5
  Hips, knees, ankles, shoulders, and thoracic
- Curtsy lunge (fourth exercise demonstrated) http://bit.ly/kb-wk-vid5
  Hips, knees, and ankles
- Hip opener (fifth exercise demonstrated) http://bit.ly/kb-wk-vid5
  Hips
- Hip circles (sixth exercise demonstrated) http://bit.ly/kb-wk-vid5
  Hips
- Kettlebell halo (seventh exercise demonstrated) http://bit.ly/kb-wk-vid5
  Shoulders

▶ A video with all of the above movements http://bit.ly/kb-wk-vid6

The shoulders are one of the most complex joints, so I spend a considerable amount of time on the shoulders. This is the reason my shoulders have remained injury free (knock on wood).

Depending on what follows in the workout or training, I would spend more time on that area. For example, if we're doing deadlifts, I would spend some more time on the hamstrings and glutes, even doing more shoulder circles, as this also works the traps. If there are many push-ups or overhead bar work, I would spend some time on the wrists.

As I proceed I try to mimic the movements that are to come, with bodyweight first, then add some light weight. I always cover all joints, then specific muscles groups if required.

Sometimes I don't do a rigorous warm-up prior to starting the tasks at hand. This is when I program in something like 100 jumping jacks, 50 burpees at the start, and then program to slowly increase the demand on the body. Jumping jacks are great; you target the shoulders, hips, legs, and warm up the body all in one.

Other great exercises are, but not limited to:

- **Jumping jacks**; awesome for anything overhead and overall body warmth

- **Hip hinge and reach**; awesome for snatches, deadlifts, squats and anything overhead
  Add a calf raise after the reach, and you're also warming up the ankles and calves
- **Squat and pull-over**; awesome for mobility work in the warm-up, squat depth/technique and opening up the thoracic
- **Wood chopper and halo**; awesome for shoulders, mid section and rotational work

I include these in my workshops, 30 seconds per exercise and 2 to 3 rounds. 3 rounds if nothing else follows, but I'll usually do some more mobility work afterwards.

Bodyweight hip hinges and squats are always good if you do cleans, snatches, deadlifts, squats etc. warming up the hammies, quads, glutes and lubricating the hip, knee and ankle joints.

Jumping jacks, jump burpees, high knees or quick feet are always great to raise the temperature of the body and prepare for more intense exercise. But some of these are also great for overhead work, like the jumping jacks for example, as you want to raise your arms higher and higher as you get warmer. You want to achieve full lockout and pull down with the lats on every rep at some stage.

The pull-over, wood chopper and halo are great for the mid section, rotational work, shoulders, thoracic and more.

In the following video you can see them in action http://bit.ly/kb-wk-vid7, also some light kettlebell work included.

Warm-up and Mobility Exercises

The following are a few more exercises you can use for warming-up or working on your mobility.

Kettlebell arm bar for shoulder mobility and stability http://bit.ly/kb-wk-vid8

Shoulder warm-up: around the body http://bit.ly/kb-wk-vid9

Kettlebell halo: shoulder and thoracic mobility plus core stability http://bit.ly/kb-wk-vid10

Shoulder mobility: tea cup exercise http://bit.ly/kb-wk-vid11

Shoulder warm-up + mobility: shoulder rotation internal and external http://bit.ly/kb-wk-vid12

Shoulder warm up + mobility: arms in and out http://bit.ly/kb-wk-vid1

Shoulder warm up + mobility: shoulder circles http://bit.ly/kb-wk-vid4

▶ Shoulder mobility flexibility and assistance exercise http://bit.ly/kb-wk-vid13

▶ Heel touching jumping jack http://bit.ly/kb-wk-vid14

▶ Burpee, tricep push up into overhead squat http://bit.ly/kb-wk-vid15

▶ Shoulder mobility and stability: kettlebell windmill http://bit.ly/kb-wk-vid16

Generic warm-up

Some of the workouts will have a warm-up listed and others won't, above I've given you information to create your own warm-ups and following is a generic warm-up you can use for those workouts that do not have one listed.

- 10 jumping jacks
- 5 jump burpees
- 5 squats

Repeat 8 times or for 4 to 6 minutes.

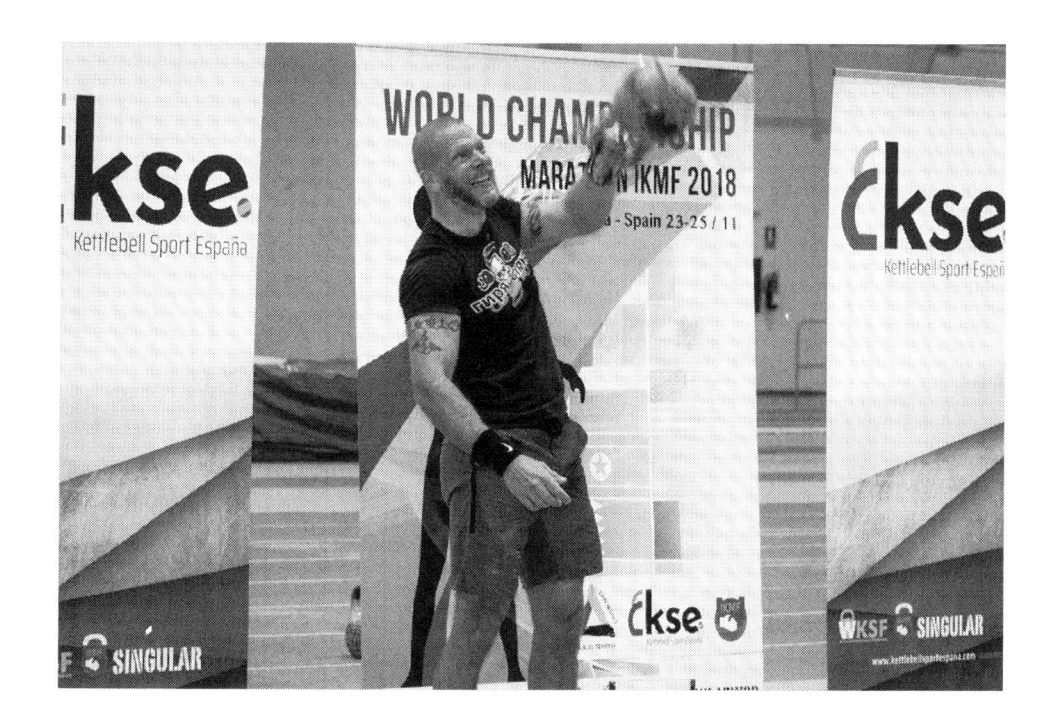

Easter egg
20% discount on the book *Master The Kettlebell Press*, use coupon code: **B78JL3FG4M**
www.cavemantraining.com/shop/ebook/master-the-kettlebell-press/

Kettlebell Workouts

Before you get stuck in the workouts. A workout is not a program. A program is something written or adjustable to you with your goals in mind. A program is written so that you progress, receive adequate rest/recovery, work the right muscle groups, etc. All these kettlebell workouts have a goal, either strength, endurance, cardio, flexibility, and so on. But to make them work for you when you pick random ones each time and are training several times a week, you need to start thinking about how it affects you, what the goals are, what muscles are worked, whether you did cardio or strength, and you need to start planning, but most importantly, listening to your body.

You can design your own program from these by picking 2 or 3 favorites and keep track of the progress you make. If it's an AMRAP workout, you aim to get more rounds out over time, then you aim to go heavier, but to a certain point only, fast workouts should really not be done with super heavy weight, so there will be a limit to how heavy you get up to with AMRAPs. With slow and controlled strength workouts you can focus on increasing the weight over time, like for example, do the workout for 4 weeks with the same weight, give it a break for a week, increase the weight, and continue this process over time.

With endurance you can break a 10 minute workout into 40 seconds work and 20 seconds rest, do the same until it get easy, then increase the work time and decrease the rest time till you're at 10 seconds rest per minute, then decrease sets from 10 sets to 4 sets of 2 minutes work and 30 seconds rest, increase work time and decrease rest time, continue until you're at 2 sets and finally at 10 minutes unbroken. Over time you can increase the weight and repeat the process.

If there is a workout with 100 reps for time, take that workout and only do 40 for time, take note, do the same again, aim for 50, next time aim for 60, till you comfortably reach 100 and increase weight to repeat the process.

Scale your workouts. If there are deadlifts programmed and you lack flexibility, then elevate the weight or change the deadlifts to hang lifts to work on your range. If there is a workout with 2 x double kettlebell press, convert it to 2 x one kettlebell press on one side and 2 on the other, continue to work like this until you reach double bell work over time.

The point being, learn how to do your own programming for progression with the workouts provided. Get smart, invest in your training.

Weights. I will list some of the weights used but describe is as light, medium, or heavy. What is light for one is heavy for another. To figure out what you should use you should look at your 1RM (1 rep max) shoulder press. I'll take the shoulder press as the general indicator but will let you know if the 1RM of another exercise is expected. 1RM means your heaviest 1 rep that you can do with good form and technique.

Light = 0% to 33%
Medium = 34% to 66%
Heavy = 67% and up

To pick a heavy weight you would go by your 1RM, if your 1RM is for example 24kg/53lbs then you would divide that by 100 and times it by 80 for example, where 80 represents a number of 67% and up. The result would be (24 / 100 = 0,24) * 80 = 19,2kg which you would round to the nearest number you have in kettlebell weight. But remember, listen to your body, if the workout calls for heavy and that heavy is not working for you at this moment in time, go lighter.

Duration. For the duration I will list just the duration of the workout itself and either skip details of warm-ups and cool-downs or provide a suggestion. So, an 8 minute workout would be listed as 8 minutes but you need to add your warm-up and cool-down time.

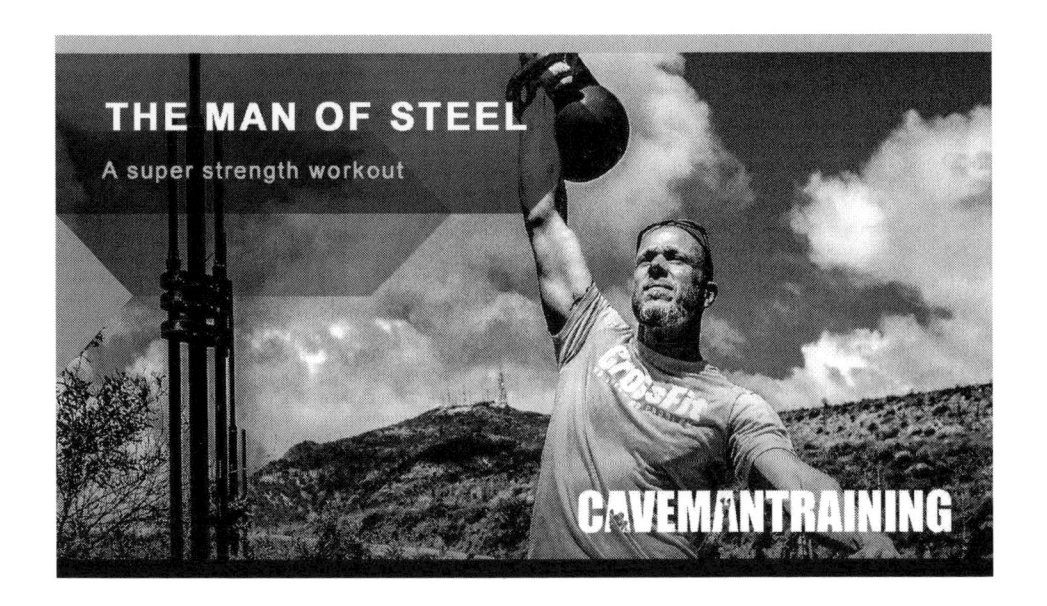

THE MAN OF STEEL WORKOUT

Level: Intermediate

Weight: Heavy

Kettlebell(s): (or 1 if you just do the workout)

Type: Strength and mobility

Duration: 40 minutes

Other: Full-body, legs, shoulders, back, chest; slow

▶ workout go.cavemantraining.com/kbwc-vid1

▶ stretching go.cavemantraining.com/kbwc-vid2

One of the best kettlebell strength workouts!

This is literally one of the best and my favorite strength workouts. It covers everything, full-body. It's performed super slow, which makes it super intense. This workout is to be performed super slow, as slow as possible with the heaviest weight possible, all while maintaining good form & technique during the full range of motion.

Warm up approx 10 minutes, workout 30 to 40 minutes, 5 minutes rest, 5 minute finisher, 5 minute mobility work, and 10 minutes stretching. You can skip the finisher and mobility work if you've only got an hour.

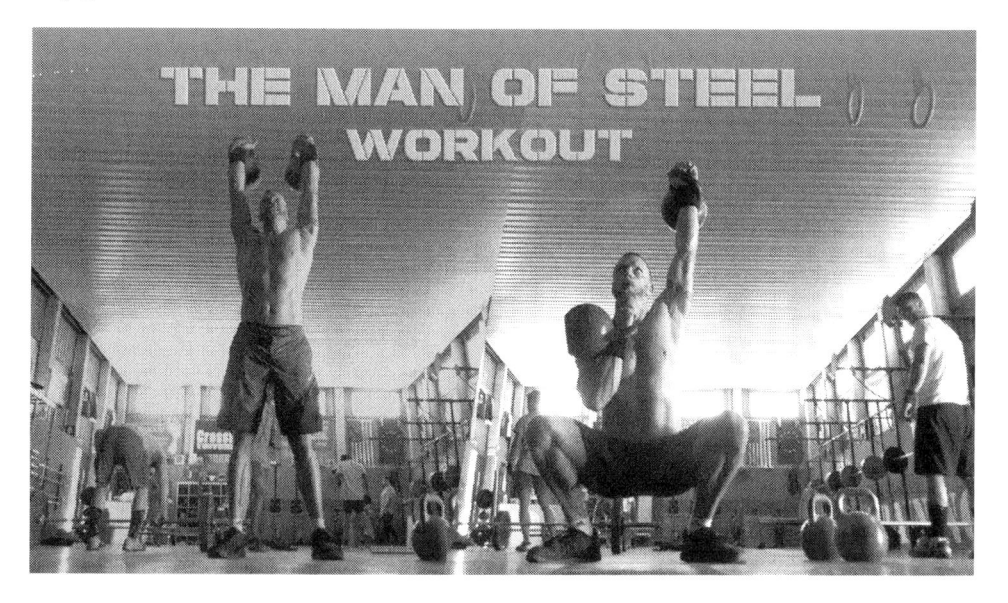

The workout is as follows:

- → Dead swing clean
- → Squat
- → Press

Combo to be performed on the left and right side.

- → Chin-up
- → Pull-up
- → 2 x chest push-up

All performed with just bodyweight.

- → 2 x tricep push-up

➜ 2 x bent-over dead row (left/right)

⊚ 5 rounds

Pick the right weight so that you can perform the full range of the exercise as slow as possible, think slow-motion. If you have to perform the exercise fast, then you picked the wrong weight. You'll fatigue as you go through the rounds, reduce weight or rest more.

Five rounds took me about 30 to 40 minutes. I used a 32kg /70.5lbs kettlebell, but you need to use whatever works for you, whether that is 8kg or 40kg, choose wisely for results. Ditch the ego lifting.

Combo

Let's dig into the specifics of the exercise combos. **For the first combo** you'll be needing a good rack for the squat, you'll be taxing the core during the slow squat as well as the legs. Your feet will need to be wider for the deep slow squat. Once you come out of the squat adjust your feet for the press, pause, this is not a push press. Tighten/tense everything and start your slow press, full overhead lockout in perfect alignment, push your head and chest through so that you get a nice straight joint line-up side-on: ankles, knees, hips, shoulders, elbow, and wrist. On the way down there is no dropping, control the bell from overhead back into the rack. If you can't maintain a position where the shoulders stay high and the hips go low then you need to work on your squat technique and ROM first before adding weight and going slow.

You perform the combo on the left and right side.

The second combo is a chin-up, pull-up, and chest push-up. For the chin-up you want to start hanging with the head through, not back. Employ a supinated/underhand grip (palms facing you). Start pulling and end with the chin as high as possible up above the bar. Keep the rest of the body as still and controlled as possible. Slowly lower back down, don't release till you're back in the full hang with the head through. This all requires good shoulder and thoracic mobility, so if you do not have this yet, or do not have the strength yet, work on that first. You can do a negative chin-up, jumping up and releasing slowly, or use a resistance band with the movement. The chin-up prime movers are the elbow flexors, biceps, brachialis, and brachioradialis, plus the rear delts.

For the pull-up we'll be focussing on the lats only, make them the prime mover! Employ a pronated/overhand grip (palms pacing away from you). Think about pulling your elbows into your hips, think about pulling the bar towards your chest. Focus on the forearms doing nothing but holding on to the bar, refrain from elbow flexion as much as possible. Again, you can do the same as for the chin-up, use negative or resistance bands to progress with this exercise.

For the chest push-up we'll be focusing on the chest, the pectoral muscles for the prime mover. You'll want your elbows away from you as close to a 90 degree angle between your elbow and ribs, but go by how your shoulders feel. Think about pulling the elbows in, rather than pushing away, as soon as you start pushing away you'll be engaging more delts. Try and isolate your muscles, Mind-muscle-connection (MMC). Everything needs to be tight, packed chest and shoulders during the movement, hips and knees locked. Kiss the floor and come back up.

Take a little rest to give the core a break.

Next is the last combo which consists of the tricep push up and bent-over dead rows. With the tricep push-up, again, you want to isolate and think about the triceps, so forget pushing, think pulling, in particular elbow extension through pulling of the triceps and anconeus. Keep the elbows tucked. If you're having trouble, do negative tricep push-ups and just focus on the lowering phase as good as possible. Do 4 reps instead of two.

The last exercise is the bent-over dead row, one of my favorites to work on those nice round delts, i.e. nice and full from the front, side, and back. The great thing is, this is also a core exercise and works the glutes and hammies isometrically, otherwise your pelvis would fall forward! So, take the load of the lower back, squeeze those buttocks as tight as you can and hold, brace the core to create a nice firm and rigid structure to start rowing from. Nothing but your arm should move during the row. Row back and into the hips, don't turn this into a bicep curl by pulling towards the shoulders. Go down in weight if you find you're needing to move other body parts or you start to perform elbow flexion rather than shoulder extension. Shave those ribs on the way up and down.

The whole routine should take you about 30 to 40 minutes, not including the finisher. If you did it faster, work slower, go heavier! Muscles_under_tension.

Progressions

Replace the dead swing clean with assisted double arm clean (see fundamentals).

Perform the chin-ups with resistance bands or replace with barbell curls into bent over row. The curls work the elbow flexors and the row should would the posterior to pull the elbow to your hips and past.

Perform the pull-ups with resistance bands or replace

Replace the chest push-ups with light kettlebell chest press, either double bell or one bell two hands. Another option is to work on negatives, slowly lower and then come back up into plank via the knees.

Replace the triceps push-ups with light overhead triceps extensions. Another option is to work on negatives, slowly lower and then come back up into plank via the knees.

Modify the bent-over dead row and place the non working arm/hand on the knee for support and/or come up after one rep to give the lower back rest.

After the main workout I used a little finisher for the delts, I completed 2 rounds of 10 seesaw presses, and 8 side presses with two kettlebells. The side press was great to work the side delts, and the seesaw was great to give the delts that extra pump but also start thinking about the thoracic area.

With the seesaw press one kettlebell comes down while the other comes up. Some people confuse an alternating press with the seesaw press. Both bells need to move at the same time in the opposite direction.

Then last but not least, I did some mobility work with lightweight, double kettlebell alternating Sots press. There is so much happening in this exercise, it's an incredible exercise, you should include it in your regular training. Start with a light dumbbell, then 8kg, and work your way up slowly. Don't force this. You'll be surprised how difficult this is, but you'll love the benefits it will provide you with. Injury-proof yourself!. More info on the Sots press under *11-Day Sots Press Challenge by Cavemantraining*.

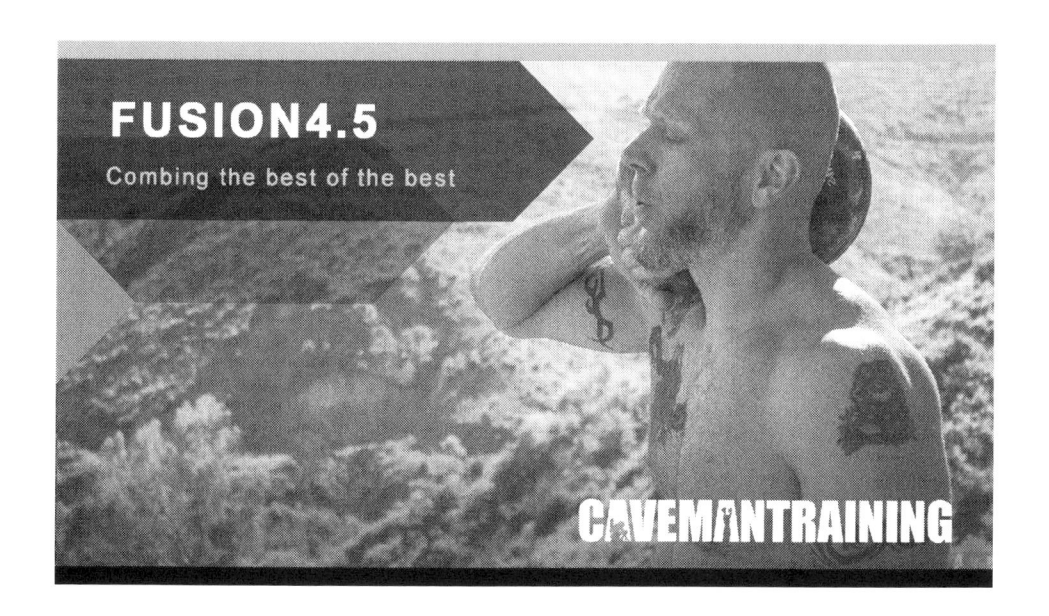

FUSION4.5

- Level: Intermediate to advanced
- Weight: Medium to heavy
- Kettlebell(s):
- Type: Strength, endurance, cardio, mobility
- Duration: 27 minutes
- Other: Full-body with emphases on the legs

workout go.cavemantraining.com/kbwc-vid3

I named this workout *FUSION4.5* as I'm bringing together several different things in one workout. I really enjoy using my rest time for stretching and mobility. I've decided to program it more for public workouts as well.

If you're still working on technique then I suggest picking a light to medium weight and stick with that. In this workout I started with 2 x 24kg/53lb first round, 2 x 20kg/44lb second and third round, 2 x 16kg/35lb for the rest of the rounds.

Fusion as in the workout combines bodyweight exercises, strength, endurance, and stretching.

Warm up approx 10 minutes, workout 30, 5 minutes rest, and 6 minute mobility work. You've already done your stretching so you could walk away after a couple of minutes focussing on any areas you might feel are tight.

The workout is as follows:

- → 1 minute of deep squat and push-up
- → 1 minute of dead swing clean and press into the alternating overhead reverse lunge
  - Perform two reps and rest for the remainder
- → 1 minute of clean and jerk
- → 1 minute of stretching
- → 30 seconds of rest

In total 4.5 minutes per round

Repeat for 6 rounds

The second exercise, dead swing clean and press into the alternating overhead reverse lunge, is just two reps, that's all you should be able to do in one minute when you do it slow enough. To perform:

- Kettlebells dead
- Hip hinge
- Pull them back
- Clean
- Rack
- Strict press
- Keep them overhead
- Reverse lunge on one side

- Alternate and lunge on the other side
- Lower the kettlebells into rack
- Drop the kettlebells
- Hip hinge
- Backswing
- Return to dead
- Repeat

The fourth exercises are stretches, my stretches were hip and thoracic hyperextension into the pike and alternating pigeon stretch, you can choose your own. The ones I used covered everything at the front and back, especially shoulders and gluteals.

I finished with 6 minutes of mobility work with the alternating Sots press.

go.cavemantraining.com/kbwc-vid4

Progressions

Dead swing clean into the alternating overhead reverse lunge progressions:
1. Alternating reverse lunge with no added weight
2. (Any clean) Alternating reverse lunge with one kettlebell racked
3. (Any clean) Alternating reverse lunge with two kettlebells racked
4. (Any clean) Alternating reverse lunge with one kettlebell overhead (switch on the next set)

The alternative for the clean and jerk is clean and push press or break the minute up and bring the bells to ground each time to perform one dead swing clean and push press.

This is a great workout to do more than once a week and build up your strength. If you program it frequently to see progress, make sure you give it a one to two week rest after 4 weeks and deload. Give it some time to recover, work on other things, especially mobility. Then pick it back up and you should see some performance/strength increase.

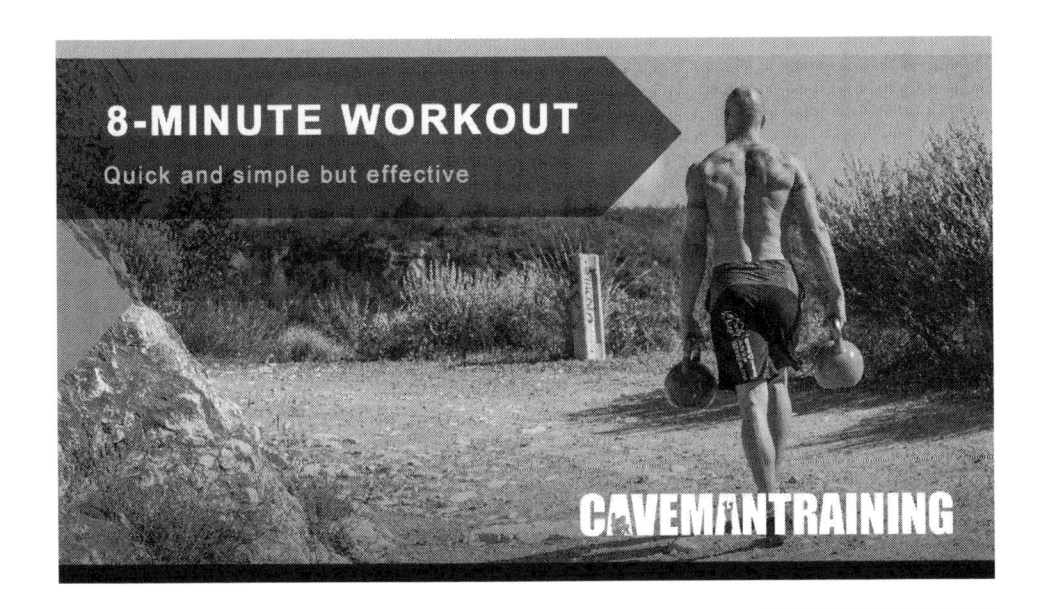

SIMPLE 8-MINUTE KETTLEBELL WORKOUT

Level: Beginner

Weight: Light to medium

Kettlebell(s):

Type: Cardio

Duration: 8 minutes

Other: Full-body

workout go.cavemantraining.com/kbwc-vid5

Come with a full-length kettlebell workout video you can work out along with. This workout is mostly lower body and some upper body, 70% lower and 30% upper. Mostly gluteus maximus and hamstrings, after that quads, calves, and shoulders. The erector spinae will also get a good workout.

30 seconds of work on one side and then switch to the other side with the last exercise being an exception.

→ 30 seconds single arm hip hinge swings

Switch
- → 30 seconds single arm hip hinge swings
- Switch and clean
- → 30 seconds squat
- Switch and clean
- → 30 seconds squat
- Switch and clean
- → 30 seconds strict press
- Switch and clean
- → 30 seconds strict press
- → 60 seconds figure of 8
- Repeat the whole sequence

🚩

Following are just some tips or cues you can use for this workout.

Swing. At the top and bottom during the swing, I focus on breathing out, as in automatically happens.

Don't follow the bell. (see fundamentals)

Squat. Shoulders high and hips low. Push the hips to the ground. If your hips are not moving down then your shoulders should not be moving down.

Press. Keep the elbows under the weight.

Figure of 8. You can replace this with around the body 30 seconds one way and 30 the other way.

Intermediate

You can make this more challenging by increasing the weight and performing more rounds. Grab a 20kg/44lb complete one round, rest 1 minute, and repeat four times to make a total workout time of 32 minutes (excluding rest).

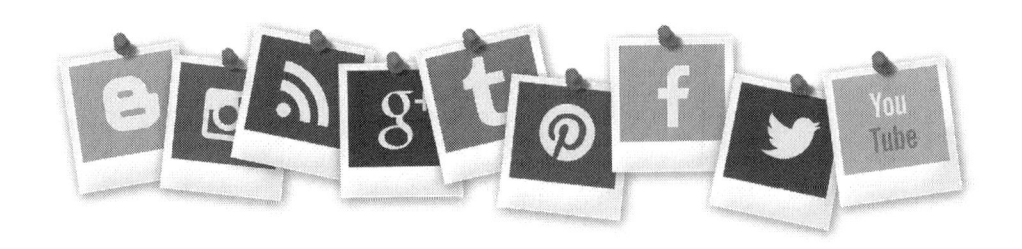

Post on Reddit, YouTube, Facebook, Instagram, or Twitter when you completed this. Hashtag #cavemantraining #workoutcompleted

If your technique is spot on and you keep the weight light then this is quite easily a workout you can do up to 5 days a week for your cardio.

QUICKSILVER

So simple but so grueling and awesome!

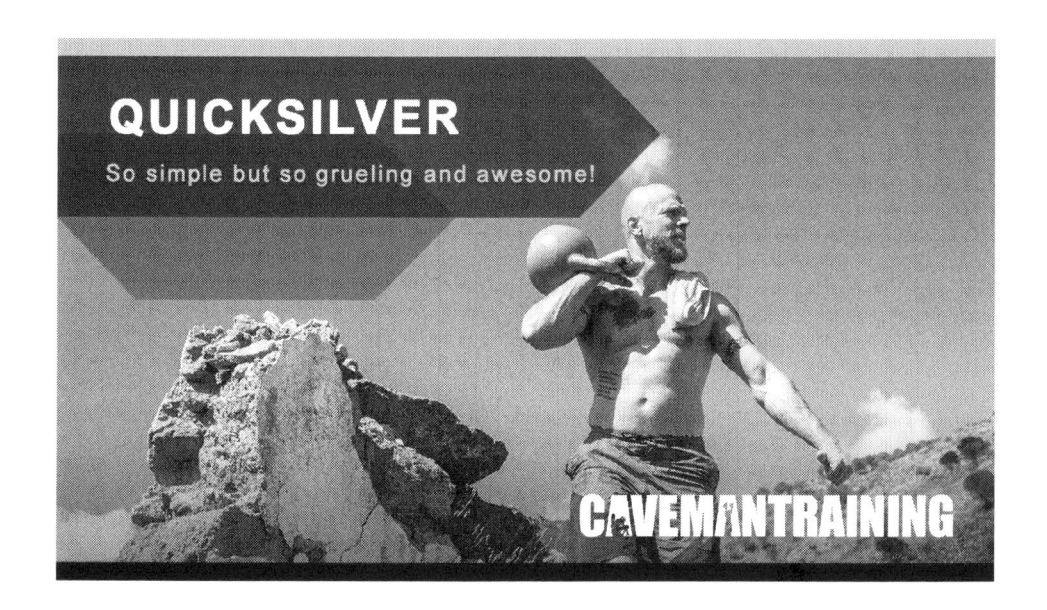

QUICKSILVER KETTLEBELL WORKOUT

- Level: Beginner to intermediate
- Weight: Medium
- Kettlebell(s):
- Type: Cardio, endurance
- Duration: 25 minutes
- Other: Full-body with focus on the trapezius and gluteus maximus; high volume; FOR TIME

workout go.cavemantraining.com/kbwc-vid7

So simple but so grueling and awesome!

Switch at will, but the switch for the clean and swing does not count as a rep. Make sure you always achieve a good rack before attempting your next kettlebell clean, don't get sloppy. The single arm swings are to be performed with a hip hinge and bell coming to chest height. The kettlebell should be of medium weight so you can move fast and get a time between 20 and 25 minutes.

The warm-up is 10 to 12 minutes, the workout up to 25 minutes, cool-down approx. 5 to 10 minutes.

- ➔ 50 hang cleans
- ➔ 50 single arm swings
- ➔ 50 half snatches

Repeat 3 times

FOR TIME

To adjust this workout to beginners just decrease the weight, reduce reps from 50 to 30 and alternate each 5 reps on the hang cleans, swings, and half snatches. If you're not familiar or confident with half snatches yet, perform a clean and push press instead.

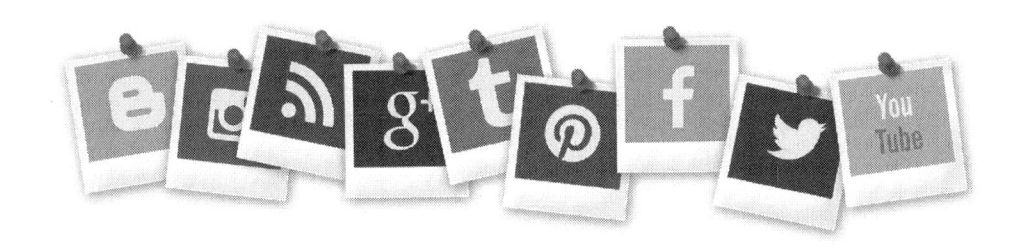

Post your on Facebook, hashtag it #cavemantraining #workoutcompleted, Reddit u/cavemankettlebells, or Instagram @realcavemantraining. Post perfect technique on your Instagram, tag us properly and we'll embed it on our website.

This is considered a high volume workout and I recommend to only do this once a week and for most people probably only once every 2 to 4 weeks.

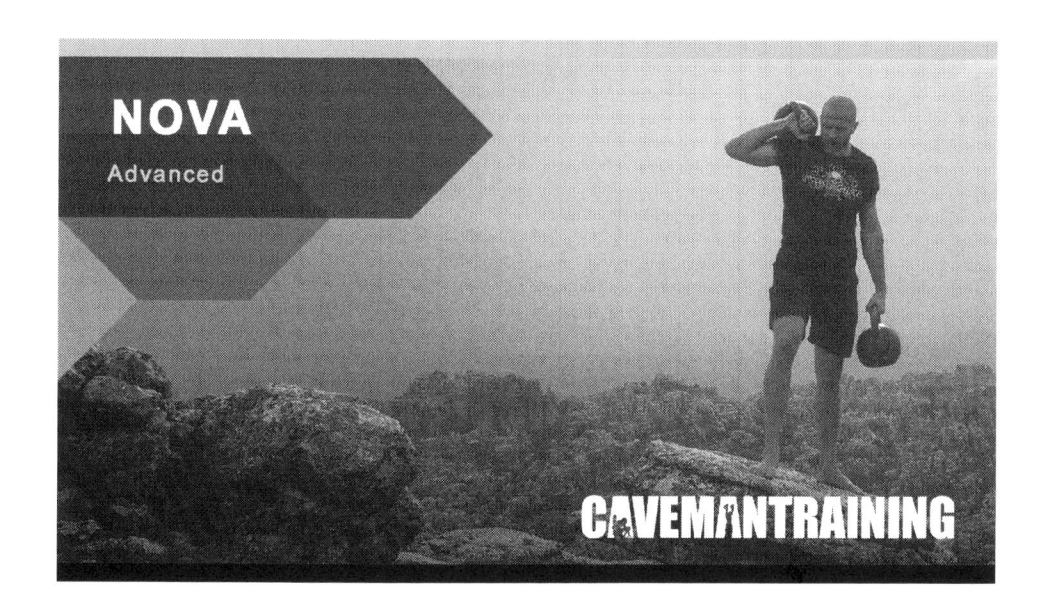

KETTLEBELL WORKOUT NOVA

Level: Advanced

Weight: Medium

Kettlebell(s):

Type: Cardio, endurance, strength

Duration: 25 minutes

Other: Full-body with focus on core, legs, shoulders, and back; buy-in; FOR TIME

workout go.cavemantraining.com/kbwc-vid8

This is Nova, an advanced kettlebell workout.

You buy in with 50 CrossFit burpees and then proceed to the main task with is 10 rounds FOR TIME of 6 double kettlebell half snatch and 3 overhead deadlifts each side.

The whole workout should take about 18 to 25 minutes.

→ BUY IN with 50 CrossFit Burpees

Perform only once

➜ 6 double bell half snatches

➜ 3 overhead squat deadlifts each side

🔄 Repeat 10 times

⏱ FOR TIME

🚩

♂ Rx is 2 x 16kg/35lbs for male

♀ Rx is 2 x 12kg/26lbs for female

You need good squat depth and shoulder flexibility to perform the overhead deadlift. With the kettlebell overhead squat deadlift one side works to keep something overhead, while the other works to lift something. Both sides of the back are doing something completely different (opposites). On one side you need to pull the scapula down, the other up, one side works more the lat, the other the upper trapezius. Extreme tension required during the full movement. There is so much going on in one move, certainly not a beginners move, nor one for those with bad mobility. Triceps, traps, lats, erector spinea, glutes, quads, abdominals, could go in, in effect an extreme full-body exercise. When has a full-body exercise with unilateral qualities not been good? An exercise that challenges every fiber in you…

Is it functional? Would you ever be in a position like this outside of the gym? Maybe if you're pulling a drowning cat out of the river while keeping your baby high and dry! But who cares, enough with all the functional stuff, not everything needs to translate to functional, some things are just fun, difficult, working on strength, on flexibility, mobility etc.

This movement requires extreme finesse, now, don't tell me that CrossFit does not do kettlebell exercises that require finesse, otherwise the TGU would not be done! When the TGU came out, people were probably thinking the same thing as when they saw "OVERHEAD SQUAT DEADLIFT" and laughed. But 3 years from now they all might be doing this exercise when Dave Castro tells them so (if they compete).

Why so specific with the naming, it looks silly! It might look silly, but I tend to err on the side of caution, just in case someone would try to do this hip hinge style! It ain't going to happen, this is a deadlift (lifting a dead non-moving object) while keeping another overhead, it can only be done squat style.

To scale to intermediate

Scaling for the overhead deadlifts is racked deadlifts and increase reps to 4.

Scaling for the double bell half snatch is one bell 3 each side or double bell clean and jerk or clean and push press.

To scale to beginner

Scaling for the overhead deadlifts is single kettlebell deadlifts and increase reps to 4.

Scaling for the double bell half snatch is one bell 3 each side clean and press.

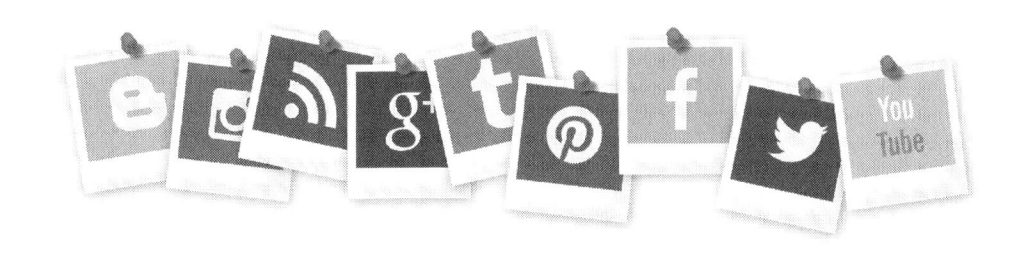

Ask your questions on Facebook, Instagram, or Reddit.

Join our groups:
fb.com/groups/KettlebellTraining
fb.com/groups/crossfit.wod.and.programming

Post your results for Nova when you completed this awesome kettlebell workout.

Tag #cavemantraining #workoutcompleted, Facebook @Cavemantraining, Instagram @realcavemantraining, Reddit u/cavemankettlebells

This kettlebell workout rips into the core muscles and is one I would recommend to perform every 1 or 2 weeks.

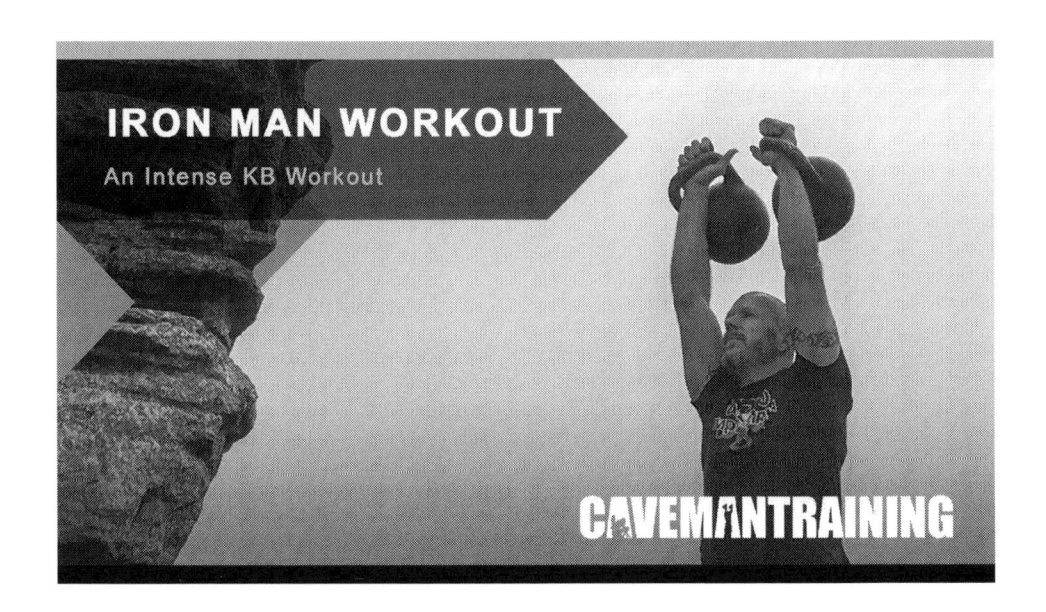

IRON MAN KETTLEBELL WORKOUT

Level: Intermediate

Weight: Medium

Kettlebell(s):

Type: Cardio, endurance, strength

Duration: 35 minutes

Other: Full-body with focus on shoulders, core, and legs; AMRAP; buy-in

workout go.cavemantraining.com/kbwc-vid18

This is the Iron Man workout, an intense KB workout.

The workout consists of a 100 kettlebell swing buy-in followed by a 30-minute AMQRAP of military press, hang clean, and squat with two kettlebells.

The whole workout should take about 35 to 40 minutes.

➔ BUY IN with 100 double arm kettlebell swings

Perform only once

- → Military press
- → Hang clean
- → Racked squat

AMRAP 30 minutes

Yes, 30 minutes is a lot, so, pick your weight wisely, these are thirty minutes of quality work, we want as many quality reps as possible (AMQRAP). This workout is all about pacing and taking appropriate rest.

This workout is truly a full body workout but in particular, it will hit your deltoids, the whole area around the shoulder blades, the hip abductors and adductors, obliques, quadratus lumborum, and so much more.

AMQRAP

AS MANY QUALITY REPS/ROUNDS AS POSSIBLE

#CAVEMANTRAINING

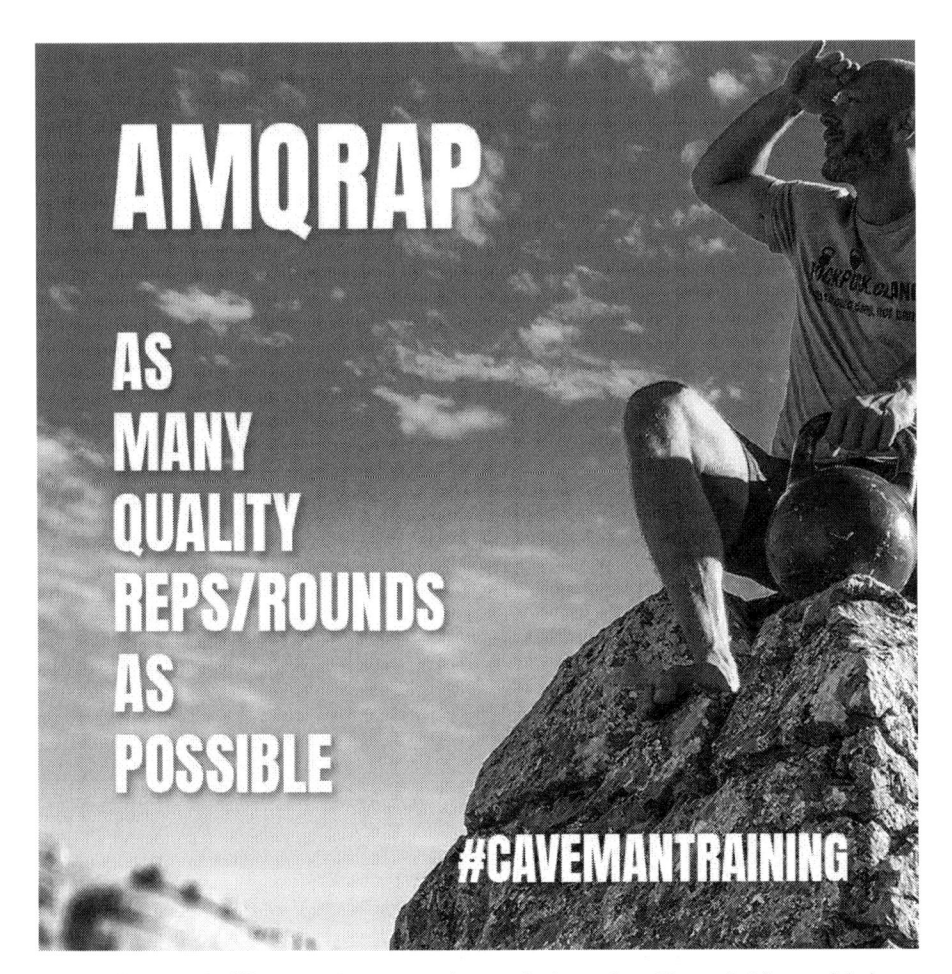

Yes it sounds like AMCRAP and I made it up but I'm sticking with it.

Structure

- Workout
- Warm-up
- Buy-in with 100 double arm kettlebell swings
- Start your 30-minute timer and perform
  - Military press
  - Hang clean
  - Racked squat

- Cool-down and stretch

Are the biceps used in this workout?

Yes, the elbow flexors are used as stabilizers during the military press. As you're pressing up and to the side the stabilizers will need to work to keep the forearm vertical, in fact, even the triceps are working. I mention this as you might be wondering the next day why you're feeling your bi's and tri's, plus it's a fun fact.

Military press

A true military press, no matter what you heard, seen, or been taught, is a standing press with the heels close together and the hands wide on a bar, or when using kettlebells/dumbbells going out and up laterally with focus on working the lateral deltoids.

The advantage of the military press

Due to the feet being closely together you're removing stability, stability is great to focus on heavy presses, but challenging stability also helps press heavier because moving the heels together requires more core stabilization, and as we all know, a strong core is key to pressing heavy.

Why is it called military press?

There are several thoughts on why it's called the military press, one being; because this variation of the overhead press used to be the general indicator or test of one's strength in the military. The other being; the heels are together like standing to attention and the press itself could be seen as a salute.

Why is the military press harder?

The military press requires a lot more core stabilization than a normal press where the feet are wider for a stable base. A lot of work goes into the stabilization underneath the weight which makes this lift a lot harder than a normal shoulder press. Secondly, the press is driven more by the lateral deltoids which are usually less conditioned. In everyday life when we lift stuff over our head it's usually directly up, hence, not an angle we're conditioned for, neither from the gym as most presses focus on the front. The side press usually gets a bad rap because it easily produces injury, which is not due to the press itself but due to not properly progressing or choosing the right weight. The side press/military press is a movement you should include in your training if you want awesome shoulders.

Military press standards

- Heels together (or with minimal space between them)

- Knees and hips locked
- Weight racked
- Elbows under the weight
- No momentum
- Strict press overhead till elbows are locked

Seated military press

There is no seated military press. There is a seated side press.

Staggered military press

You can do the military press with a staggered stance as well, this is where one foot is in front of the other and making the stability even more challenging. You can lift the heel of the back foot slightly off the ground to make the stance easier to achieve.

If you choose the weights correctly then you can do this workout 2 times a week. Definitely a benchmark workout but never when sacrificing form. Benchmark your weight and time, write it down and improve over time. Make sure the time is achieved with a solid 100% technique and adequate rest.

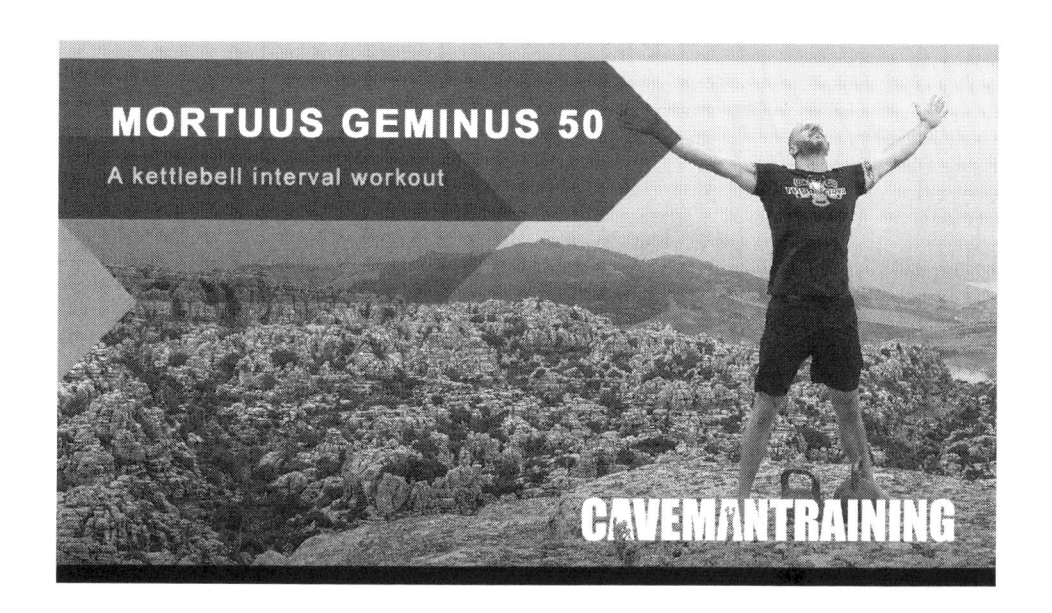

MORTUUS GEMINUS 50

Level: Intermediate

Weight: Medium

Kettlebell(s):

Type: Cardio, endurance, strength

Duration: 8 minutes

Other: Full-body with focus on the legs and back; interval

workout go.cavemantraining.com/kbwc-vid19

A kettlebell interval workout.

You need two kettlebells for this interval workout and you'll be performing an exercise every 12 seconds for a total of 8 minutes. I used 2 x 16kg/35lbs. It's mostly a lower-body workout if you do your swing snatches right and power them up with your hip extensors. The back will also be working hard.

The choice for the workout name, I tell you, it gets pretty hard sometimes coming up with something that's original. In this case I took the Latin words for DEAD and DOUBLE, added 50 as that's how many reps are done in total.

To complete this workout you need to be able to:

1. Dead swing
2. Half snatch
3. Work with two kettlebells

The workout:

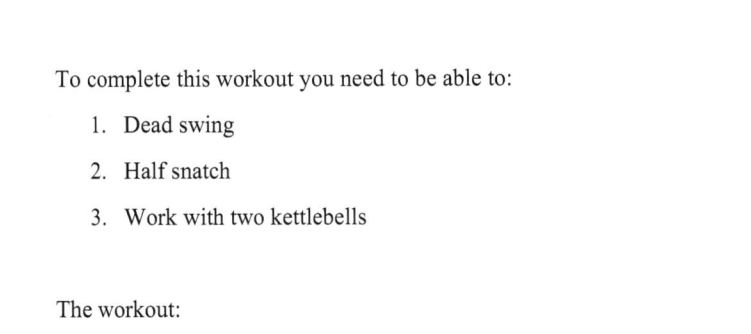

➔ 40 x 12 seconds to perform dead swing half snatch

⏱ Total workout time: 8 minutes.

🔄 40 x 12 seconds can be seen as 40 rounds

🚩

Every 12 seconds you perform one repetition. **The first 10 rounds you add an additional half snatch.** I increased the reps at the start to get that heart rate up right away, starting with just one rep would give you too much rest and make it too easy. So, with those first 10 reps you'll work that heart rate up and then should sort of stay in that zone when switching to just one rep.

In other words first 10 rounds:

- Rep #1
    - Dead
    - Backswing
    - Swing into snatch
    - Drop into rack
    - Drop into backswing
- Rep #2
    - Swing into snatch
    - Drop into rack
    - Drop into backswing
    - Return to dead

After that, round 11 to 40 is just:

- Dead
- Backswing
- Swing into snatch
- Drop into rack
- Drop into backswing
- Dead

Download the pre-programmed timer here you'll need the workout timer app installed before you can run this.

Timer: www.cavemantraining.com/workout-timer/timers/Mortuus-Geminus-50.json

App: workouttimer.app/

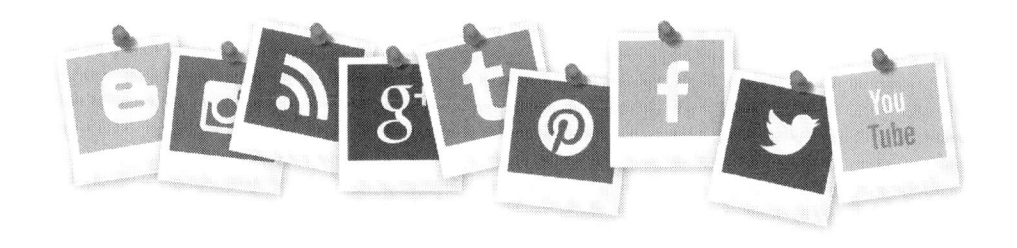

Hashtag: #cavemantraining #workoutcompleted

Instagram: @realcavemantraining

Facebook: @cavemantraining

Progressions and modifications

If you wanted to work on your endurance with this workout then you would for example start with an interval that currently works for you, perhaps that's 20 seconds, 16 seconds, etc. whatever it is, record it and use it. Then over time you can decrease the intervals to 10s, 8s, and eventually perform 8 minutes unbroken. This is a great way to increase your endurance gradually.

To adjust and progress to the full workout you can start with 1 kettlebell and perform the same sequence as programmed but swap hands on each round. You can progress with complexity by starting with dead swing clean and push press until you feel comfortable with that exercise. Once you feel comfortable with the clean and push press you invest time into learning to snatch, the quickest instructions I can give is to think about more explosive and higher clean into a press out. If you want to learn the ins and outs of the snatch check out the book Snatch Physics on Amazon, Cavemantraining, or iTunes.

To make this workout more advanced, reduce the rest time, increase reps, and/or have a 2 minute rest after completing the full cycle once and repeat again, making the workout time a total of 16 minutes.

You can easily do this workout up to 5 days a week for your cardio if you pick the right weights.

DAVID KEOHAN
A workout with a friend

CAVEMANTRAINING

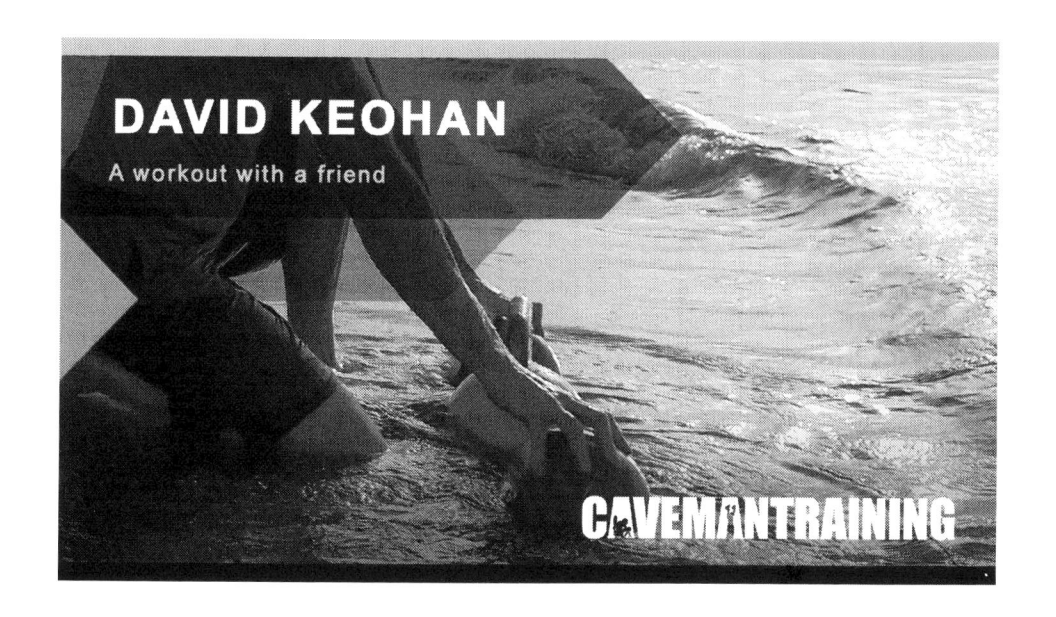

DAVID KEOHAN KETTLEBELL WORKOUT

Level: Intermediate to advanced

Weight: Medium

Kettlebell(s):

Type: Cardio, endurance, strength, flexibility

Duration: 25 to 30 minutes

Other: Full-body; FOR TIME; AMRAP

workout go.cavemantraining.com/kbwc-vid20

I designed this workout to 'try' and impress an amazing kettlebell athlete and put him to the test. David Keohan is someone who truly turned his life around and is achieving amazing feats, feats most of us can only dream of. To you and me 10 minutes of lifting two kettlebells is already an amazing feat (hell), to this man 10 minutes is nothing, to this man 30 minutes is nothing, to this man… well, you should read for yourself how berserk this man goes when you give him two kettlebells. go.cavemantraining.com/kbwc-link1

"I was clinically obese and suffered from high blood pressure, acid reflux, and was diagnosed asthmatic. I was never a sporty person growing up and only got into sport of any kind at 32 years of age when I started running. Oh, and it turned out I wasn't actually asthmatic I was just REALLY unfit!"

Yes, this is a kettlebell workout book, but part of my objective is to try and inspire people, and I believe this story can do that. Help share go.cavemantraining.com/kbwc-link1

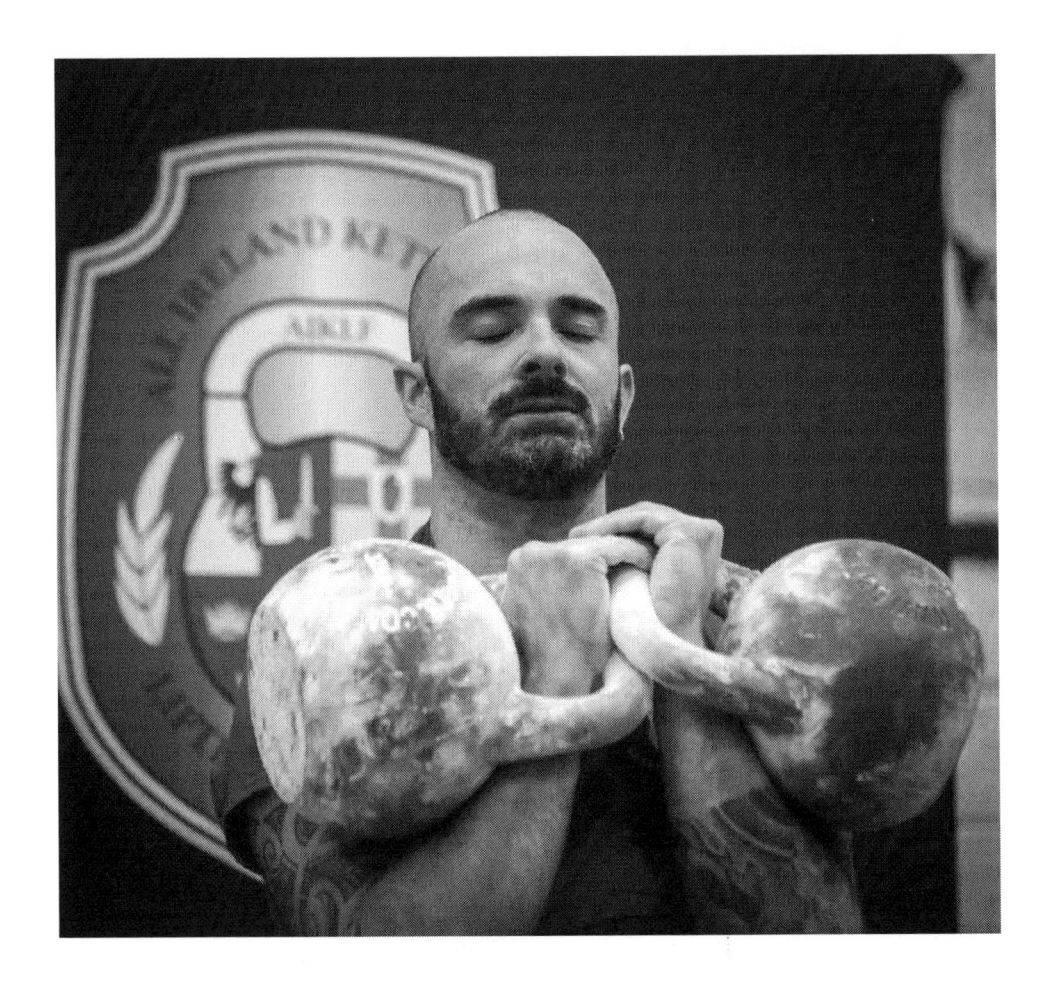

The workout we completed is as following:

⏱ **4 min AMRAP**

→ deadlift

→ hang clean

→ strict press

switch at will

🕒 2 min rest

⏱ **8 min AMRAP**

→ dead clean and squat

→ dead snatch and oh squat

→ swing snatch and reverse lunge

switch at will

🕒 2 min rest

→ 100 single arm swings

→ 100 half snatch

⏱ **FOR TIME**

℞ Rx 1 x 16kg/35lb

I recommend to perform the following lifts with a squat rather than a hip hinge:

- Deadlift
- Hang clean
- Dead clean
- Dead snatch

The following exercises to be performed with a hip hinge:
- Swing snatch
- Single arm swings
- Half snatch

This is a workout you pull out every two weeks to put your whole body to test.

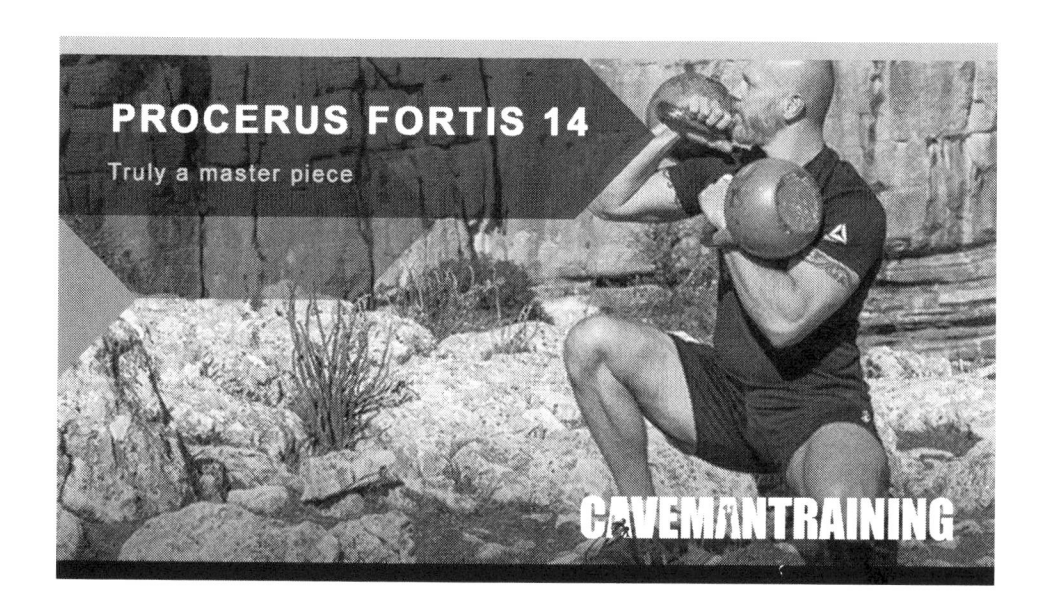

PROCERUS FORTIS 14

Level: Intermediate to advanced

Weight: Medium

Kettlebell(s):

Type: Strength

Duration: 14 minutes

Other: Full-body with focus on triceps, shoulders, upper back, and legs; EMOM

workout go.cavemantraining.com/kbwc-vid21

The perfect kettlebell workout.

This workout requires two kettlebells, is 14 minutes in duration, and is a full-body workout for intermediate to advanced level of kettlebell training. You should have good overhead mobility, be able to clean, strict press, and most of all have the strength and stability to perform an overhead reverse lunge.

This kettlebell combination is designed to get the maximum benefits from the workout. This workout will be getting it's own book as a progressional strength program. Stay tuned. The name is Latin, *Procerus* for overhead, *Fortis* for strong, and 14 for the duration.

A good 10 minute warm-up, 14 minutes kettlebell workout, and 6 minutes stretching, makes a total of 30 minute session.

The warm-up:

- 10 calf raises
- 10 Curtsy lunges each side
- 10 hip hinge into overhead with calf raise
- 10 alternating dynamic pigeon pose
- 10 deep squat working on dorsiflexion into knee extension
- 10 alternating reverse lunge with a twist
- 10 offset shoulder rolls
- 10 arms overhead Hindu squat
- 10 neck circles each way
- 10 thoracic flexion into extension
- 30 to 40 jumping jacks
- 10 alternating thoracic rotations

The areas worked but not limited to with this workout are:

- Back
- Shoulders
- Triceps
- Quadriceps
- Calves
- Gluteals

The workout is **14 minutes EMOM** (think 14 rounds). Every minute on the minute you perform 2 reps of the following kettlebell combo with two kettlebells:

→ Clean
→ Strict press
→ Alternating overhead reverse lunge

The first set starts dead from the ground and the second set is continuous. Put the weights down and rest for the remainder of the minute. You want to go so slow that you have about 20 to 15 seconds of rest per round. If you find yourself resting for longer then you're missing out on the effects this workout is supposed to have, go slow, time it correctly. If you find that you can't hold the weight overhead nor slowly lower it, then you've gone too heavy.

♂ Rx for males is 2 x 16kg/35lbs

♀ Rx for females is 2 x 12kg/26lbs

But as always, form and technique first, weight and reps second.

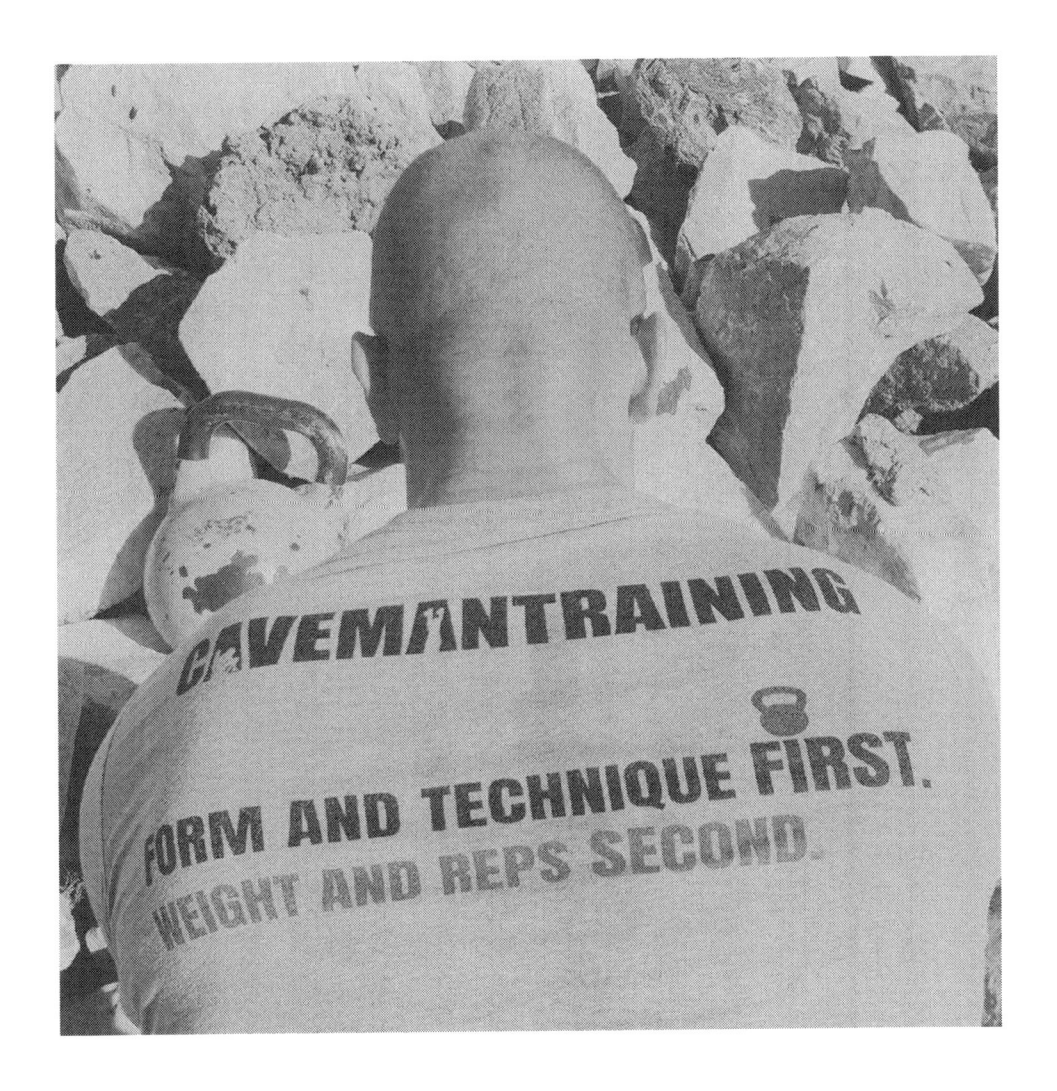

Step-by-step:

1. Dead start
2. Hinge
3. Space between you and the bells
4. Pull the bells into the backswing
5. Clean the bells up into a good rack
6. Create tension and strict press

7. Keep the weights overhead
8. Keep pressing up throughout the movement
9. Reverse lunge on one side
10. Keep the weight on the front leg
11. Come back up through the strength of the front leg
12. Repeat on the other side
13. Slowly lower the weights into rack (take advantage of the eccentric phase)
14. Do not drop the weight into rack
15. Drop into backswing
16. Clean with a swing
17. Strict press
18. Alternating reverse lunge
19. Rack
20. Drop
21. Return to dead
22. Rest
23. Repeat on the next minute

The **Procerus Fortis 14** is a great full-body kettlebell strength workout to schedule in your weekly training for serious results. Some benefits and attributes of this workout are:

- Unilateral leg work
- Leg strength
- Shoulder strength (press concentric and eccentric)
- Back strength
- Shoulder mobility
- Tricep strength (isometric)
- Leg stability
- Psoas stretch
- Shoulder stability
- Core strength

- Thoracic mobility
- Calf strength

Scaling and progressions

- Use a lighter weight
- Use only one kettlebell and switch on each round
- Reduce the reps from 2 to 1
- Reduce the total time from 14 to 10 or 6
- Increase to E2MOM
- Perform the reverse lunge with the kettlebells racked

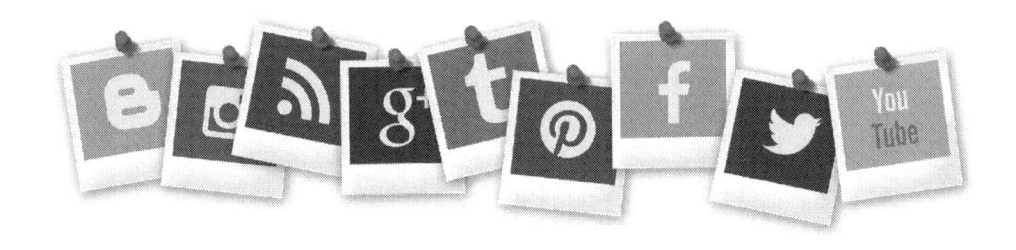

Questions on Reddit, Facebook, YouTube, or Instagram (@realcavemantraining). Don't forget to post after you've completed the workout.

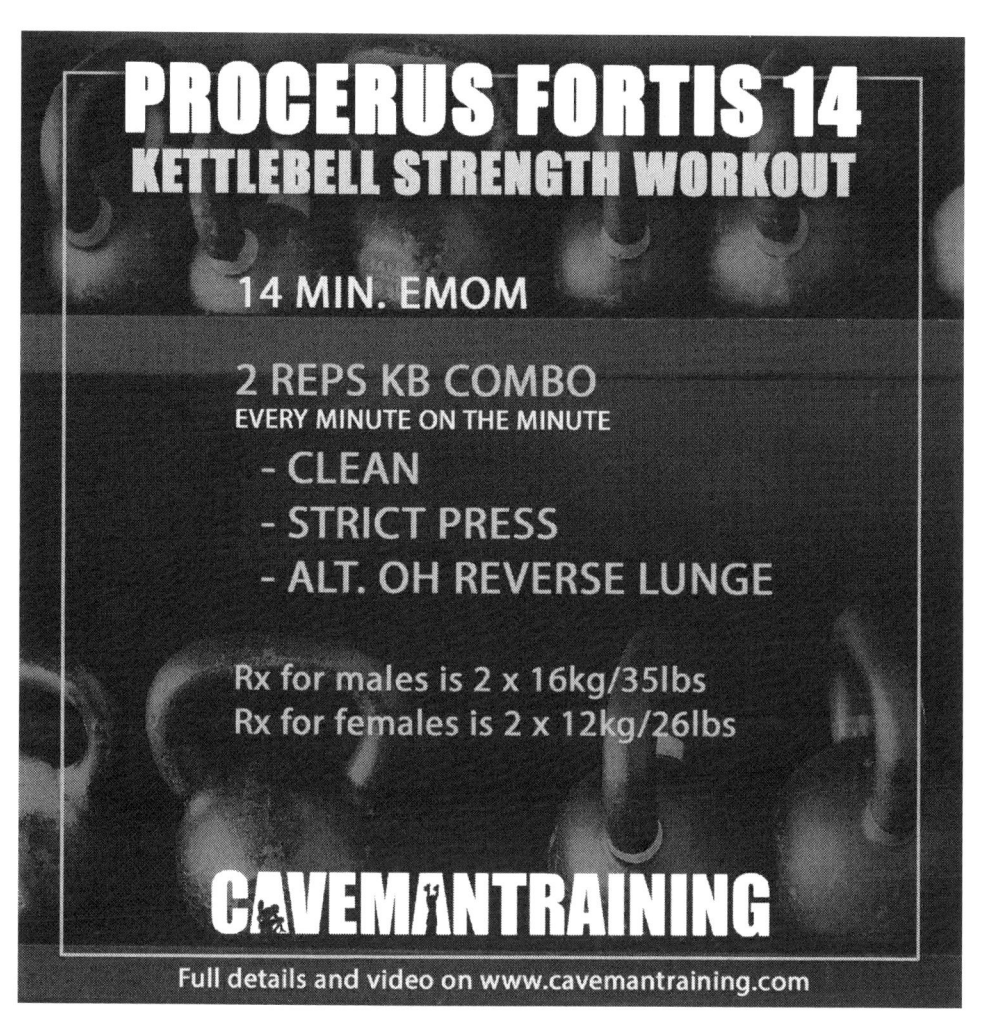

PROCERUS FORTIS 14
KETTLEBELL STRENGTH WORKOUT

14 MIN. EMOM

2 REPS KB COMBO
EVERY MINUTE ON THE MINUTE

- CLEAN
- STRICT PRESS
- ALT. OH REVERSE LUNGE

Rx for males is 2 x 16kg/35lbs
Rx for females is 2 x 12kg/26lbs

CAVEMANTRAINING

Full details and video on www.cavemantraining.com

Share from Instagram go.cavemantraining.com/kbwc-link2

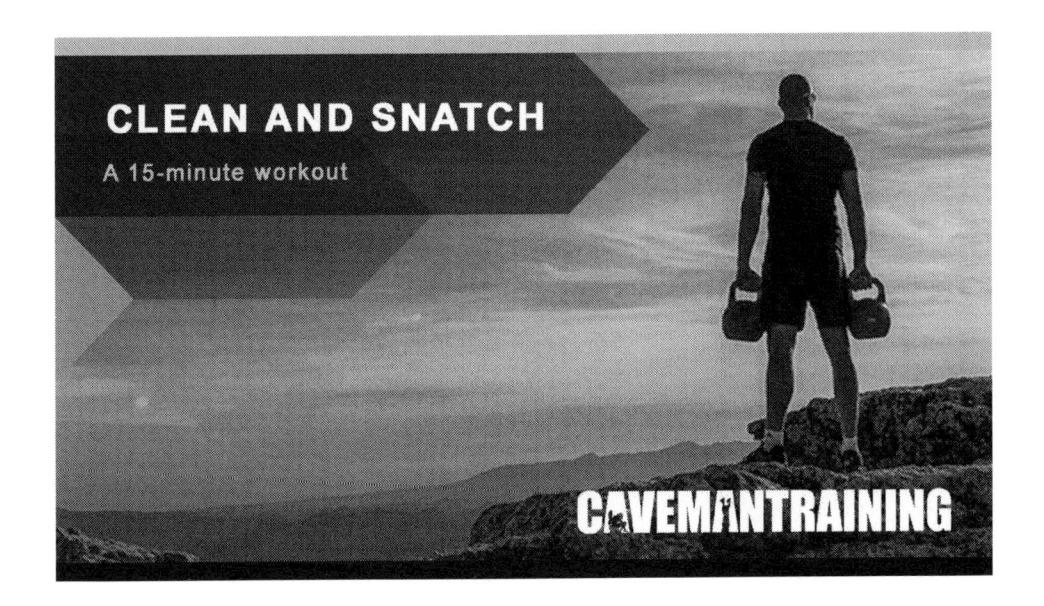

CLEAN AND SNATCH WORKOUT

Level: Intermediate

Weight: Medium

Kettlebell(s):

Type: Cardio and strength

Duration: 15 minutes

Other: Full-body with focus on the lower-body; FOR TIME

workout go.cavemantraining.com/kbwc-vid22

A 15-minute workout.

This workout consists of cleans and snatches. The key is to make sure that kettlebell doesn't bang on your forearms or shoulders upon each rep. Perfecting your clean takes time and is not something I can cover in this book, I have covered the subject to prevent bruising, banging, and ripping of hands in the book Master The Kettlebell Clean. The quickest tip I can give you is, open up, insert and catch the weight before it bangs.

This kettlebell workout takes about 15 minutes to complete and consists of the following kettlebell exercises:

- → 2 x kettlebell dead cleans
- → 2 x kettlebell hang cleans
- → 2 x kettlebell swing cleans
- → 2 x kettlebell full snatches

Left + right = 1 round. Perform 8 rounds.

Rest 3 minutes and perform another 6 rounds.

Both the dead and hang clean should be performed with a squatting movement where as the swing clean and snatch should be performed with a good deep hip hinge.

To adjust this workout for beginners, reduce the reps just 1 and take more time to perform each rep, i.e. perform the rep, pause and focus on the rep to come. Once you master the exercise you can increase intensity.

To make this workout more advanced you can work with two kettlebells, I would recommend to change the weight from medium to light to medium.

This is a work you can do 2 to 3 times a week, just make sure you have your technique spot on as you don't want to be putting up with the banging of the kettlebell on your wrist.

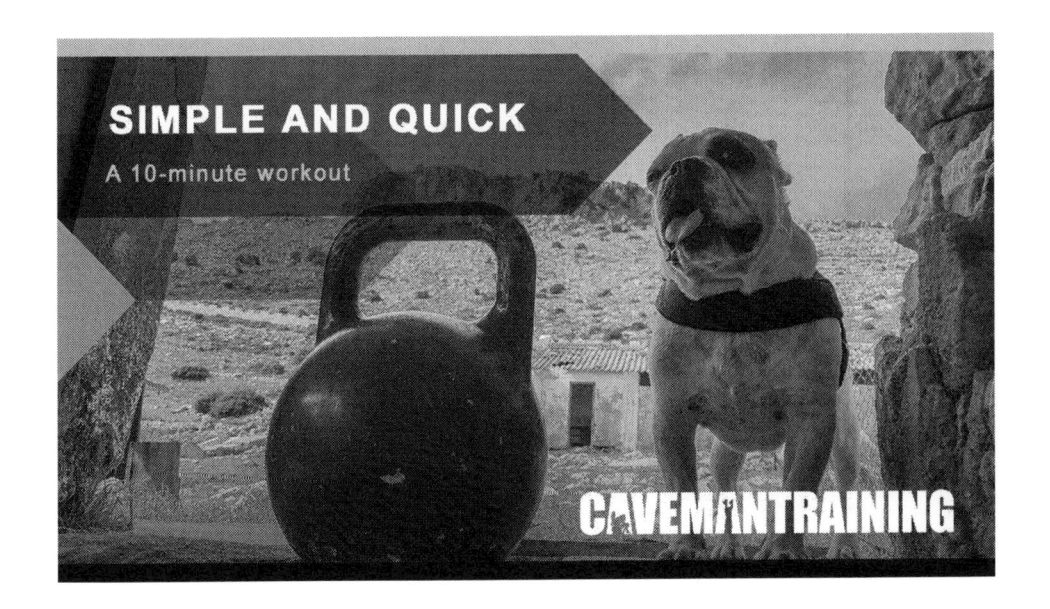

10 MINUTE KETTLEBELL WORKOUT

Level: Intermediate to advanced

Weight: Medium

Kettlebell(s):

Type: Cardio, strength, and flexibility

Duration: 10 minutes

Other: Full-body with focus on the lower and upper-body; FOR TIME

workout go.cavemantraining.com/kbwc-vid23

A 10-minute workout.

Just a simple quick 10-minute kettlebell workout that will get your heart rate up and burn some serious calories. The overhead squat is quite challenging and it requires good shoulder, thoracic, hip, knee, and ankle mobility. A great drill to work up to the overhead squat is squatting in front of a wall with one arm up and switching on each rep. This will take time.

The kettlebell workout is as follows:

- ➔ 4 x dead clean
- ➔ 3 x swing clean
- ➔ 2 x racked squat
- ➔ 1 x snatch to overhead squat

Left + right = 1 round. 1 round should take you about 1 minute to complete.

Complete 10 rounds and post on our Facebook.

With the dead clean you want to use the squat movement and with the swing clean you want to hip hinge. Make sure you implement clearly different movement patterns for each and accentuate each one.

You can modify this workout to beginner level by just putting the kettlebell down on the ground after the two reps of racked squat, stand up, and perform an overhead squat with just the arms in the air. Don't force anything, understand that the overhead squat is very much a back exercise. Push that chest out, work on thoracic and shoulder flexibility while maintaining good pelvic alignment (inline with the spine).

Some videos for the overhead drills to improve your overhead squat mobility as mentioned above.

wall squat mobility drill go.cavemantraining.com/kbwc-vid24

overhead squat progression go.cavemantraining.com/kbwc-vid25

This is a workout you can include in your training 2 to 3 times a week.

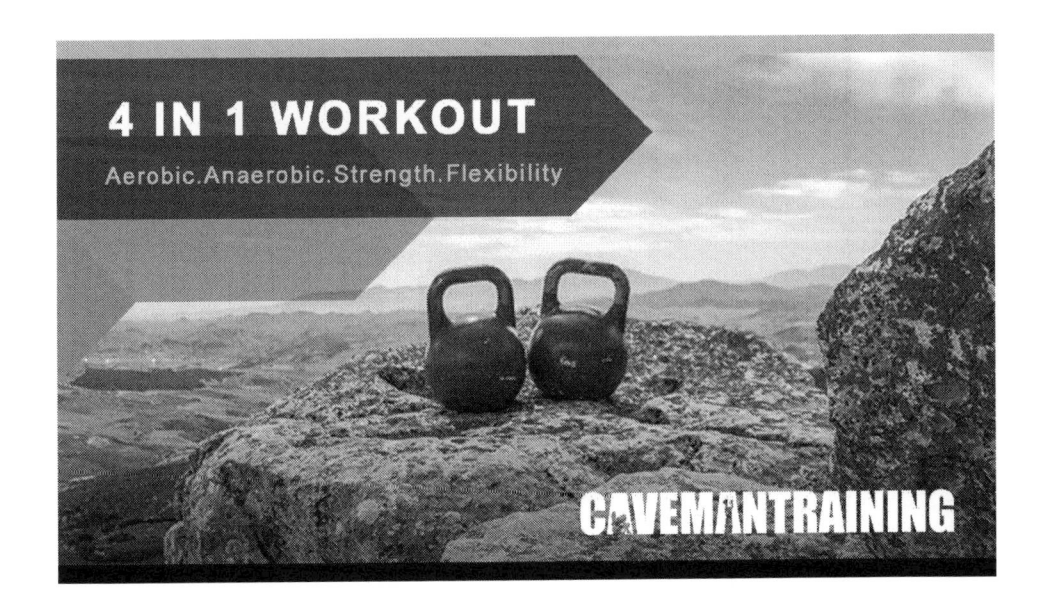

4 IN 1 KETTLEBELL WORKOUT

Level: Intermediate

Weight: Medium

Kettlebell(s):

Type: Cardio, strength, and flexibility

Duration: 30 minutes

Other: Full-body; training; EMOM; AMRAP

workout go.cavemantraining.com/kbwc-vid26

A versatile workout.

This workout was designed to incorporate aerobic, anaerobic, strength, and flexibility in one, to demonstrate the effectiveness of the kettlebell and our Cavemantraining kettlebell workouts.

This kettlebell workout is a full body workout that has four tasks:

→ **4 minutes** of alternating kettlebell swings

　AMRAP

　2 minutes rest

→ **4 minutes** of kettlebell strict press

　AMRAP (switch at will)

　2 minutes rest

→ **8 minutes** of a kettlebell combo squat and hang snatch

　EMOM (switch each minute)

　4 minutes rest

→ **3 to 5 rounds** of kettlebell exercises for flexibility and mobility

FOR TRAINING

Rx weight

Male 16kg/35lb

Female 12kg/26lb

The objective of the alternating swing in the first task is to provide an **aerobic** effect and warm the body up for what's to come, that doesn't mean you can skip your warm-up, it just means you'll have an additional warm-up. I programmed alternating so that the weight provides sufficient resistance (for one arm) and the grip can last longer, possibly the full 4 minutes.

The kettlebell strict press in the second task is for **strength**, shoulders and core, yes, you're also working your core in the strict press for stabilization and to provide a stable base to press from.

The kettlebell combo in the third task is carefully designed to tax the **anaerobic** system with a squat followed with a hang snatch. You can't get any more compound than that! There are 8 minutes in this EMOM, you perform 8, 10, or 12 reps depending on your fitness, and for the first 4 minutes, you perform that amount per minute. If you complete the reps before the minute is up, you rest for the remainder of that minute. After 4 sets you reduce the reps by 2, so, if you started with

10, you do 8 for the last 4 minutes (per minute). Decide whether you're ready for 8, 10, or 12 before you start, and also keep in mind that you want at least 10 seconds rest before the next minute. To perform:

- Rack
- Squat
- Drop into hang
- Snatch the weight overhead
- Drop into rack
- Repeat

The last task is the windmill and overhead reverse lunge, of course, either of those is also great for strength, but they're programmed for their effects on flexibility and mobility, in particular, shoulders and hips. The reverse lunge is great if you push the hips forward on the back leg to get deep into the hip flexors (front).

So, with this kettlebell workout, you're getting maximum bang for your buck and get a cardio workout on different levels, a strength workout, and a mobility workout all in one.

4 IN 1 KETTLEBELL WORKOUT

4 MIN. ALT. KB SWINGS
2 MIN. REST
4 MIN. STRICT PRESS
2 MIN. REST
8 MIN. EMOM KB COMBO
- RACKED SQUAT
- HANG SNATCH
4 MIN. REST
3 TO 5 ROUNDS OF
10 ALT. WINDMILL
10 ALT. OVERHEAD REVERSE LUNGE

CAVEMANTRAINING

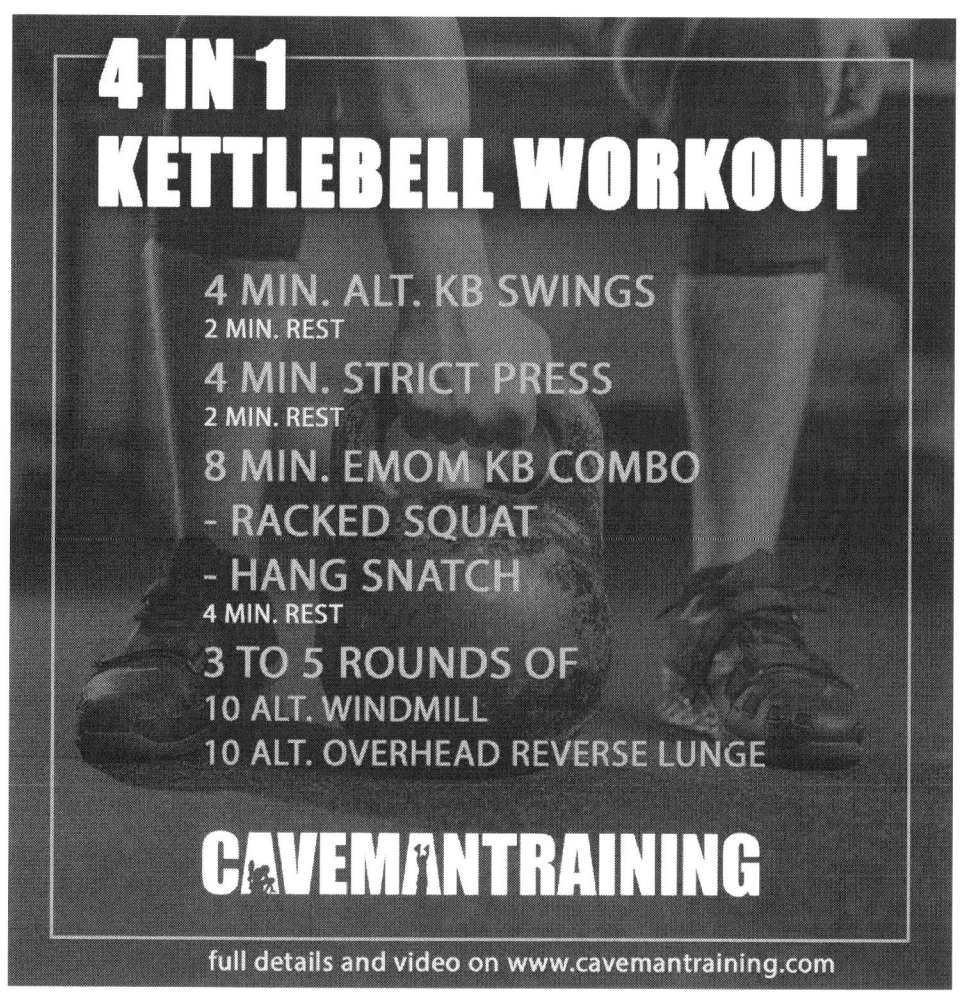

full details and video on www.cavemantraining.com

Share the workout go.cavemantraining.com/kbwc-link3

Main muscles worked:

- Deltoids
- Erector spinae
- Glutes
- Quadriceps
- Trapezius
- Calves
- Hamstrings

- Obliques
- Abdominals
- Hip flexors
- And many more …

Pre-programmed Timer

Download the pre-programmed timer for this workout. You'll need the Cavemantraining Workout Timer from Google Play. Below is a screenshot of the timer structure, it's all ready for you to download and run, it can't be any easier than this. https://play.google.com/store/apps/details?id=com.cavemantraining.variable.workout.timer

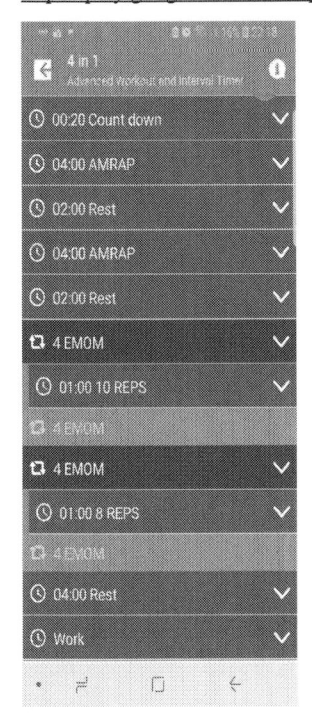

Download the timer here or see all pre-programmed timers available. You need to have the workout timer app installed.

https://www.cavemantraining.com/workout-timer/timers/4-in-1-Kettlebell-Workout.json

https://www.cavemantraining.com/workout-timer/workout-timers/

https://play.google.com/store/apps/details?id=com.cavemantraining.variable.workout.timer

> "The greatest creation will be what you make of yourself."
>
> *Heather Mamachu*

CAVEMANTRAINING

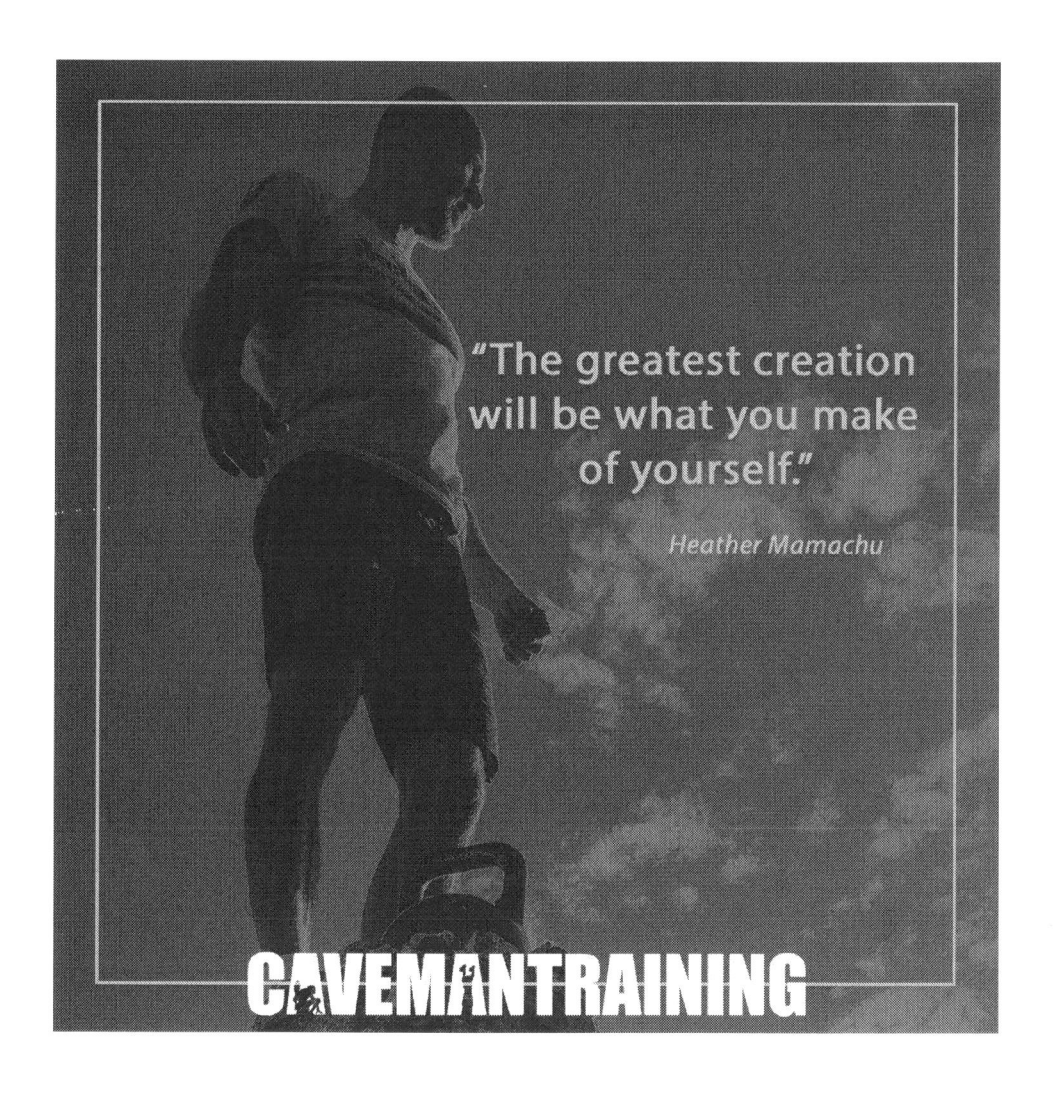

This is a workout you can program in your training 1 to 2 times a week. It's a great workout to include at least once a week to test yourself from every angle. Definitely a benchmark workout.

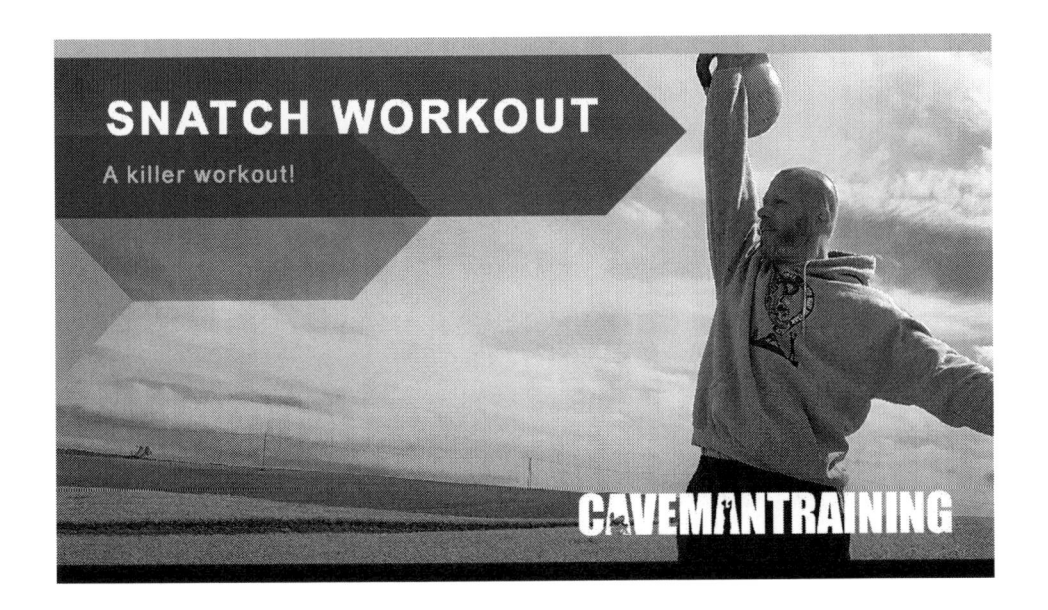

KETTLEBELL SNATCH WORKOUT

Level: Intermediate

Weight: Medium

Kettlebell(s):

Type: Cardio and strength

Duration: 35 to 40 minutes

Other: Full-body with a focus on legs and cardio; FOR TIME; AMRAP

workout go.cavemantraining.com/kbwc-vid27

A killer workout.

Snatches and sprints for three AMRAPs and then a FOR TIME task. I programmed adequate rest with a rep scheme that allows you to go all out for the duration of the tasks.

The tasks are:

→ 4 hang snatches on each side

→ 50m sprint

⏱ 6 min **AMRAP**

⏲ 3 min rest

→ 4 full swing snatches on each side

→ 40m sprint

⏱ 6 min **AMRAP**

⏲ 4 min rest

→ 8 double bell half snatches

→ 30m sprint

⏱ 6 min **AMRAP**

⏲ 4 min rest

→ 6 double bell half snatches

→ 20m sprint

◎ 10 rounds

⏱ **FOR TIME**

Rx 1 x16kg/35lb 2 x 16kg/35lb

The hang snatch is from hang directly into overhead and dropped back into the hang. The path it travels is straight up and down. Use a squatting movement to snatch the weight up overhead in one fast and explosive movement. You can dip under the weight but come into full extension before you drop into the next rep. You perform 4 on one side and then switch with a hang clean to perform 4 reps on the other before you start your sprint.

The full swing snatch starts from racking position into backswing directly overhead and into a drop that goes into backswing to repeat. A full snatch is where the weight goes from overhead into the full drop, a half snatch is where the weight goes from overhead into racking position before it drops into the next rep.

The double kettlebell half snatches start dead on the ground for the first rep into backswing, snatched overhead, dropped into racking position for the next backswing and snatch.

With any of the snatch variations you want to use your lower body to power the movement, with the hang this movement is a squat, and with the swing the movement is a hip hinge. You want to power the kettlebells up so high that the shoulders need to do as little work as possible.

Download the timer here. You need to have the workout timer app installed.

https://www.cavemantraining.com/workout-timer/timers/Kettlebell-Snatch-Workout.json

https://play.google.com/store/apps/details?id=com.cavemantraining.variable.workout.timer

The snatch is a full body exercise that delivers amazing effects. The snatch can be used to increase cardiovascular endurance, muscular endurance, strength, flexibility, core stability, explosive power, and much more. The snatch truly works each and every major joint in the body, ankles, knees, hips, shoulders, elbow, and wrists. For strength, you can't deny the major areas that will improve, such as, latissimus dorsi, deltoid, triceps, erector spinae, abdominals, gluteals, hamstrings, calves, hip flexors, quadriceps, lumbrical muscles, and many more. All these properties make it the king of kettlebell exercises, an exercise everyone should include in his or her training.

This is a full on workout that is great to include at least once in your training every week.

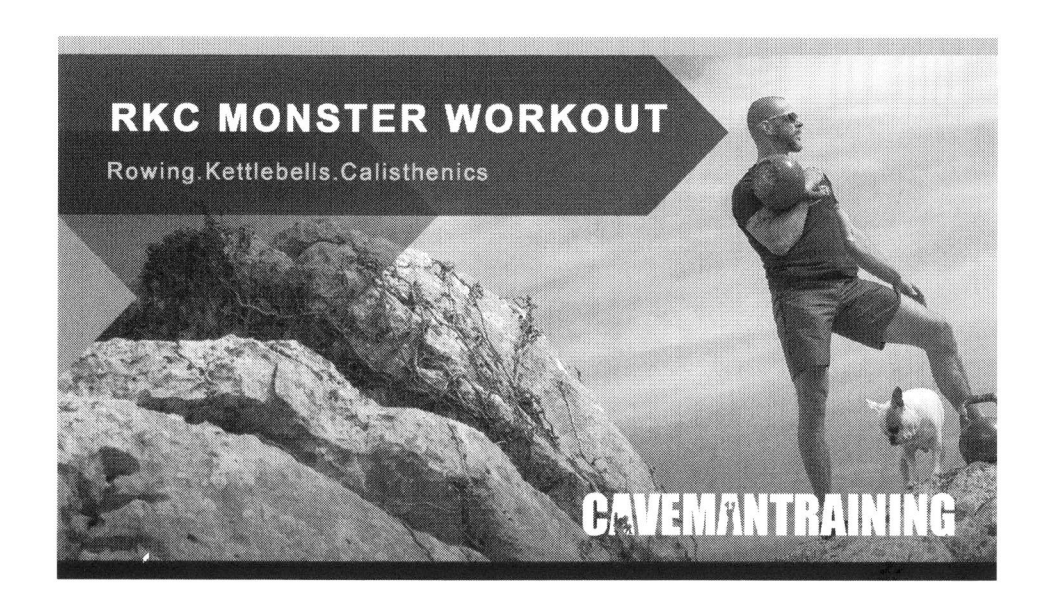

RKC MONSTER WORKOUT

Level: Intermediate

Weight: Medium to heavy

Kettlebell(s):

Type: Cardio, strength, and power

Duration: 25 to 30 minutes

Other: Full-body with a focus on the upper back and legs; FOR TIME; AMRAP

workout go.cavemantraining.com/kbwc-vid28

Four tasks to complete.

This is a monster workout involving rowing, kettlebells, and calisthenics. Two tasks FOR TIME and two for AMRAP.

The tasks are as follows.

Task 1

- → 100 calorie rows or a 1.5k run
- **FOR TIME**

Task 2

Kettlebell combo:

- → Dead clean
- → Dead snatch
- → Swing snatch
- → Overhead reverse lunge

Switch at will

8 minutes **AMRAP**

Rx 24kg/53lb for men and 20kg/44lb for females

Task 3

- → 4 x push-ups 'any'
- → 2 x pull-ups
- → 4 x squats
- → 2 x chin-ups

8 minutes **AMRAP**

Task 4

- → 100 double arm kettlebell swings
- **FOR TIME**

Rx 24kg/53lb for men and 20kg/44lb for female

The kettlebell combo goes from dead to racking (dead clean), racking to dead, dead to overhead, overhead to racking, racking to swing, swing to overhead, reverse lunge, racking and back to dead.

The push-ups can be any push-up variation you prefer, chest, triceps, or hybrid. The pull up is performed with the focus on the lats and the palms should be wide apart facing away from you when holding on to the bar. The chin-ups are the opposite, you want the palms facing you approximately inline with your shoulders, and the chin should come above the bar.

You can only do this workout on your own due to the design (FOR TIME, AMRAP, AMRAP, FOR TIME) of the workout, but it can be done in a group if each person has a smartphone and the *Cavemantraining Workout Timer*, and it's a lot of fun in a group. After you install the app timer on each phone all you need to do is download the pre-defined timer for this workout and everyone is ready to go.

Download and install the timer here.
https://www.cavemantraining.com/workout-timer/timers/RKC-Monster-Workout.json

A great benchmark workout to pull out every 4 weeks and see how you've improved.

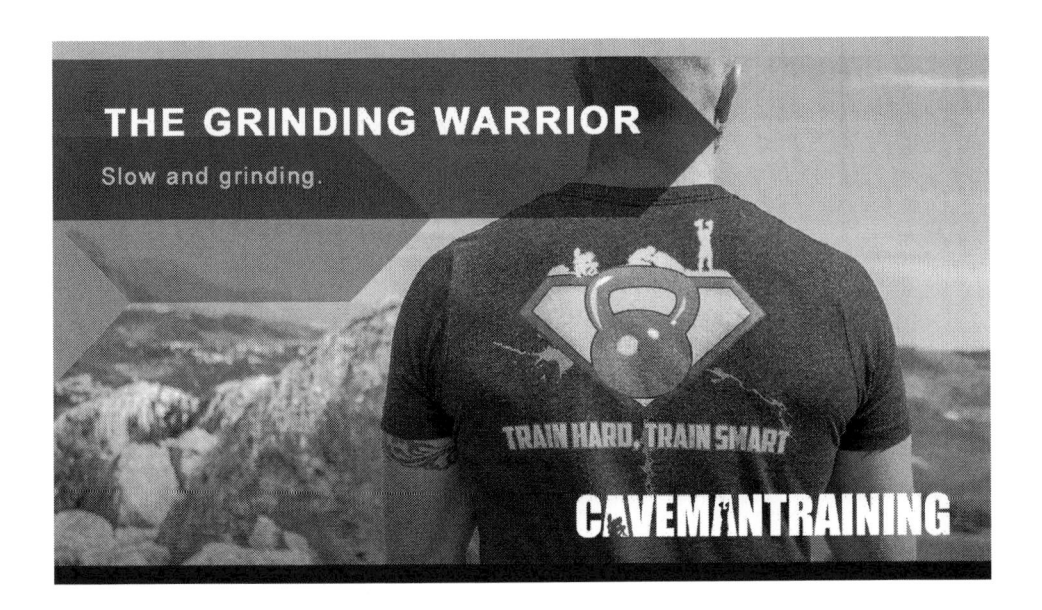

THE GRINDING WARRIOR

Level: Intermediate to advanced

Weight: Medium

Kettlebell(s):

Type: Strength and flexibility

Duration: 22 to 25 minutes

Other: Full-body, training, slow

workout go.cavemantraining.com/kbwc-vid29

Do something that your body will thank you for.

This workout is all to be performed slow and grinding. Focus on perfecting the movements. 2 rounds with one kettlebell and the last two rounds with two kettlebells. Beginners should perform the workout without weight.

The video includes a warm-up, no special effects or titles, just the warm-up and workout. You could use it to work out at the same time as watching the video, I cut the rest breaks, so you would have to pause the video at that stage and press play when ready to resume the workout.

2 rounds with one kettlebell

- ➔ 5 front squats L
- ➔ 5 front squats R
- ➔ 5 windmills L
- ➔ 5 windmills R
- ➔ 5 bent press L
- ➔ 5 bent press R
- ➔ 5 cossack squat R
- ➔ 5 cossack squat L

Repeat with two kettlebells. Use a medium weight that is safe for you. I used two 16kgs/35lbs.

🚩

These movements are quite advanced when it comes to flexibility. You can progress to these movements with no weight used at all. Your second stage would be to add a very light weight, you can even use light dumbbells. The bent press however is always best performed with some heavier weight add resistance which improves the pull and come under.

The bent press is an exercise made popular by strongwomen and strongmen such as Eugen Sandow, Arthur Saxon, and Louis Cyr in the 19th century. Unfortunately the exercise is no longer popular, even though it has incredible benefits. But…

The exercise is making its come back. (I have to admit that I'm against the name of the exercise)

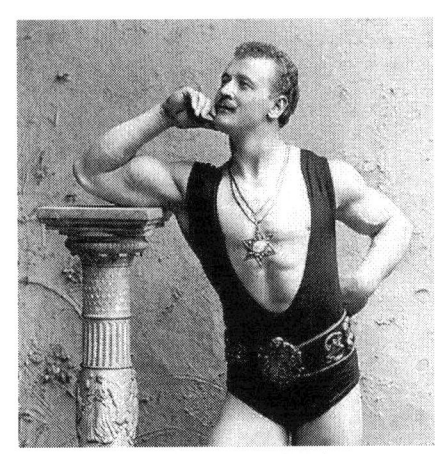

Strongman *Eugen Sandow*

The problem with the exercise is that many people don't understand its objectives, they press from an angle they're not conditioned for; first off, it's not a press, hence my resistance against the name; second, they're not conditioned, lacking thoracic mobility, hip mobility, core strength, lat strength etc.

The bent press is an exercise everyone should be incorporating in their training, it's awesome for so many things:

- Thoracic mobility
- Flexibility
- Core strength
- Shoulder mobility
- Shoulder strength
- Improved posture
- Injury prevention
- Kyphosis prevention (rounding of the back)
- Improved breathing
- Stability and much more

It's also great to get heavier weight overhead and focus on the down-phase of the overhead position, i.e. increase your pressing strength.

When I say everyone I mean every, it's great for people who sit behind the computer all day, it's great for Crossfitters to improve overhead mobility, shoulder strength and much more, it's great for

Brazilian Jiu Jitsu practitioners, not much to be said other than the word ROTATION. Above all, good thoracic mobility will help prevent injury, i.e. a stiff thoracic spine will require you to employ other areas less suitable for certain moves, and creating potential for injury.

It Is NOT a Press

Unlike the name suggests, it's not a press and something I'm personally not happy about, but I've covered that in plenty of articles. Quick recap, the Bent Press in summary is performed as follows:

1. Rack
2. Thoracic rotation
3. Push the hips back
4. Pull the elbow down
5. Bent
6. Come under the weight
7. Lock out
8. Come up
9. Shoulder rotation
10. Neutral stance
11. Rack and repeat

▶ bent press go.cavemantraining.com/kbwc-vid30

One can come under the weight in different ways, one leg locked and other bent, or bending both knees and turn it more into a squat under.

SAFETY AND PROGRESSION FIRST

I know this exercise looks cool and you'll probably want to grab a heavy weight right now and try it out, DON'T! … unless you're already conditioned in this area, do not attempt this move straight away, it requires progression. Work on your flexibility first, hamstrings especially, work on shoulder strength, work on rotation with just bodyweight, work on the movement without weight, then slowly increase the weight over time.

Because of the super qualities this workout provides you with it makes it a great workout to include once every week or at least once every two weeks. You can include it more often but you have to adjust the weights accordingly.

KILLER. KILLA. WORKOUT

A gasping for air workout.

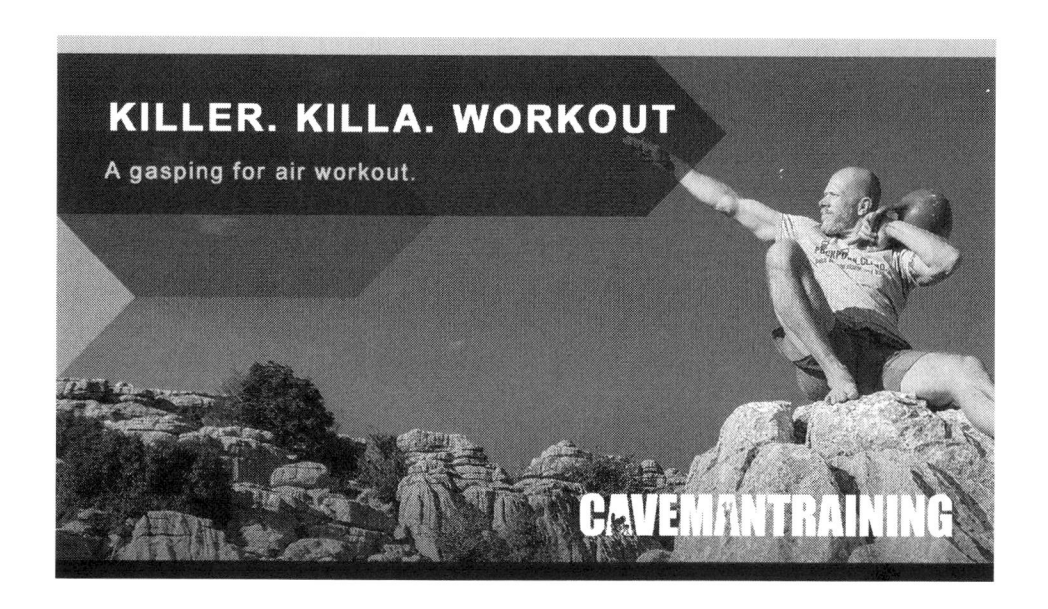

KILLER. KILLA. WORKOUT

Level: Intermediate

Weight: Medium to heavy

Kettlebell(s):

Type: Cardio and strength

Duration: 30 to 40 minutes

Other: Full-body; buy-in; FOR TIME

workout go.cavemantraining.com/kbwc-vid31

This cardio workout is an absolute killer.

If you like a gasping for air workout, this is it. You buy in with 100 calories on the assault bike, 80 for females.

Then you proceed with 12 rounds of:

→ 4 alternating snatch into overhead reverse lunge

- ➔ 4 push ups 'any'
- ➔ 8 calories on the assault bike (6 for females)

Rx for the snatch is 20kg for male and 16kg for female.

If you don't have a bike, replace the 100 cals with a 2k run, and the 8 cals each round with 60 high knees.

Standards

Snatch into overhead reverse lunge:

- Weight needs to be snatched with a hip hinge
- Overhead lockout maintained throughout the rep
- Knee gently touching the ground
- Weight lowers only after coming into full extension
- The drop is full into the next snatch on the other side
- The hand switch can be performed with a switch snatch or swing
- Last rep can be lowered into racking

Push-ups:

- Any variation allowed
- Elbow reach 90-degree flexion

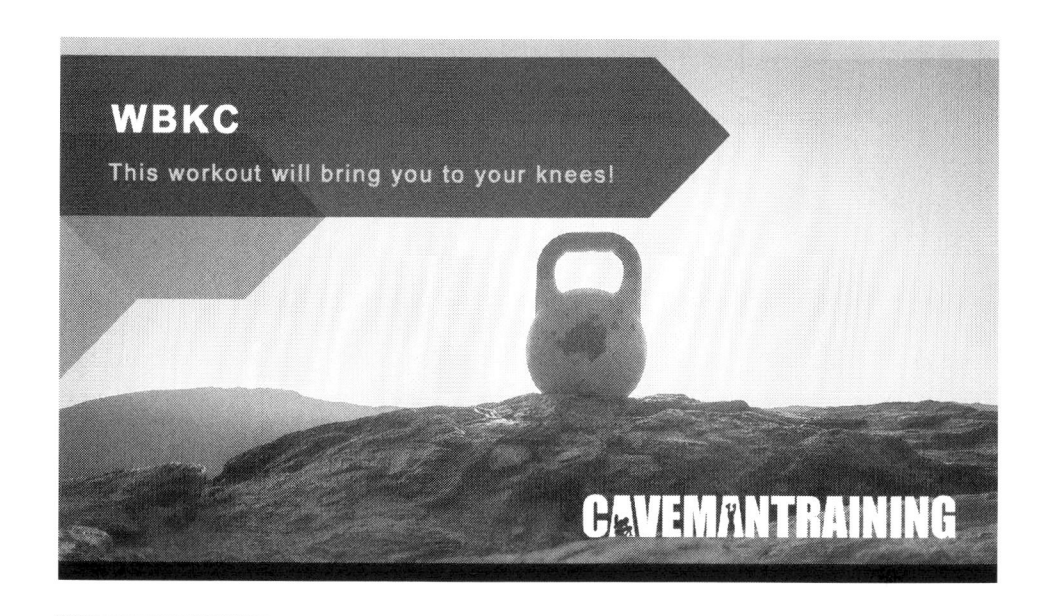

THIS WORKOUT WILL BRING YOU TO YOUR KNEES!

Level: Intermediate

Weight: Medium

Kettlebell(s):

Type: Cardio and endurance

Duration: 20 to 40 minutes

Other: Full-body; high reps

workout go.cavemantraining.com/kbwc-vid32

I baptized this WBKC. It's an absolute killer!

World's Best Kettlebell Combo consists of a half swing snatch and squat thruster. You're hip hinging, snatching, squatting, and thrusting. It gets pretty explosive and is extremely taxing on the system.

It's simple though, take on the challenge and perform 100 **FOR TIME**.

→ 100 x half snatch and squat thrusters with double kettlebell

🚩

If you need to rest, rest. Of course, your objective is to complete it as fast as possible with minimal rest but good form and technique.

The squat is judged on hips below knee line, the thrust has to be one movement, i.e. not coming out of the squat, pause, and press. To be completely honest, if you want a good thruster, you can't program 100, but as long as your movement is continuous/powerful from squat into overhead, we'll count it as a thrust, You can hang snatch if you like, hell, you can dead snatch if you want, but those variations are way more taxing than the swing snatch. You come into racking after the snatch, hence half snatch, and lower straight away into the squat.

Like it or hate it, complete it, post on our YouTube, Facebook, or Instagram when completed. Rx is 2 x 16kg/35lb for male, and 2 x 12kg/26lb for female.

Worlds Best Kettlebell Combo

This is by far the worlds best kettlebell combo you'll come across, it consists of two highly effective exercises, namely the squat thruster and the king of kettlebell exercises the snatch, half snatch to be exact. The combo is performed with two kettlebells.

I'm using a half snatch (back into racking rather than full drop) because it makes the combo flow nicely as you'll be in racking position ready to go right into your squat thruster.

- Clean once
- Rack
- Squat
- Thrust
- Press out
- Lock-out
- Drop
- Rack
- Drop

- Back swing
- Up swing
- Bell to body proximity
- Pull
- Press out
- Lock-out
- Drop
- Rack
- REPEAT

What is a thrust? The dictionary says: push suddenly or violently in a specified direction. The keyword is push, we don't want to be pressing, we want to use the lower-body to push the weights up, press those heels into the ground and come up as quick as possible immediately following through with the kettlebells, then press out if needed.

How to use this awesome kettlebell combo in different ways?

Training

Use about 60% of your 1RM to perform 10 reps of the combo followed by 5 chin-ups. 6 rounds and take a minute rest after each round.

EMOM (interval training)

10 minutes every minute on the minute perform work. First 5 minutes 6 reps at the start of the minute with a lighter weight and rest the remainder of the minute. From the 6 minute mark you increase the weight, decrease the reps and perform 4 reps.

Power (training)

Go heavier and use about 80% of your 1RM to perform low reps with adequate rest. 4 good solid reps followed by 2 minutes rest. 4 rounds.

Challenge yourself!

If you want to challenge yourself, work with two different weights, you get all the fun of working with two kettlebells and also get more unilateral qualities through the uneven weights and the body having to compensate for that. Did you know that snatching with one kettlebell is actually harder than snatching with two kettlebells? If you snatch with one kettlebell you'll probably see differences between right and left, use two kettlebells and in most cases they won't show.

This is a workout you should program in your training every 4 weeks and use as a benchmark workout. Set a time and record it the first time you complete it, beat the time on subsequent goes, once your time does not increase drastically anymore, go up in weight and start again.

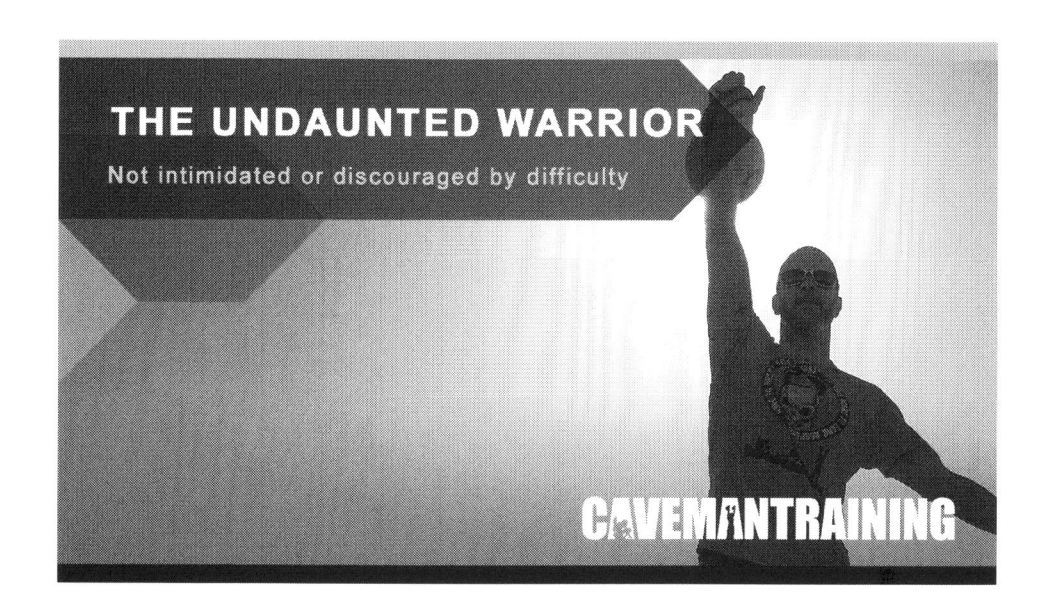

THE UNDAUNTED WARRIOR

Level: Intermediate

Weight: Medium

Kettlebell(s):

Type: Cardio and endurance

Duration: 30 to 40 minutes

Other: Full-body; high reps; Concept2; chipper

workout go.cavemantraining.com/kbwc-vid33

I love this workout!

You need a Concept2 rower and 2 kettlebells. If you don't have a rower, you can replace the 100 cal rows with 100 kettlebell swings (it's actually easier, so, do 150 if your swing is good).

- → 100 cals on the rower
- → 50 burpee squat dead lifts
- → 50 bent-over rows
- → 50 suitcase dead lifts

⏱ FOR TIME

🚩

℞

♂ Rx for male is 2 x 16kg/35lb and rower on max resistance

♀ Rx for female is 2 x 12kg/26lb and rower on medium

If you're doing swings instead of rowing

♂ Rx for male is 1 x 24kg/53lb

♀ Rx for female is 1 x 20kg/44lb

Form and technique first! Come out of the bent-over position (hip flexion) before your gluteals give up and your back starts to round, straight back at all times!

Hips low and shoulders high on all those squats.

Bring the weight dead to the ground each time.

Have fun, and post your results on our YouTube, Facebook, Instagram, or below.

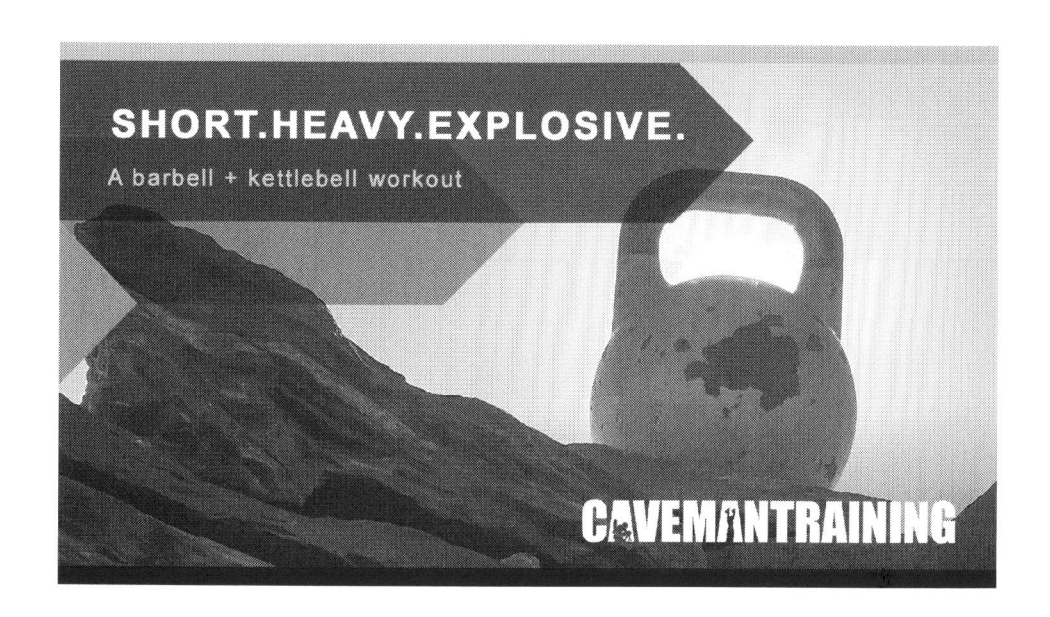

SHORT, HEAVY, AND EXPLOSIVE.

Level: Intermediate

Weight: Heavy

Kettlebell(s):

Type: Cardio and endurance

Duration: 12 minutes

Other: Full-body; low reps; barbell; AMRAP

workout go.cavemantraining.com/kbwc-vid34

A barbell + kettlebell workout

The workout is short, just 12 minutes AMRAP, that's all you need to walk away feeling like you accomplished something today. This workout includes a barbell as my training philosophy is that one should be good at and include everything that attributes to a better version of yourself. The barbell has it place. The alternative for the barbell clean and squat is the kettlebell clean and squat.

Start with a full body warm-up. Perform some light barbell cleans, kettlebell jerks, and kettlebell swings. Find about 60% to 70% of your 1RM on the barbell and kettlebell. Or use the following Rx if you don't know or don't want to find it:

- 60kg/132lbs barbell
- 32kg/70.5lbs kettlebell

The rep scheme is:

→ 2 x barbell clean + squats

→ 2 x dead swing clean + jerks on each side

→ 4 x kettlebell single-arm swings on each side

12 minutes AMRAP

The single arm swings are not something that is seen a lot in CrossFit. It's such a great exercise, especially with heavy weight, the torque requires full core activation and resistance, i.e. great to work the core.

If you don't have access to a barbell you can use two 20kg/44lb or two 24kg/53lb kettlebells to perform a racked squat.

Scaling and progression for beginners

This workout can quite easily be turned into a beginners workout with the following:

→ 2 x single kettlebell clean and squat

→ 2 x dead swing clean + push press on each side

→ 4 x kettlebell single-arm swings on each side

12 minutes AMRAP

For weight start with something light and complete the workout 1 or 2 times a week over a period of 4 weeks. Take one week rest and increase the weight. Continue to do so until you're at a heavy weight.

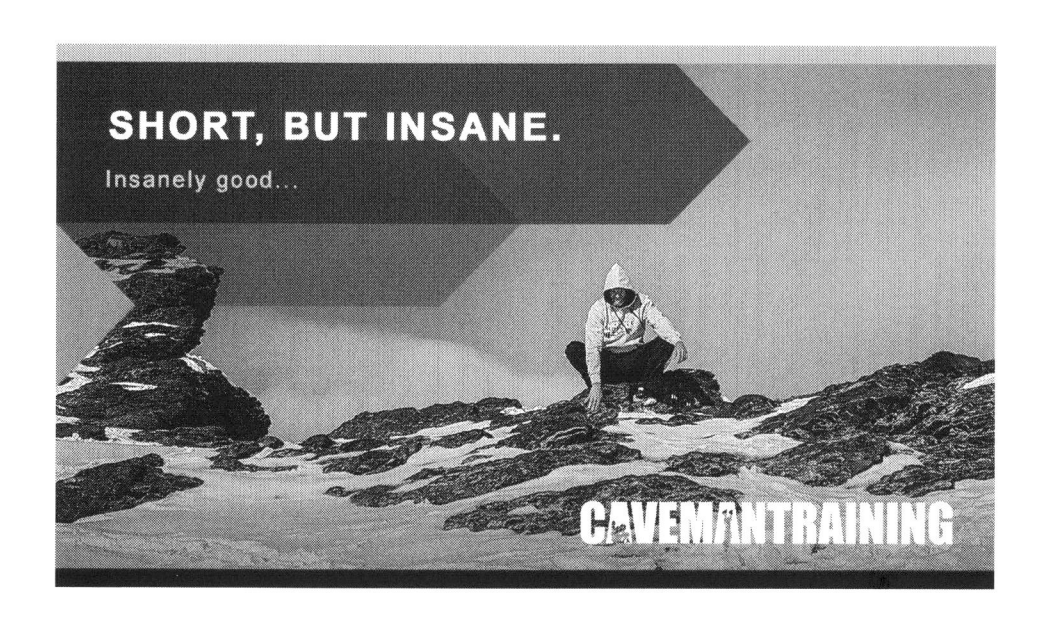

SHORT, BUT INSANE.

Level: Intermediate

Weight: Heavy

Kettlebell(s):

Type: Strength and power

Duration: 20 to 25 minutes

Other: Full-body; short

workout go.cavemantraining.com/kbwc-vid35

Insanely good.

This workout is short, or rather, the tasks are short and have few reps, but the weights are heavy, hence the reason I kept the reps low. This is two rounds of short fast bursts of explosiveness. Finishing with pure strength, strict pull-ups, and triceps push-ups. All FOR TIME.

→ 6 CrossFit burpees

→ 4 double kettlebell swings

→ 4 dead snatch each side

🔄 4 rounds

⏱ 3 minutes rest

Repeat twice.

Finish with:

→ 25 strict pull-ups

→ 25 triceps push-ups

🚩

℞

♂ Rx male 2 x 20kg/44lbs

♀ Rx female 2 x 16kg/35.2lbs

Standards:

- **CrossFit burpee**
    - Neutral standing position
    - Hips to the ground
    - Chest touching the ground (bottom of sternum)
    - Hands near the shoulders (tricep push-up)
    - Come back up
    - Feet flat on the ground
    - Jump up
    - Clap above the head
    - Vertical position
- **Swings**
    - Hip hinge movement

- Kettlebells swinging with the bells coming behind the legs
- At the top of the swing the bells should reach chest height

- **Dead snatches**
  - Weight dead on the ground without movement
  - One uninterrupted explosive pull to overhead
  - Coming into full extension
  - One split second the bell is motionless overhead
  - The bell is returned into proper racking
  - The bell is returned to dead via a controlled deceleration

- **Wide grip overhead pull-ups**
  - The arms create a 'Y'
  - Fully hanging start with elbows extended
  - Chin above the bar
  - Controlled decent to hang

- **Triceps push-ups**
  - Hands under elbows
  - Elbows reach an angle of 90 degrees
  - The elbows and shoulders remain in one straight vertical line till towards the feet (not flaring out)

I've said it before, and I'll say it again, these are called kettlebell dead snatches, if we really want to get picky, they're called half dead snatches. The weight is snatched dead from the ground each time and returned into racking to dead. The word 'dead' means nothing else but the weight being dead on the ground upon each rep. It does not mean the weight needs to be deadlifted, nor that it should be a hip hinge.

It's not redundant to put this in the exercise name. CrossFit has the Snatch (which is really a dead snatch) and the hang snatch. Because the dead snatch is so popular, it's shortened to just the purest form of the exercise name. The purest form of an exercise is the exercise itself, not its variations or how it's performed:

- **Pull-ups**

    Pulling yourself up

- **Push-ups**

    Pushing yourself up

- **Snatches**

    A fast and explosive movement in which equipment goes from lower directly to overhead

- **Squats**

    A movement in which the hips move towards the ground and the knees come forward

- **Swings**

    A movement in which a piece of equipment moves back and forth

Etcetera, none describe the variation or the way it's performed.

Now, let's describe the actual variation of a couple of exercises:

- **Dead snatch**

    Could also be half dead snatch with squat under

- **Dead lift**

    Could also be hip hinge dead lift or squat dead lift, etcetera

- **Dead clean**
    Could also be dead clean with squat under

- Wide grip overhand pull-up
- Chest push-up
- Hybrid push-up
- Triceps push-up

Naming becomes important when dealing with the public or teaching different variations.

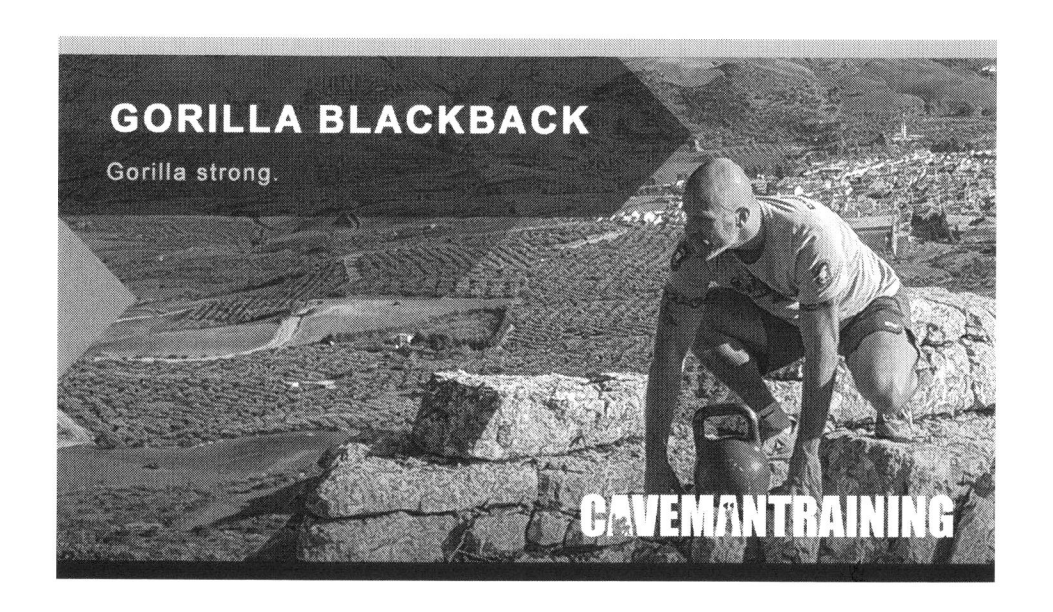

GORILLA BLACKBACK WORKOUT

Level: Advanced

Weight: Medium

Kettlebell(s):

Type: Strength

Duration: 20 minutes

Other: Full-body; low reps; AMRAP

workout go.cavemantraining.com/kbwc-vid36

Gorilla strong.

For those that have been following *Cavemantraining* for a while, they know the Silverback Workout which was designed in 2016 and redone in 2018. A 20-minute AMRAP with low reps and medium weight.

This is the new workout, which features exercises like Gorilla Rows and Gorilla Curls. Let's get stuck into it.

The workout:

- ➔ 4 x gorilla rows
- ➔ 4 x gorilla cleans
- ➔ 4 x gorilla curls
- ➔ 4 x renegade rows deadlift

⏱ 20 MINUTES **AMRAP**

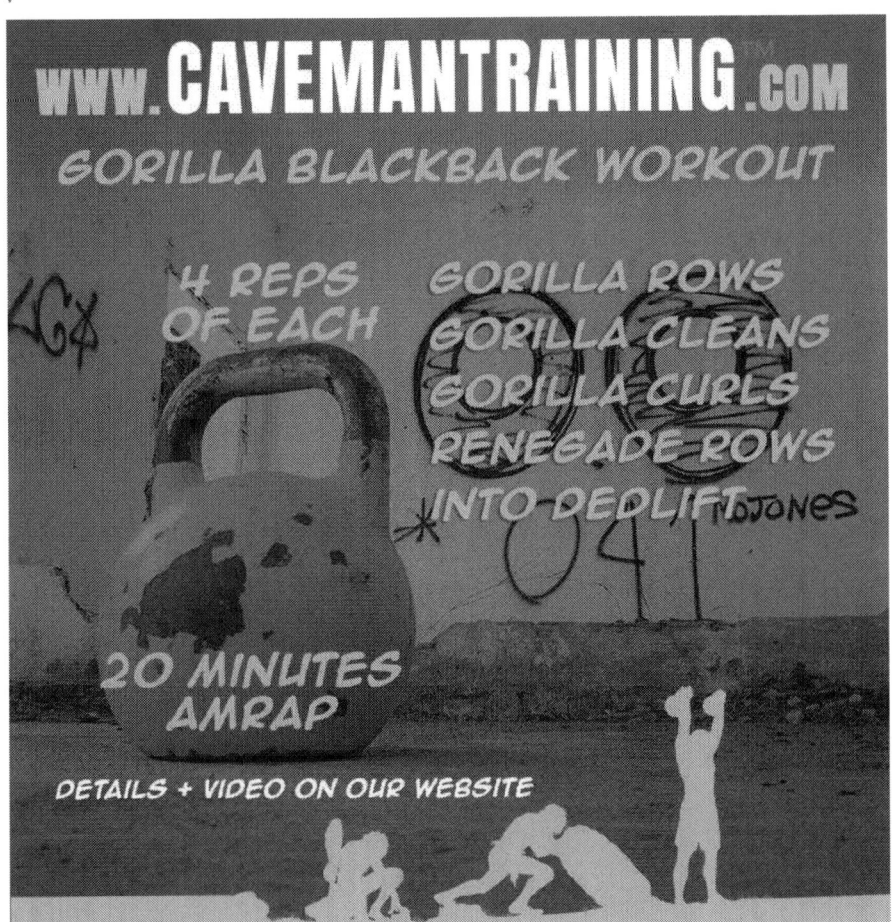

🚩

Share go.cavemantraining.com/kbwc-link4

Use two kettlebells of medium weight. The curls are the exercises upon which you need to base your weight, i.e. you might be able to perform all other exercises with two 24's/53lb but you struggle to maintain even close to a proper curl with that, it ain't the weight to be using. The curl is also the exercise with which you run the most risk of tendon issues. So, check your ego at the door and pick the weight based upon the Gorilla Curls!

Kettlebell Gorilla Rows

Come into a hip hinge with the hips pushed back and the back parallel to the ground. Lean on one kettlebell as you work with the other. Row into the groin, we want to target the rear deltoids, so, row back and focus on the forearm being relaxed.

Kettlebell Gorilla Cleans

These are my favorite cleans and are covered further in this book.

Kettlebell Gorilla Curls

As with the rows, you want to come into a hip hinge with the hips pushed back and the back parallel to the ground. Lean on one kettlebell as you work with the other. You want the elbows to flare out to the side and bring the hand towards the middle of the chest. Don't employ a tight grip, just let the handle loosely rest in the gorilla grip. Try and refrain from moving anything else but the elbow and elbow flexors.

Gorilla grip go.cavemantraining.com/kbwc-link5

Renegade Rows Deadlift

While in a plank position, row one side into the hips, row the other, this is usually one rep, but we're also going to add a deadlift to the exercise. Kick the feet back in with the feet landing flat next to the kettlebells just on the outside and perform a deadlift. Return to plank position and repeat.

ROSES AND BABIES 96

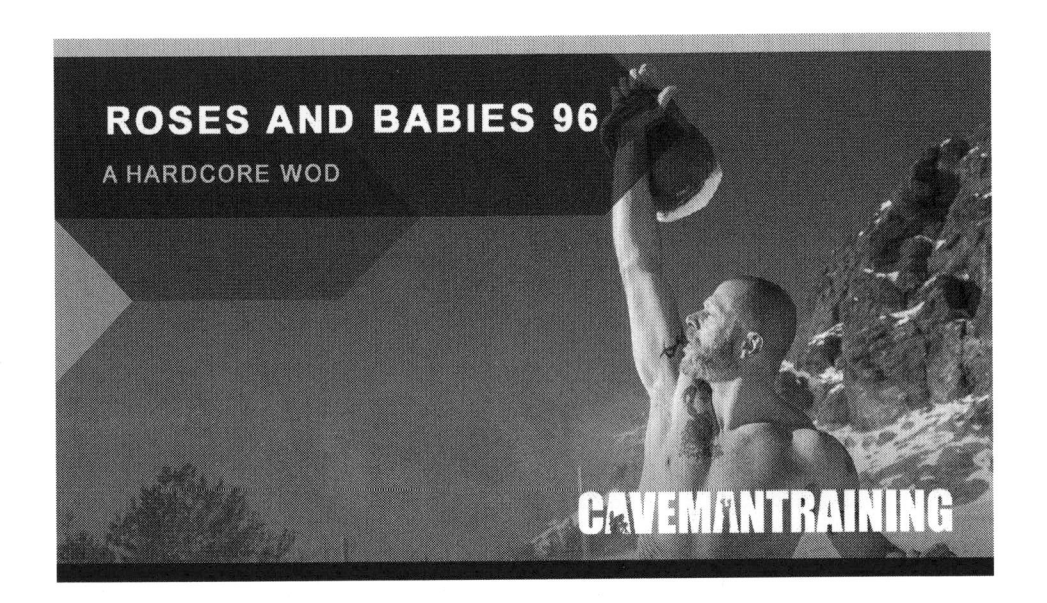

Level: Intermediate

Weight: Medium

Kettlebell(s):

Type: Cardio

Duration: 20 to 30 minutes

Other: Full-body; Concept2; partner workout; interval; FOR TIME

workout go.cavemantraining.com/kbwc-vid37

A HARDCORE PARTNER WOD

Look, I could not stand to use another name like *Workout From Hell 96*, *Torture Workout 96*, or *Killer Workout 96*, so I went the complete opposite way, and the first thing that came to mind when thinking about this workout was roses and babies. Behold, I present to you…

An awesome partner workout, Roses and Babies 96 FOR TIME

Enjoy!

Just 4 exercises and easy to remember cals or reps to complete, here it is:

- ➔ 8 calories on the rower
- ➔ 8 calories on the assault bike
- ➔ 8 kettlebell swings
- ➔ 8 half kettlebell snatches

Swap with your partner after all four exercises are completed. Partner counts reps and also reminds the number of cals to burn, for example, the first person will do 8 cals on both the rower and the bike, then the next person will start at 8 and go to 16 on both, the next will be 24, and so on. Pretty simple, but when you're doing this intense WOD, sure as eggs you'll forget, and you don't want to be burning any extra calories!

12 rounds in total or the same as 96 cals/reps a station. 6 rounds each, one person rests while the other works, you're going to need it. This WOD is FOR TIME. We recorded our time with the *Cavemantraining Workout Timer* on Google Play, check it out, you're not going to find anything better for your workouts.

A partner WOD is a great form of interval training, you do some work and then you rest while your partner works. Just make sure you're not paired with a machine for a partner or you won't be getting much rest. If partner workouts are new to you, let me run you through it one more time:

Athlete 1 starts

- 8 calories on the rower (count shows 8 at end)
- 8 calories on the assault bike (count shows 8 at end)
- 8 kettlebell swings
- 8 half kettlebell snatches

Athlete 1 rests

Athlete 2 starts

- 8 calories on the rower (count shows 16 at end)

- 8 calories on the assault bike (count shows 16 at end)
- 8 kettlebell swings
- 8 half kettlebell snatches

Athlete 2 rests

Athlete 1 starts

- 8 calories on the rower (count shows 18 at end)
- 8 calories on the assault bike (count shows 18 at end)
- 8 kettlebell swings
- 8 half kettlebell snatches

This pattern continues till you reach 96 for rower, bike, swings, and snatches. 12 rounds in total or 6 rounds each.

Another awesome workout to pull out of the bag every 4 to 6 weeks. You can't use it as a benchmark unless you get the same partner. If you do not have a partner and want to do this workout then simply do one test round, if that takes 60 seconds, then you rest 60 seconds for every time a partner would go. It's actually harder on your own as in reality the rest will become longer when working with a partner, i.e. as they fatigue they will get slower, giving you more rest.

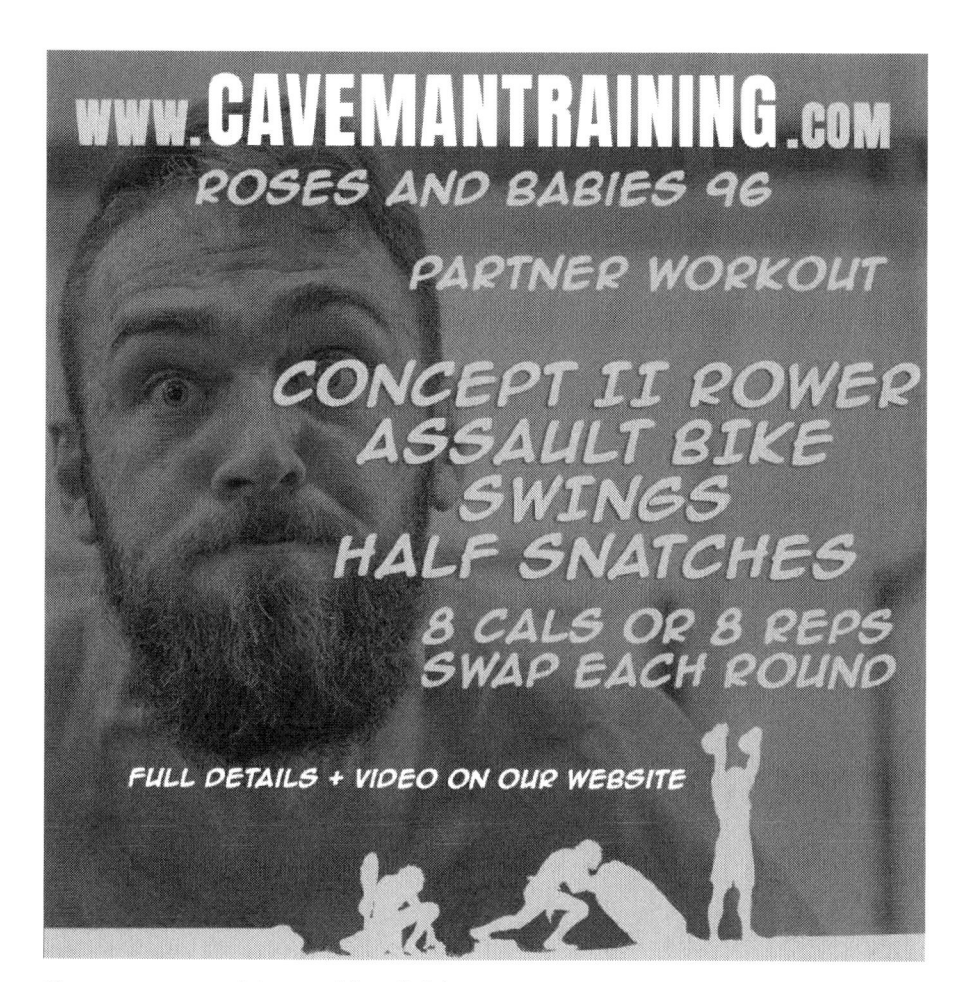

Share go.cavemantraining.com/kbwc-link6

RX weights are:

Male

32kg/70lbs for swings

2 x 16kg/35lbs for half snatches

Female

24kg/53lbs for swings

2 x 12kg/26 for half snatches

Standards:

- Swings
  - ☐ Bell to chest height
  - ☐ Bell visible behind the knees
- Snatches
  - ☐ Full overhead lockout
  - ☐ Into racking
  - ☐ Into backswing with bells visible behind the knees

If you don't have a rower or bike then replace with 60 jump rope for each, i.e. instead of 8 cals on the rower perform 60 jump rope, instead of 8 cals on the bike perform 60 jump rope.

You can scale this workout for beginners by reducing the weight on the swings to ½ and swapping the snatches for either single or double kettlebell clean and push press (see clean and jerk further in this book).

DROP SET SHOULDER WORKOUT

For strong and good looking shoulders.

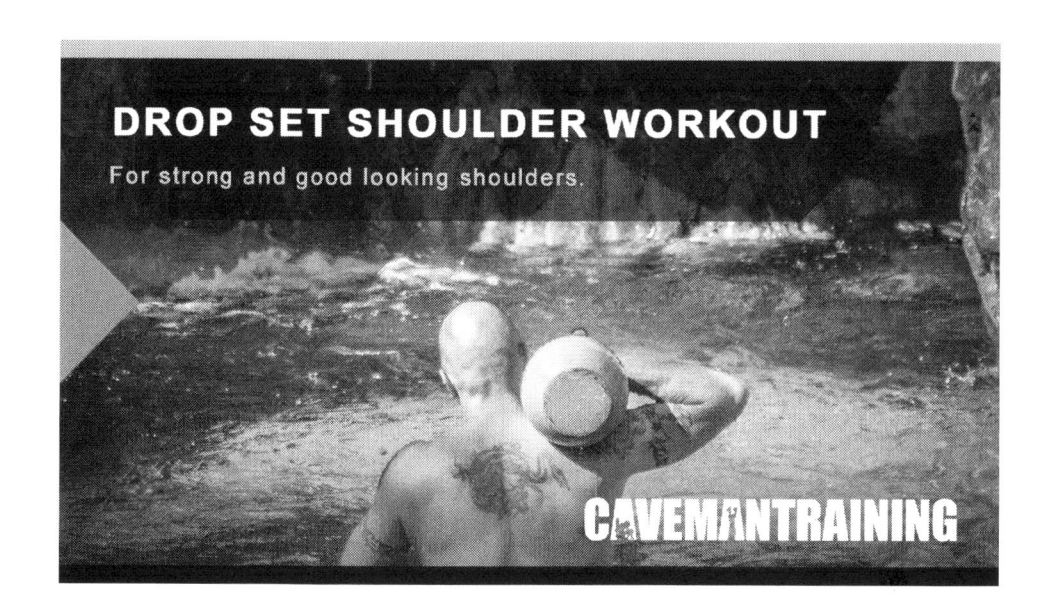

KETTLEBELL DROP SET SHOULDER WORKOUT

Level: Beginners

Weight: Heavy

Kettlebell(s):

Type: Strength

Duration: 24 to 30 minutes

Other: Shoulders and triceps; upper-body; slow

workout go.cavemantraining.com/kbwc-vid38

For strong and good looking shoulders.

This workout focusses on the deltoids/shoulders and triceps. Your workout should start with a good shoulder warm-up, if you have a mace, you should use it for some swings mixed with other bodyweight warm-up exercises.

Once you're nice and warm, start your workout with the drop set of kettlebell dead clean and strict shoulder presses. Take your time with each press, perform as slow as possible, do both sides and rest when required. If you want to add another muscle group to your workout then perform up to 6 triceps push-ups after doing a press on the left and right side. Adjust the number depending on your triceps strength, you don't want to gas your triceps for the press.

Go as slow as possible, there is no rushing in this workout, it's not an AMRAP or FOR TIME, take your time. I took about 15 to 20 seconds per rep on each side, 40 to 50 seconds in total and followed up with 6 good triceps push ups, then I rested for about 1 minute before moving to the next lower weight. Let's say 2 minutes for one weight, I had 4 weights set out which would be about 8 minutes. 2 to 4 minutes rest and repeat.

It sounds like it would not be very taxing, but you need to make sure that you're going really slow on the up and down phase, and most importantly, you want to start your first weight at about 90% of your 1RM.

If you're doing just one drop set you can go to failure on each weight before dropping down. If you're planning on doing two sets, keep some strength in the tank and/or make sure you rest enough after your first set. You might not be able to start with the heaviest weight on your second set, just start with your second one.

I used the following weights, 32kg/70lb, 28kg/62lb, 26kg/57lb, and 24kg/53lb.

After the workout, I spend some time on mobility with light kettlebells performing thoracic rotational presses and Sots presses. (see thorax workout for the spiral/rotational press and further in this book for the Sots press).

To press heavy, you need to know how to kettlebell clean safely and effectively. If you don't have a mace, buy one, or use kettlebell halo's (see further in this book). go.cavemantraining.com/kbwc-vid39

This workout is suitable for beginners because what is 1RM for one does not have to be 1RM for another. Meaning, if your 1RM is currently 16kg, no problem, go with 16, 12, 8, 8, or even 12, 8, 8, 8. But keep the pace **incredibly** slow.

This is definitely a workout you should repeat often if you want to gain upper-body strength. You could do this once or twice a week. Increase the weight once your heaviest weight becomes easy to press. You measure progress by your heaviest weight, i.e. if your first go at this is with 24, 20, 16, 16 for example, then 24 is what you record with the date, then the date you upped to the next weight, and so on. It's not a workout you want to overdo, and after 6 weeks you want to give deload and give it one to two weeks while focussing on something else, especially mobility and flexibility. This would be a great combination with the Magnus Dorsi workout.

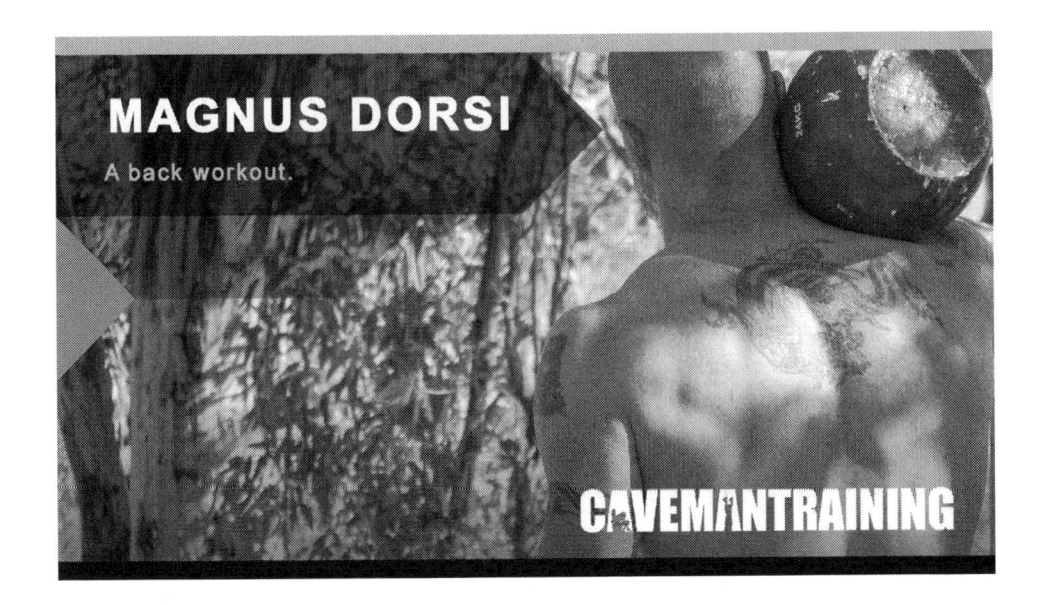

MAGNUS DORSI

- Level: Beginners
- Weight: Heavy
- Kettlebell(s):
- Type: Strength
- Duration: minutes
- Other: Back; slow

▶ workout go.cavemantraining.com/kbwc-vid40

An awesome workout for a great back.

This is one of the best back workouts you can do at home. You can do it with one kettlebell, or up to three if you have them. In my training I spend quite some time on the back.

I used two kettlebells in this workout, a 32kg/70lb and a 28kg/62lb. After a couple of rounds, I went down to 28kg for the rows but stuck with the 32kg for the shrugs. Let me run you through the workout:

- → 2 x wide rows (90 degrees)
- → 2 x hybrid rows (45 degrees)
- → 2 x narrow rows (0 degrees)
  Repeat on the other side
- → 6 x shrugs
  Repeat on the other side
- → 6 x wide grip overhand pull-ups

Use a TRX if you don't have a pull-up bar at home (see further down).

Repeat for 5 to 6 rounds. I spend over an hour on the warm-up, workout, and mobility.

🚩

It's also a great back workout to use for drop sets, i.e. if you have heavy enough kettlebells, you can start with your heaviest, then drop to a lighter one each round.

There should be plenty of rest, you can rest after doing one side, after a set, but definitely rest after a round.

If you look at the video you'll notice I adjust my stance for every 2 reps of the row. When going wide you need a good wide base, then in a bit for the hybrid, and feet close together for the narrow row. The degrees or distance is in relation from the elbow to the ribs, i.e. 90 degrees would be a 90-degree angle between the elbow and ribs.

The wide row requires progressing, so be careful, you might want to start with 6 narrow ones for a while, then include hybrid, then include the wide rows. The wide rows require good lat activation to protect the shoulders. You'll also want to use a lighter weight for the wide rows if you're just starting. Seriously, this angle is great to work from, but also dangerous for those who don't have great MMC or are just starting out.

You need to first master the hip hinge before you attempt the bent over dead row, this is a must to protect your lower back.

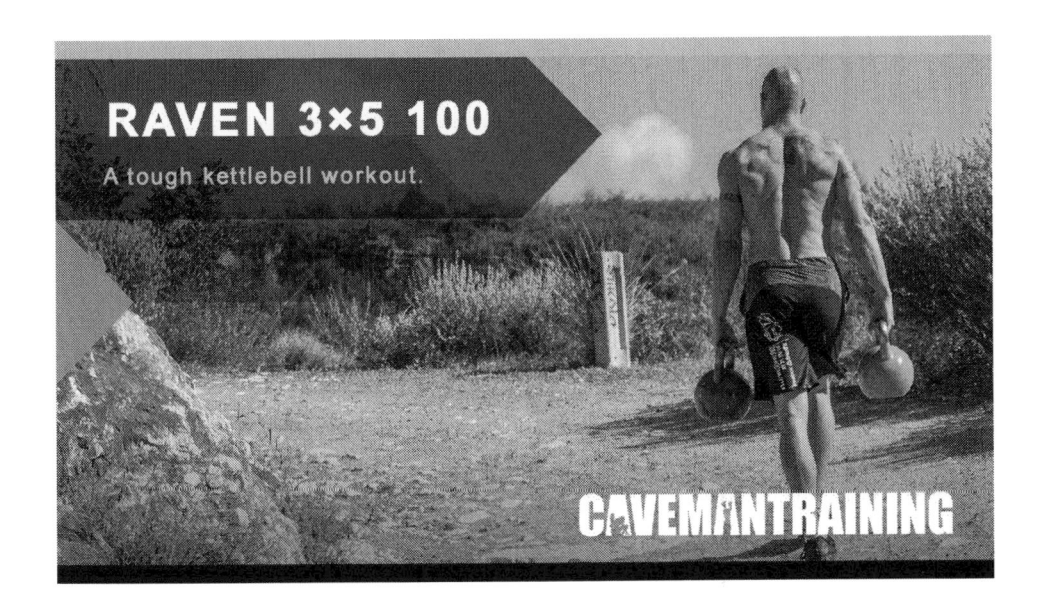

RAVEN 3×5 100

Level: Intermediate

Weight: Medium

Kettlebell(s):

Type: Cardio, strength, and endurance

Duration: 25 to 30 minutes

Other: Full-body with focus on legs, chest, and shoulders; AMRAP; FOR TIME; unbroken

workout go.cavemantraining.com/kbwc-vid41

A tough kettlebell workout

This workout has four short enough tasks with ample rest in between to allow you to go all out. 3 times 5 minutes of work followed by a 100 rep task for time.

First task:
→ 5 jump burpees

→ 5 full snatches on each side

⏱ 5-minute **AMRAP**

⏱ 2-minute rest

℞ Rx weight:

♂ Male 1 x 16kg / 35.2lbs

♀ Female: 1 x 12kg / 26.4

Second task:

→ 5 dead swing clean into squat

→ 5 chest push-ups

⏱ 5-minute **AMRAP**

⏱ 2-minute rest

℞ Rx weight:

♂ Male 2 x 16kg/35lb

♀ Female: 2 x 12kg/26lb

Third task:

→ 1 minute half snatch UNBROKEN

→ 30-second rest (skip on last round)

🔄 5 rounds

⏱ 2-minute rest

Rx weight:

♂ Male 2 x 16kg/35lb

♀ Female: 2 x 12kg/26lb

Final task:
→ 100 dead clean and strict press

FOR TIME

Rx weight:

♂ Male 1 x 16kg/35lb

♀ Female: 1 x 12kg/26lb

Movement standards

- **Jump burpee**

    Plank into jump with hands above head and looking ahead

- **Full snatch**

    Swing movement into full overhead lockout

- **Dead swing clean into squat**

    Weight dead on the ground upon each rep

    Clean into full extension

    Elbows touching inside of thighs

    Coming into full extension

- **Chest push-up**

    Elbows at least at a 45-degree angle from the ribs

Elbows coming in line with the shoulders

Back into elbow full extension

- **Half snatch**

    Swing movement into full overhead lockout

    Into full racking position

- **Alternating dead clean and strict press**

    Weight dead on the ground

    Cleaned into full racking position

    Strict press with no momentum

    Back into full racking position

    Dead to the ground

    Alternate

Task 1,2, and 3 are scored as one, and task 4 is scored separately, i.e. an athlete can win at both.

Task 1 and 2 is 1 point per rep, and task 3 is 2 points per rep.

UNBROKEN means that the kettlebells can't be put down, rest is in racking or overhead position. No points counted if the full 60 seconds are not completed.

To scale this workout for beginners you can change the full snatches in the first task to clean and push press. The dead swing clean into squat for the second task can be done with one kettlebell or just keeping one kettlebell racked and add 2 additional reps. The half snatches in the third task can be changed to one kettlebell and switching at will. The dead clean and strict press can be changed to a swing clean and press. The dead clean is not that complex but squat depth is usually lacking with beginners and the hip hinge (swing) will be more suitable for safety purpose, especially when we're dealing with high reps.

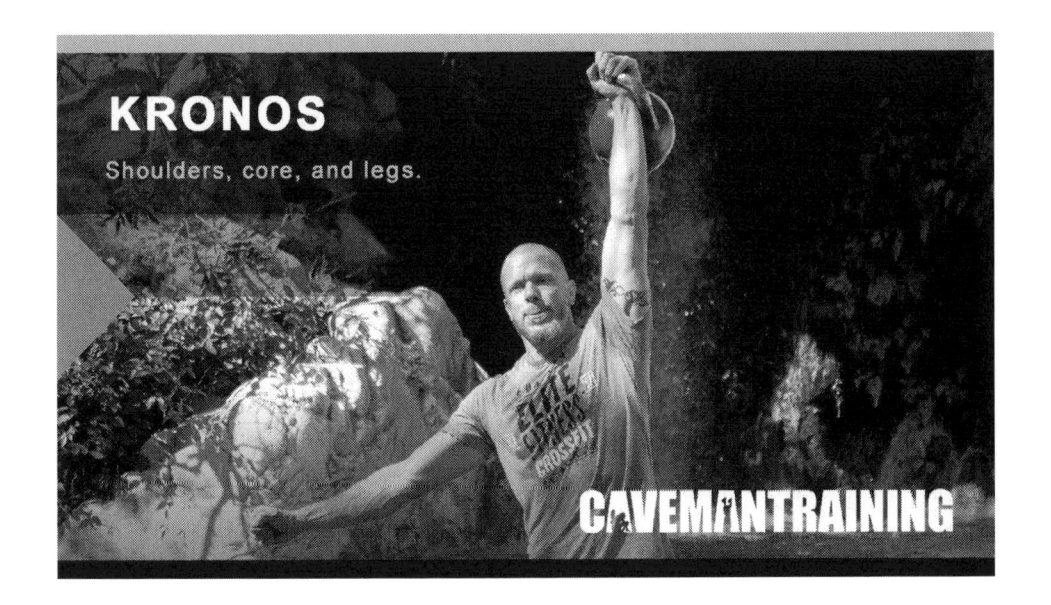

KRONOS WORKOUT

Level: Beginner to intermediate

Weight: Medium

Kettlebell(s):

Type: Strength, flexibility, and mobility

Duration: 30 to 45 minutes

Other: Full-body with focus on rotation, shoulders, core, and legs; slow

workout go.cavemantraining.com/kbwc-vid42

Shoulders core and legs

This is KRONOS, Kronos works the shoulders, thoracic, and legs. One kettlebell required. A great workout for strength and mobility.

FIRST PART

→ Bent-over dead row

→ Bent-over dead row and rotate

→ Deadlift (hip hinge)

Perform the sequence 5 times on one side. Performed on both sides equals one round.

Complete 8 rounds in total.

SECOND PART

→ Clean

→ Spiral press

Perform the kettlebell combo 5 times on one side. Performed on both sides equals one round.

Complete 6 rounds in total.

THIRD PART

→ Racked cossack squat

Performed five times on one side. Performed on both sides equals one round.

Complete 4 rounds in total.

You can rest when you need to, this is not an AMRAP, consider it training. The weight should be medium.

KRONOS WORKOUT

- BENT-OVER DEAD ROW
- BENT-OVER DEAD ROW AND ROTATE
- DEADLIFT (HIP HINGE)

REPEAT 5 TIMES ON ONE SIDE. PERFORMED ON BOTH SIDES EQUALS ONE ROUND. COMPLETE 8 ROUNDS IN TOTAL.

- COSSACK SQUAT

PERFORMED FIVE TIMES ON ONE SIDE, PERFORMED ON BOTH SIDES EQUALS ONE ROUND. COMPLETE 4 ROUNDS IN TOTAL.

1 KETTLEBELL

- CLEAN
- SPIRAL PRESS

5 TIMES ON ONE SIDE, PERFORMED ON BOTH SIDES EQUALS ONE ROUND. COMPLETE 6 ROUNDS IN TOTAL.

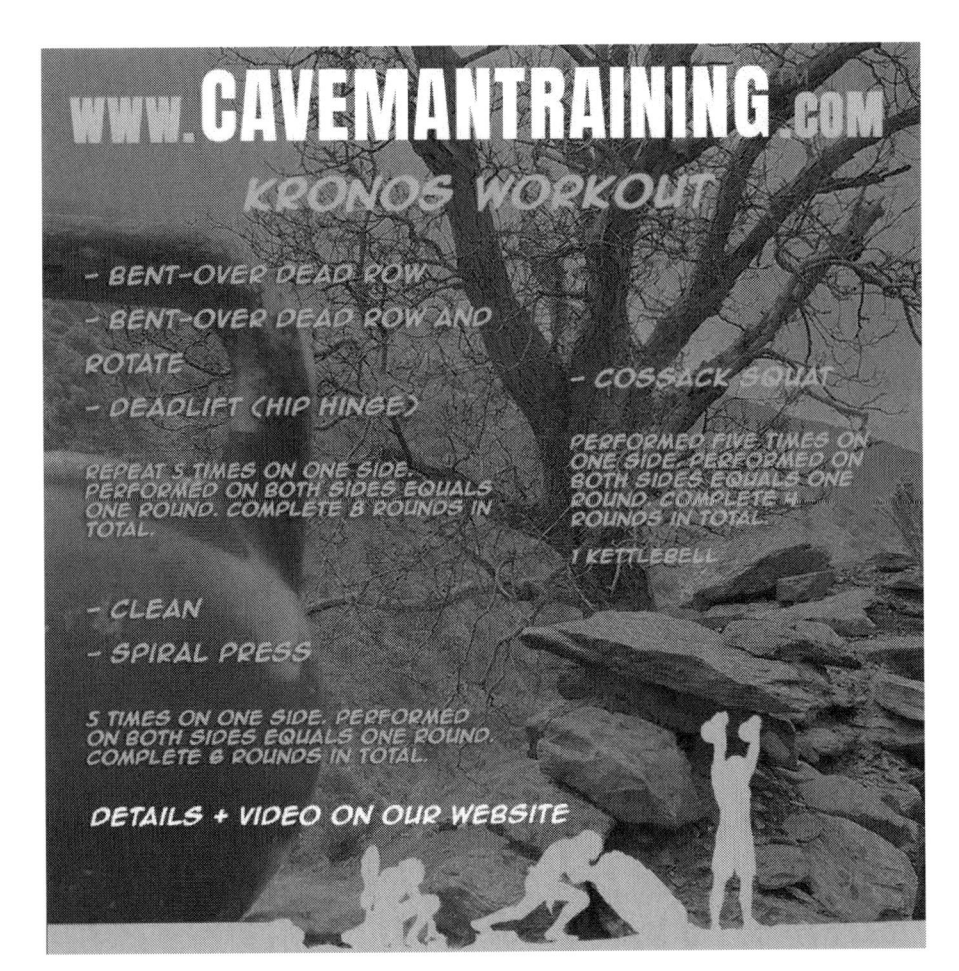

DETAILS + VIDEO ON OUR WEBSITE

https://www.facebook.com/coach.taco.fleur/photos/a.1487054661565231/2364456623825026/

Attention: The main area in which you could experience issues is the lower back. Use your hip extensors to raise the weight, and use them to stay in the static bent-over position. The workout is 5 times the sequence of bent-over rows and deadlift, but you should rest in between those if you feel your gluteals are getting fatigued.

Exercise 1: Bent-over dead row

The kettlebell should be placed under the shoulder once you're in hip flexion (bending over), you do not want to reach out for it. You also return the weight where it started. Brace the core before rowing. Row into the hips, if you're uncomfortable rowing between the legs, try the feet close together and row on the outside. Focus on the rear deltoids, i.e. you do not want to feel it in your elbow flexors.

Exercise 2: Bent-over dead row and rotate

This exercise is practically the same as the first, apart from it having thoracic rotation. Thoracic rotation is excellent to include in your training, but start with small steps and build up. More than likely you've not trained in this area before, so pay attention.

Exercise 3: Deadlift hip hinge

The weight starts dead under the shoulders and is then lifted through a deadlift hip hinge style, meaning, the knees don't come forward. You can also deadlift squat style, but our focus for this exercise is the gluteus maximus.

Exercise 4: Clean and spiral press

With this press, you start rotation at the thoracic and pressing at the same time. The path of the kettlebell follows a spiral pattern. Unlike other presses, you can look at the weight when it's in the top position, you actually want to follow it as you press to get more rotation at the spine happening. Usually, we slightly rotate the opposite side in racking as well, today we'll transition in the clean. The great thing about this press is obviously the rotation that you get, but also the different angle the deltoids are worked in.

Exercise 5: Cossack squat

This exercise is not a beginners move and you need to already have some good flexibility and strength to attempt this. It's almost like pistol squat, but with the other leg resting on the ground. You're doing the work with the one leg, the other is just for balance and getting a good hamstring stretch. Like with the squat, you want to stay as upright as possible, as a matter of fact, everything for the squat applies on the one side. Hold the racked kettlebell on the side which your leg is straight.

Having a hard time finding a workout timer that is flexible enough to handle any AMRAP, circuit, or FOR TIME workout? Get the Android app now and run the Cavemantraining workouts by downloading free timers.

Any questions? Don't forget to join our online discussion forum where anyone can ask questions about the workouts, or training general. https://www.facebook.com/groups/unconventional.training/

There is not much complexity in this workout, but the progression/regression for beginners to the cossack squat would be reverse lunges instead of the cossack squat. With the spiral press you simply don't create a lot of thoracic rotation but ease in to it over time. The bent-over rows are not that complex either, it will just come down to back and gluteal strength, come out of the position upon each rep until you feel you've mastered the bent-over position (static hip hinge).

It's a great workout to include in your training every week or every other week, but that will also depend on what your goals are. If you train mostly slow and for strength plus mobility then this is a good workout to do more often.

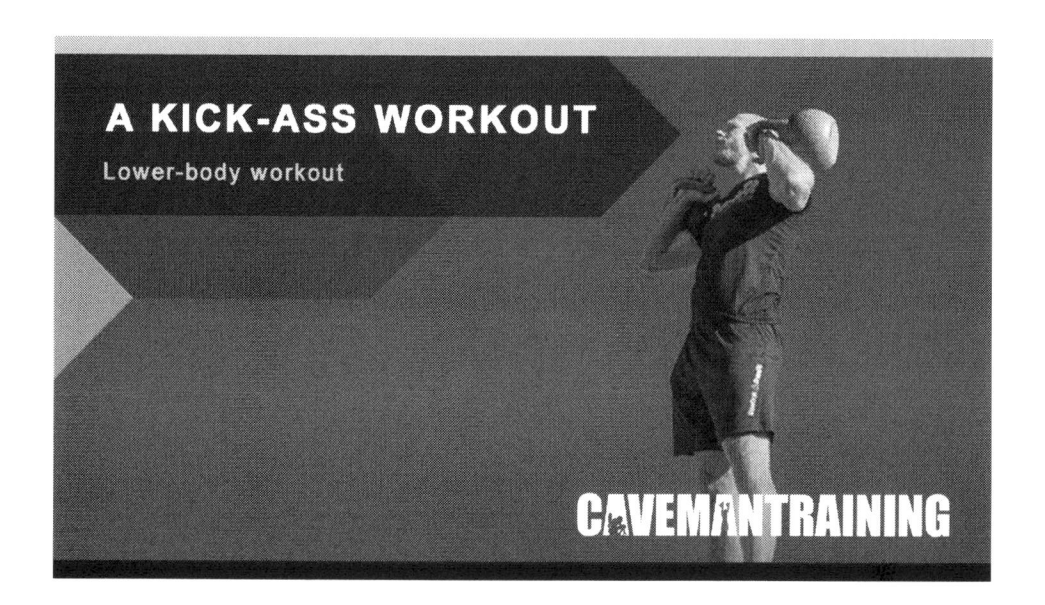

A KICK-ASS LOWER-BODY KETTLEBELL WORKOUT

Level: Intermediate

Weight: Light to medium

Kettlebell(s):

Type: Strength and endurance

Duration: 3 minutes

Other: Full-body with focus on the legs, shoulders, and triceps; stability; high reps

workout go.cavemantraining.com/kbwc-vid43

Make sure you're up for it!

This is a kick-ass lower body kettlebell workout that's not for the faint of heart. First, let me start by saying that the overhead reverse lunge is not a beginners move, especially with 100 reps to complete. So, make sure you're up to this task before attempting it.

I kept it super simple for this lower body kettlebell workout, just two awesome exercises, or kettlebell combos to be exact.

→ 100 overhead reverse lunge
→ 100 Dead swing clean and squat

With the overhead reverse lunge, you want to complete as many reps on one side as possible, this is for several reasons:

Stress the triceps

Work on muscular endurance

Improve your overhead work

Complete the task faster if doing this FOR TIME

Increase overhead stability

I got to about 30 on one side, I made sure I did the same amount on the other, the next set was 20 and 20. Don't sacrifice form for reps though. You need to have a full proper lockout for the rep to count. Knee needs to touch the ground, gently!

With the reverse lunge, you can slide back on the ball off the foot, or step back. If your stability is great, step back, if not, slide back. Keep the weight on the front leg at all times. If you find you're falling over to one side, make sure your feet are in line with the hips, i.e. where they started when you were in neutral standing position.

With the dead swing clean and squat, you want to make sure you get a good hike back to where the bell is between the legs and you have a nice hip hinge. Then squeeze your gluteals to come up, clean, rack, and squat deep. Hips below the knees while remaining upright.

Although the focus was on the legs with this workout, I added the overhead hold to challenge stability even more. We're working with a light to medium weight but the overhead lockout and long hold will stress the triceps. If you want more of a tricep workout from this then go more toward medium-heavy with the weight.

This is a workout you want to do every 1 or 2 weeks due to the high volume.

SIMPLE CARDIO WORKOUT

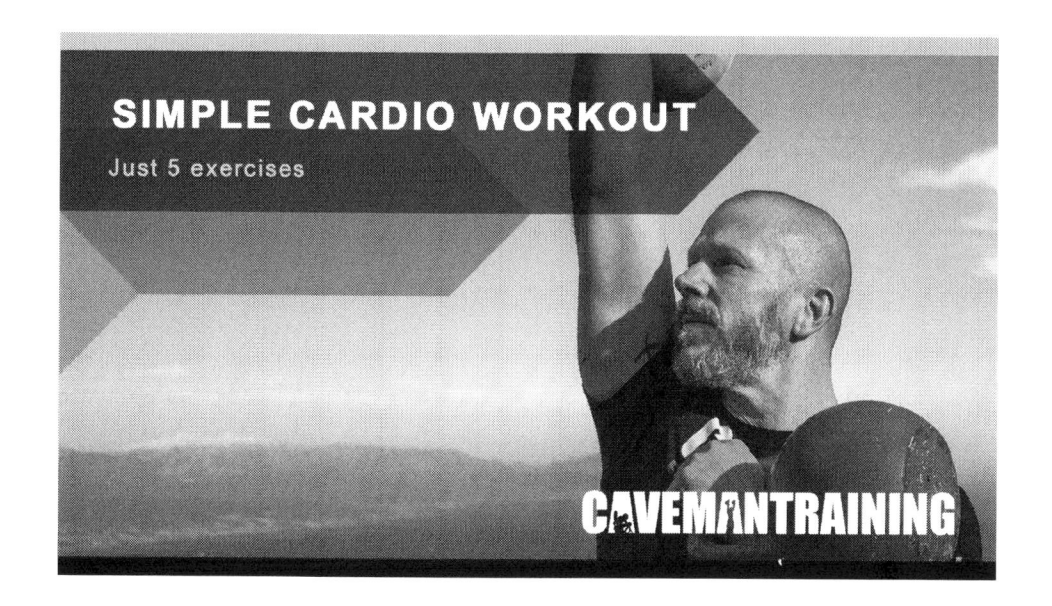

SIMPLE KETTLEBELL CARDIO WORKOUT

Level: Beginner

Weight: Light to medium

Kettlebell(s):

Type: Cardio and strength

Duration: 30 to 35 minutes

Other: Full-body with focus on the core

workout go.cavemantraining.com/kbwc-vid44

Simple but effective.

As the name implies, it's a simple kettlebell cardio workout with just 5 exercises and easy to remember rep counts.

I know you want this quick, so here it is:

→ 10 x kettlebell swing

- ➔ 5 x racked squat (10 in total by performing on each side)
- ➔ 5 x overhead press (10 in total by performing on each side)
- ➔ 5 x crush grip tricep push-ups (only 5 in total)
- ➔ 10 x cross-mountain climbers

🔄 6 rounds

⏱ 3 minutes rest

🔄 4 more rounds

🚩

1 light to medium weight kettlebell

You want to use a light to medium weight so that you don't fatigue, i.e. struggling to squat or press the weight, because you want that cardio effect, i.e. keep moving as fast as possible and complete all rounds with minimal rest.

This is a workout you could do 2 to 3 times a week for your cardio and strength. You can increase the weight over time and also plan a break of a 1 week to then pick it up again and see increased performance.

If you can find a couple of seconds to rate the book on Amazon I would really appreciate it. go.cavemantraining.com/kbwc-link19

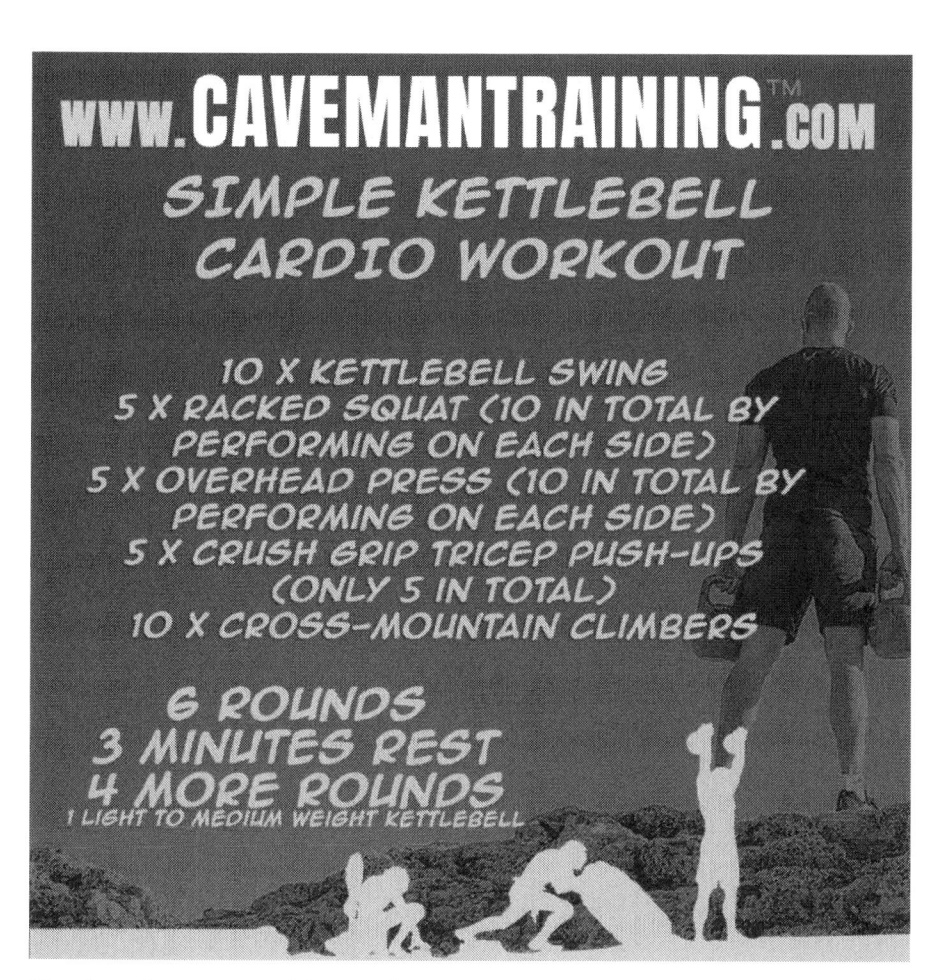

SIMPLE KETTLEBELL CARDIO WORKOUT

10 X KETTLEBELL SWING
5 X RACKED SQUAT (10 IN TOTAL BY PERFORMING ON EACH SIDE)
5 X OVERHEAD PRESS (10 IN TOTAL BY PERFORMING ON EACH SIDE)
5 X CRUSH GRIP TRICEP PUSH-UPS (ONLY 5 IN TOTAL)
10 X CROSS-MOUNTAIN CLIMBERS

6 ROUNDS
3 MINUTES REST
4 MORE ROUNDS
1 LIGHT TO MEDIUM WEIGHT KETTLEBELL

Share https://go.cavemantraining.com/kbwc-link8

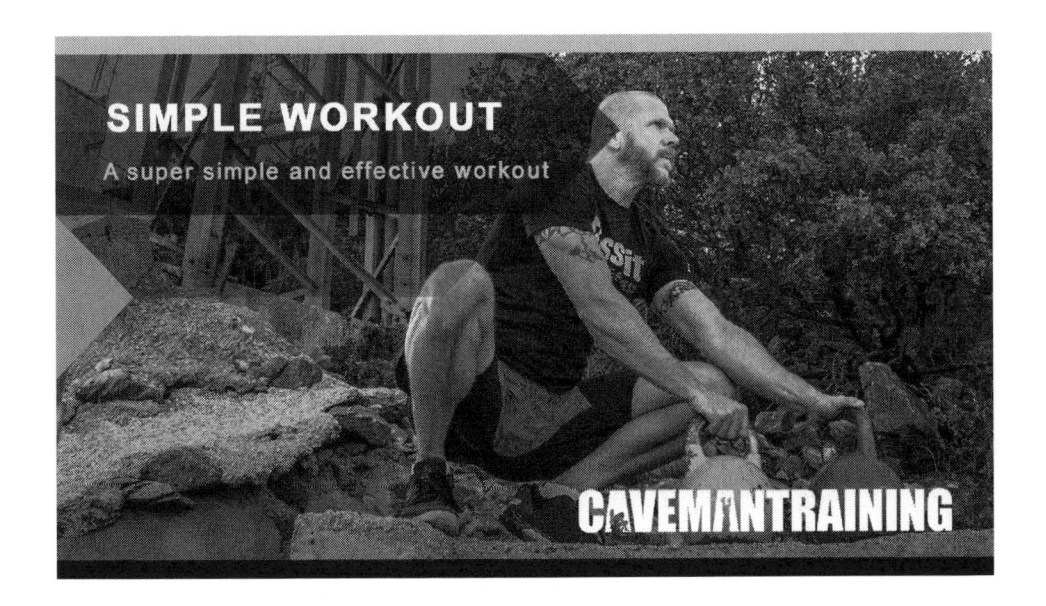

SIMPLE KETTLEBELL WORKOUT #2

Level: Beginner

Weight: Medium

Kettlebell(s):

Type: Strength

Duration: 20 to 25 minutes

Other: Full-body with focus on the legs, shoulders, and biceps

workout go.cavemantraining.com/kbwc-vid45

Flowing from one into the next.

A super simple kettlebell workout that hits full-body, performed with one kettlebell, just 5 reps for each kettlebell exercise performed one after the other with rest after each round. Complete 10 rounds.

Each exercise is performed while holding on to the kettlebell with two hands.

➔ 5 x double arm swing

→ 5 x front squat

→ 5 x shoulder press

→ 5 x bent-over row

→ 5 x bent-over curl

⏱ 30 to 60 seconds rest

🔄 Repeat 10 times

🚩

You could turn this into an E2MOM, which means you set the timer for 10 x 2 minutes and every start of the 2 minutes you perform the sequence, then you rest for the remainder of the 2 minute till you hit the next 2.

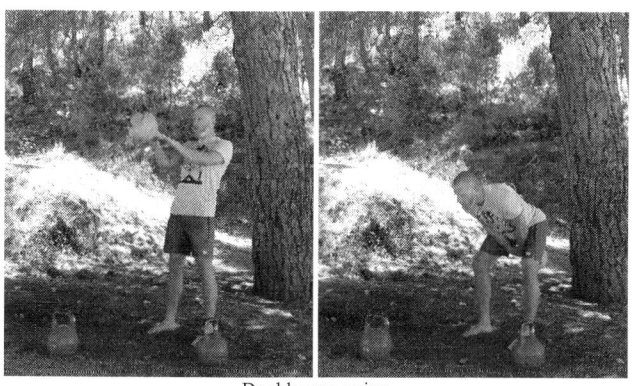

Double arm swing

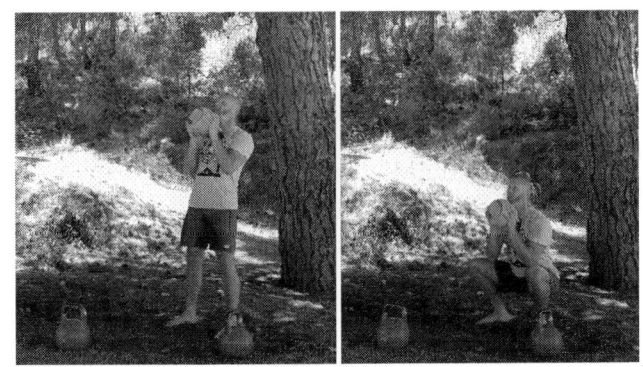

Front squat

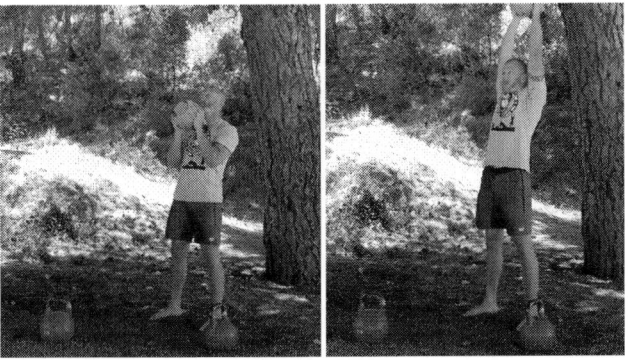

Shoulder press

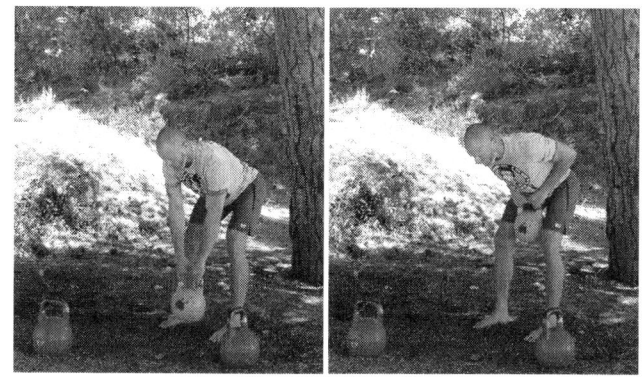

Bent-over row

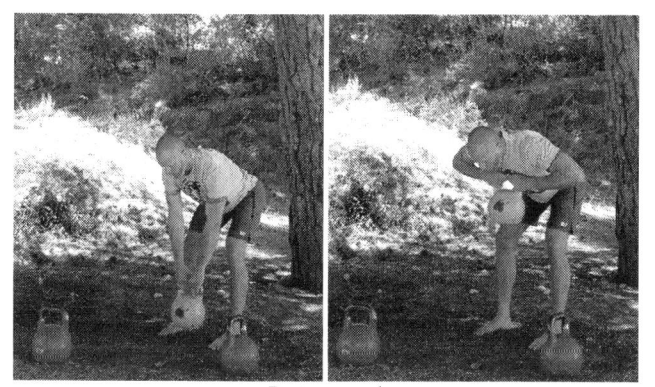

Bent-over curl

SIMPLE KETTLEBELL WORKOUT

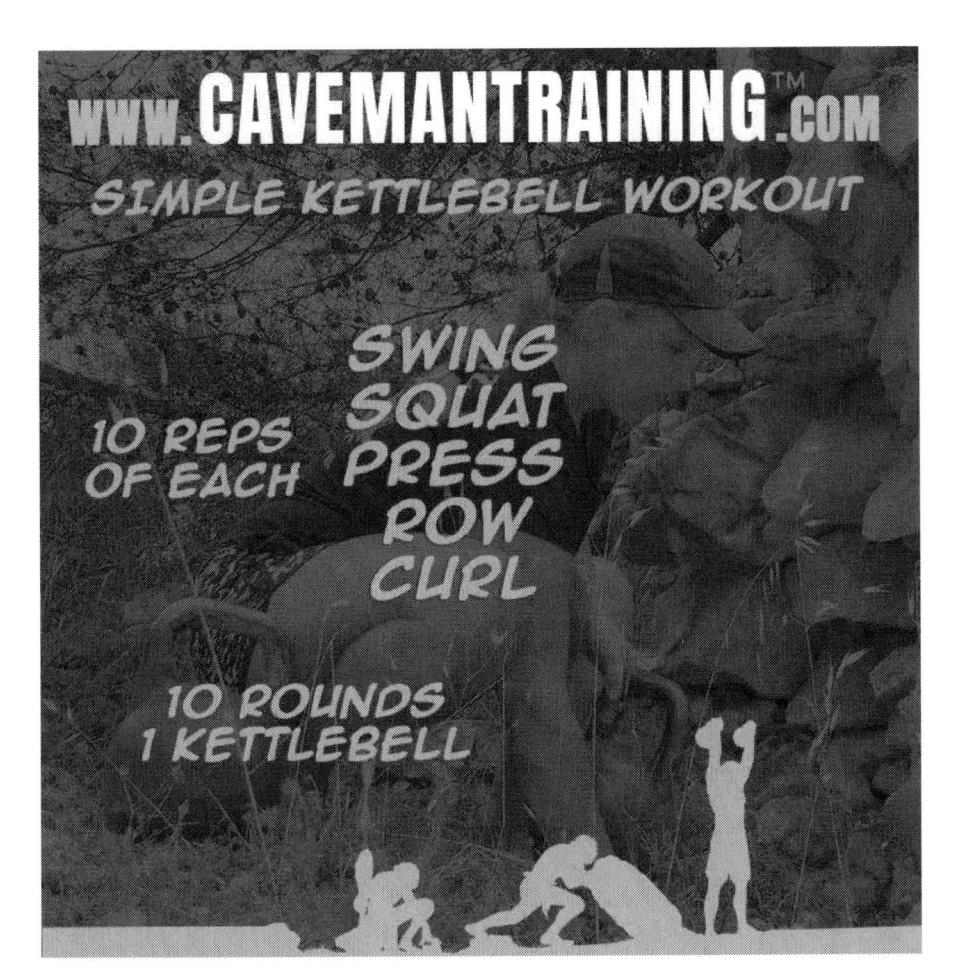

SWING
SQUAT
PRESS
ROW
CURL

10 REPS OF EACH
10 ROUNDS
1 KETTLEBELL

Share go.cavemantraining.com/kbwc-link9

Why do I advocate grips so much?

Discussing grips and making a whole book (Master Kettlebell Grips) about grips seems so unimportant, but is it? Let's give an example of why grips are so important. Take the grip in this workout for the front squat as an example. You'll often see the horn grip implemented, which is not so bad if conditioned and reps are programmed appropriately. Otherwise, this grip can play havoc on the elbow flexors, which usually comes as a surprise, after all, what did you do to tax the elbow flexors, right!? It's not immediately obvious that holding a kettlebell in racking position can tax the elbow flexors.

The horn grip requires you to keep the elbow flexors contracted during the move to stop the weight from falling forward. Let's take this workout as an example, 5 reps only, say 5 to 7 seconds per rep times 5 equals almost 30 seconds. Imagine holding up a barbell in a static curl for 30 seconds, repeat ten times, repeat over several workouts a week. This is constant stress on what could be unconditioned elbow flexors.

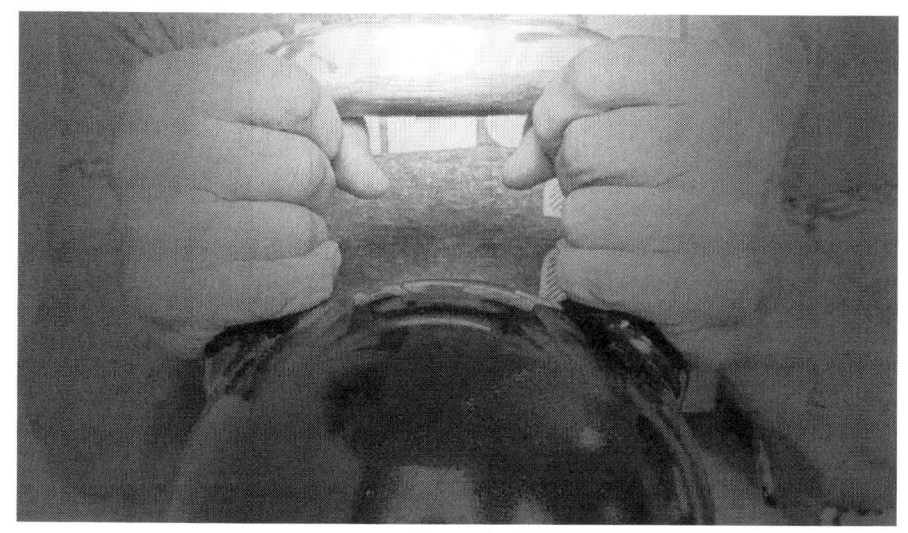

Horn grip

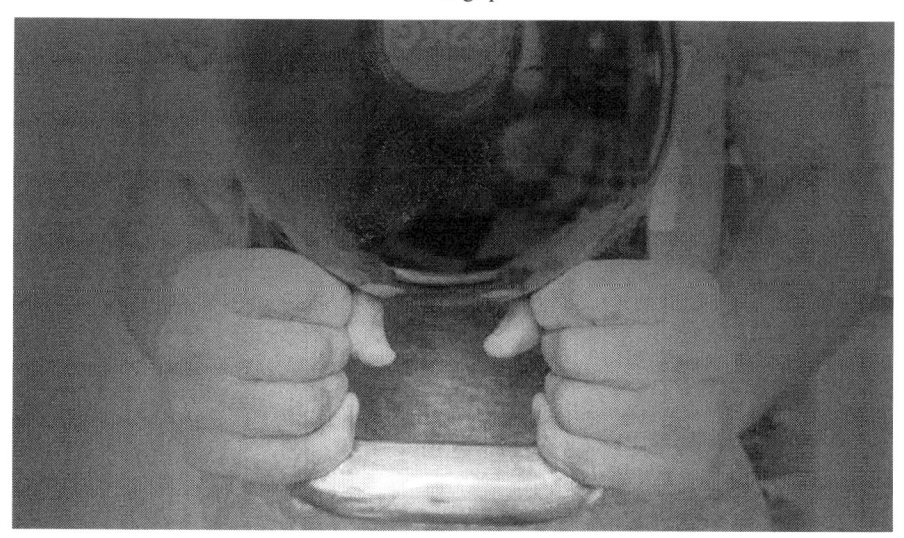

Horn grip upside down

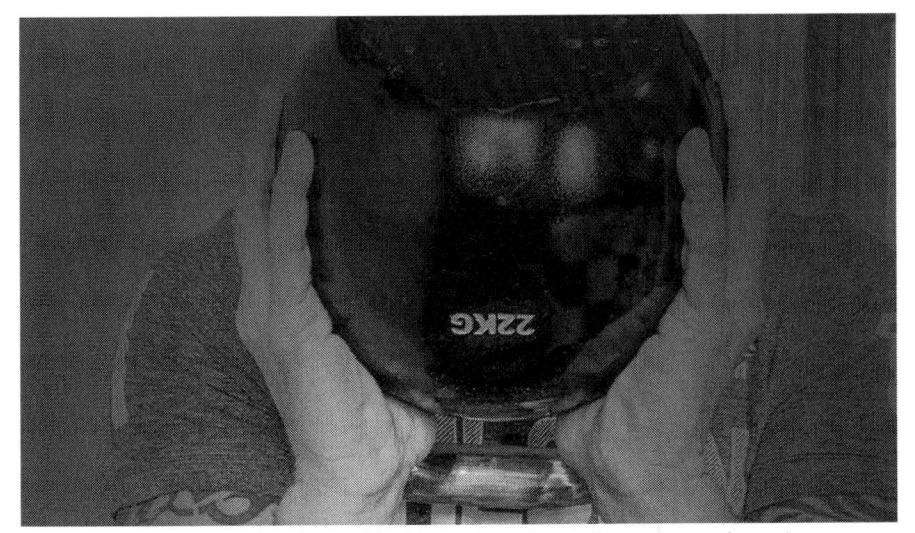

Open palm grip (grip used in this workout for the front squat and press)

Know your grips and you can transition to open hand horn grip where the bell rests in the palms and stress is taken off the elbow flexors.

The following video allows you to see a close-up slow-mo video of the first transition that's used in this workout to get the kettlebell into racking position. go.cavemantraining.com/kbwc-vid46

There is a part in this workout which I'd like to point out, you need to have good control over the hip extensors for the row and curl which are both performed in the bent-over position. The position is a static hip hinge and you need to contract your gluteus maximus, hamstrings, and adductor magus to stay in the bent-over position without putting too much stress on the lower back. Your erector spinae and other back muscles also need to stay contracted to keep the spine erect. It's perfectly fine and highly recommended that you come out of the position before you feel anything in your back, don't stay down there and put up with it. Work on your back strength over time.

This is a workout you can do 2 to 3 times a week. Make sure you're using the right amount of weight and pay attention to the two main areas which could be unconditioned, the elbow flexors and lower back. Decrease weight, rest longer, recover, and then try again with programming it once a week, then twice, and so on.

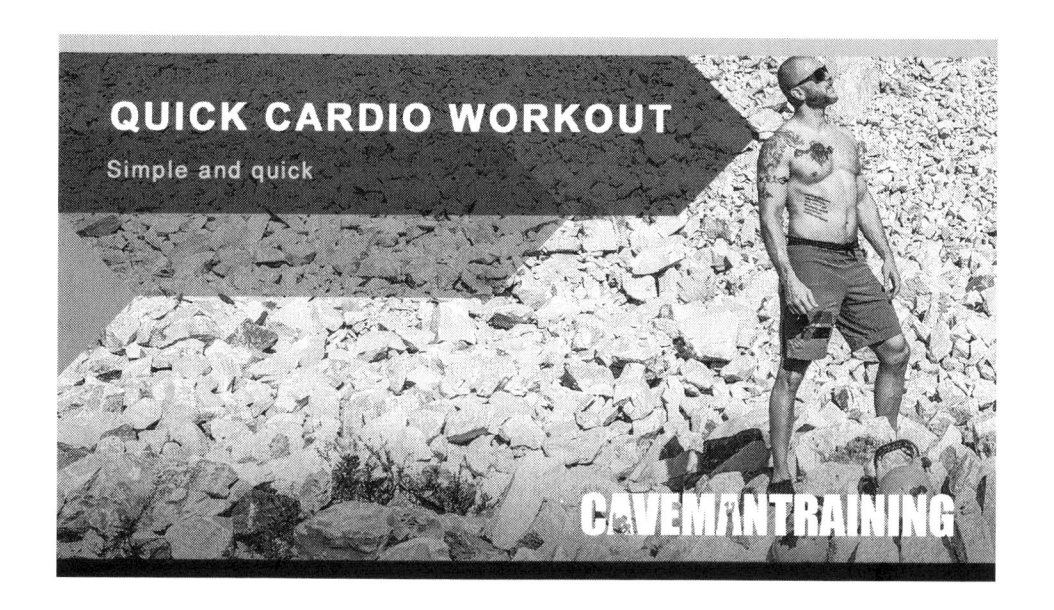

QUICK KETTLEBELL CARDIO WORKOUT

Level: Intermediate to advanced

Weight: Light to medium

Kettlebell(s):

Type: Cardio

Duration: 12 minutes

Other: Full-body; AMRAP

workout go.cavemantraining.com/kbwc-vid47

Simple and quick.

Another kettlebell workout along the lines of simple and quick. Simple as in its only four exercises and 3 reps per exercise, working only for 12 minutes. But advanced as in the movements and transitions.

You can easily do this workout on its own or you can include it in your WODs as a task to complete. The exercises are:

- ➔ 3 x reverse lunge dead cleans
- ➔ 3 x single arm swings
- ➔ 3 x jerks
- ➔ 3 x full snatches

Complete 3 reps of each. Finish one side, that's one round. Do as many as you can within 12 minutes.

You need just one kettlebell of light to medium weight because you want to be able to complete the full 12 minutes and work fast paced.

If you're a crossfitter: The workout has it all, very specific to other techniques you use with the barbell, i.e. the pull in the dead clean can be compared to the power clean, but it's just one leg you're using, so providing more benefit in your training. The swing can be used to improve your American swing, you're using one hand here, not two. The Jerk and the snatch are also in it.

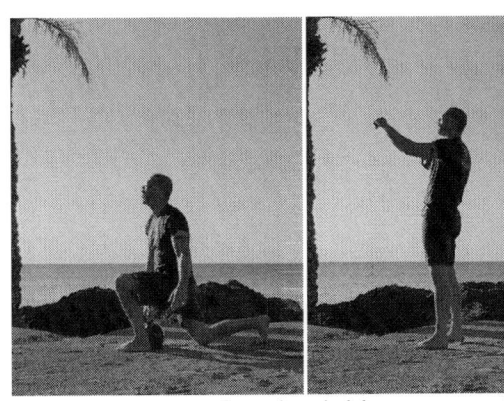

Reverse lunge dead clean

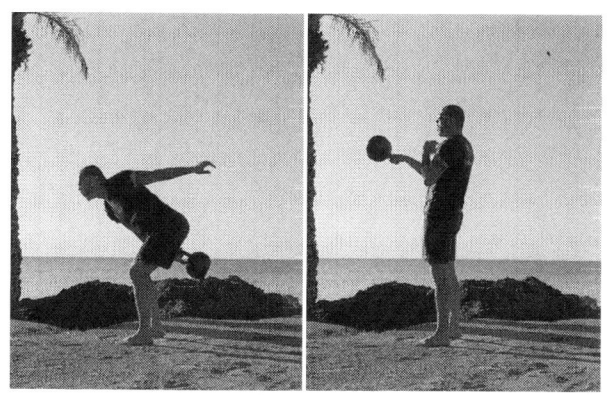

Single arm swing

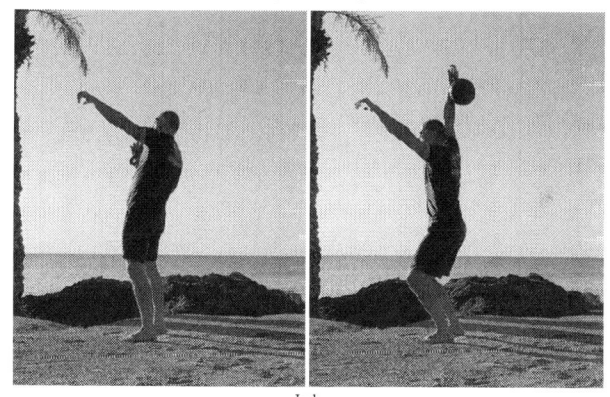

Jerk
The jerk is complex, not even 12 images would do it justice.
Make sure you check out the more detailed info on the jerk in this book.

Full swing snatch

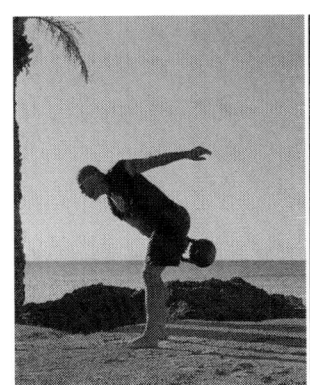

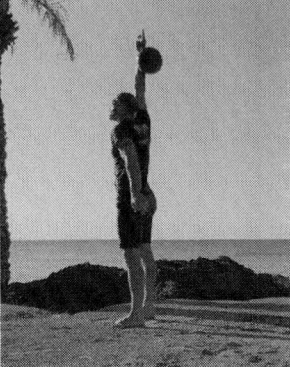

The progressions for the three exercises that are most complex would be as follows:

- **Reverse lunge dead clean**
    1. Bodyweight reverse lunge
    2. Racked reverse lunge
    3. Dead clean
- **Jerk**
    1. Shoulder press
    2. Push press
- **Full swing snatch**
    1. Single arm swing
    2. Single arm swing clean
    3. Single arm swing clean and press
    4. Single arm half snatch

So, if you want to adjust this workout to beginner level, replace the exercise with a progression from above and work on it.

This workout is short, performed with light to medium weight, and can be included in your regular training 2 to 3 times a week or more for cardio. I say cardio, but of course there is also a strength component, anytime you add resistance to your training you're working on strength.

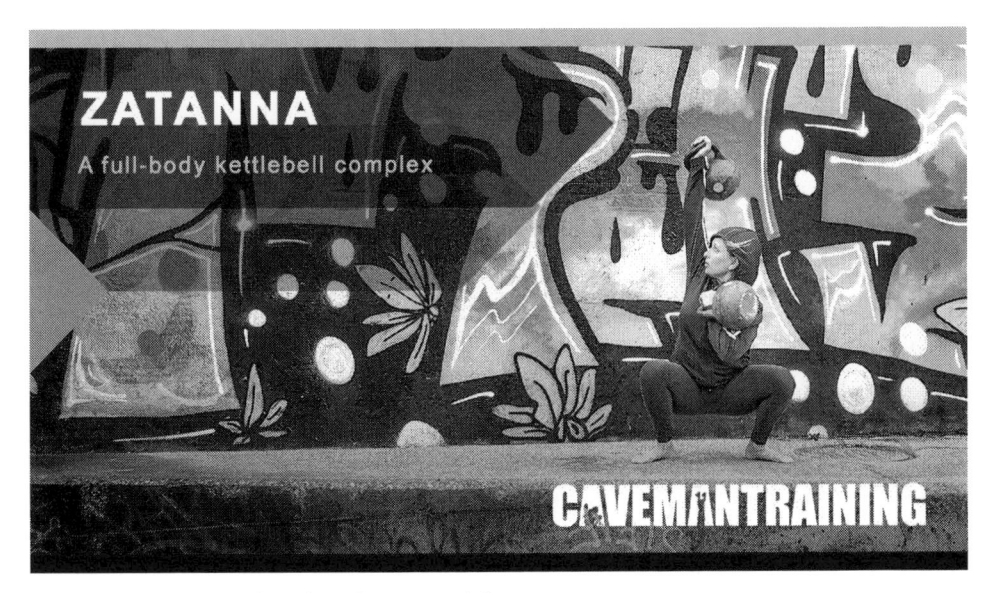

Designed by Anna Junghans from Cavemantraining.

ZATANNA

Level: Beginner

Weight: Medium

Kettlebell(s):

Type: Strength and cardio

Duration: 12 to 15 minutes

Other: Full-body; FOR TIME; complex/flow

workout go.cavemantraining.com/kbwc-vid48

A full-body kettlebell complex.

Kettlebell complexes are great to combine strength and cardio, i.e. you're moving weight but at the same time you stay active without having to put the kettlebell down. A complex/flow does require you to be comfortable with the kettlebell and transition from one exercise into the next.

- ➔ 5 x around the body (L)
- ➔ 5 x around the body (R)
- ➔ 5 x overhead press
- ➔ 5 x front squat
- ➔ 5 x Russian swing
- ➔ 4 x single arm overhead press (L)
- ➔ 4 x single arm overhead press (R)

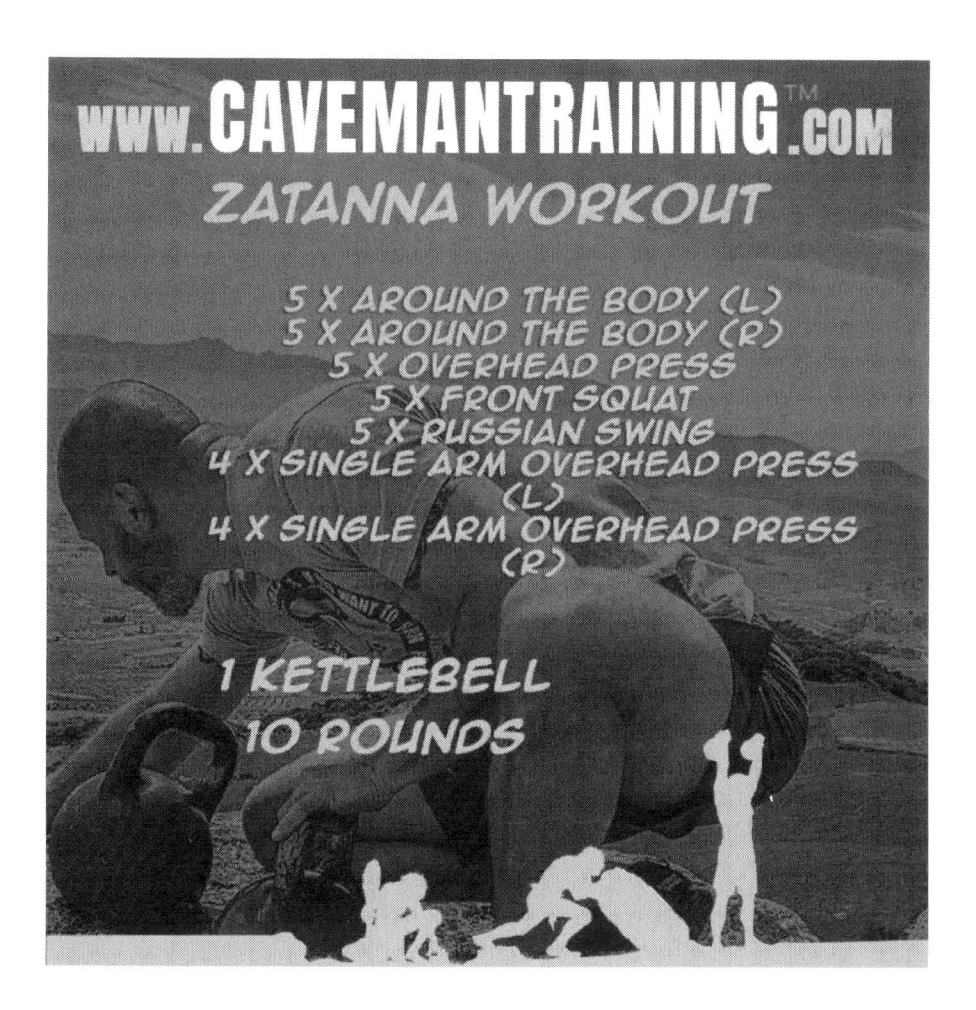

10 rounds

Share go.cavemantraining.com/kbwc-link10

After performing around the body left and right you catch the bell into one hand (the transition can be tricky) then drop and swing into a double handed swing, clean it up with open hand thumbs through the horns (download the grips pdf from our website) and go straight into your overhead presses. After your overhead press you go straight into front squats, from there you can transition into the swings after which you release one hand and perform a single arm clean to transition into the overhead press. After completing one side you transition to the other side and repeat the overhead press. Repeat the workout for 10 rounds.

Transitions

Following are the details on all transitions used in the workout.

The first transition is the catch where the kettlebell needs to stop and change direction. The catch is performed by finishing the rep with a slight curl and catching the bell with an open palm in the other hand. The kettlebell is then pushed in the opposite direction.

The second transition happens at the front after finishing the around the body, the bell comes outward at the front rather than finishing a circle, the other hand grabs the handle so that two hands are holding the handle for the backswing, transitioning into a double arm clean with open palm horn grip (thumbs around the horns).

The third transition is from swings into a one arm swing clean, transitioning from hook grip into loose/racking grip, and ready to press the kettlebell overhead.

The fourth and final transition is from one arm to the other, which is done with a swing switch, and swing clean.

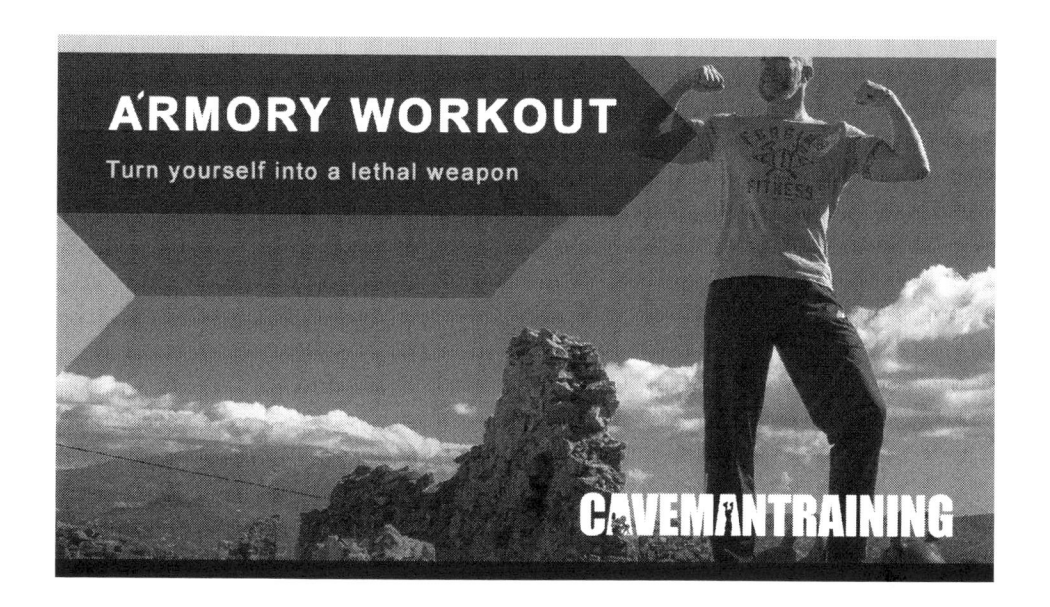

ARMORY WORKOUT

Level: Intermediate

Weight: Medium

Kettlebell(s):

Type: Strength and cardio

Duration: 24 minutes

Other: Full-body; EMOM; interval

workout go.cavemantraining.com/kbwc-vid49

Turn yourself into a lethal weapon.

This is an EMOM workout, every minute on the minute you start your task. Works as follows:

- **First minute complete:**
    → 4 x squat dead curl and press

- → 4 x single arm swings
- → 4 x full snatches

    rest for the remainder of the minute (if any)

- **Second minute:**

    → hold a static side plank for 30 seconds

    rest for the remaining 30 seconds

- Switch sides
- **First minute complete:**

    → 4 x squat dead curl and press

    → 4 x single arm swings

    → 4 x full snatches

    rest for the remainder of the minute (if any)

- **Second minute:**

    → hold a static side plank for 30 seconds

    rest for the remaining 30 seconds

- That's one round
- Perform 6 rounds which is a total of 24 minutes (23 and 30 seconds to be exact)

Your weight should be medium to heavy. Choose your weight based on the dead curl, meaning, if you can swing or snatch a 24kg but can't curl it, then that's not the right weight. You should be able to complete the following 3 exercises within 40 to 50 seconds, squat dead curl and press, single arm swings, and full snatches.

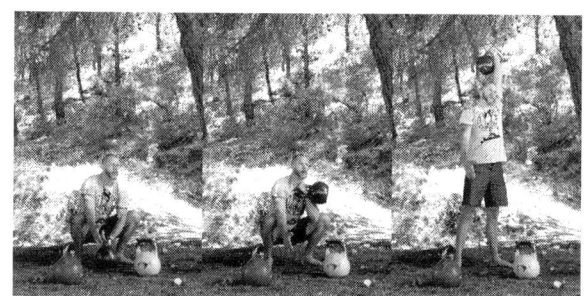

Squat, dead curl, and press combo

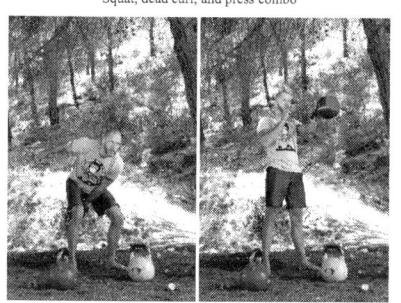

Single arm swing

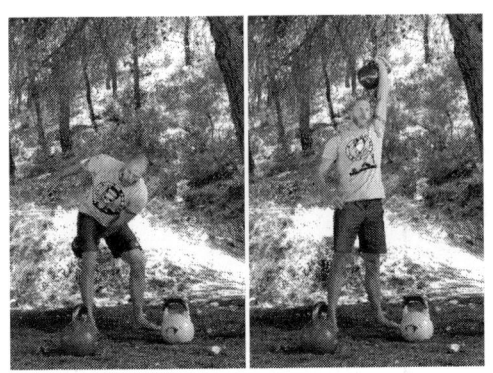

Full swing snatch

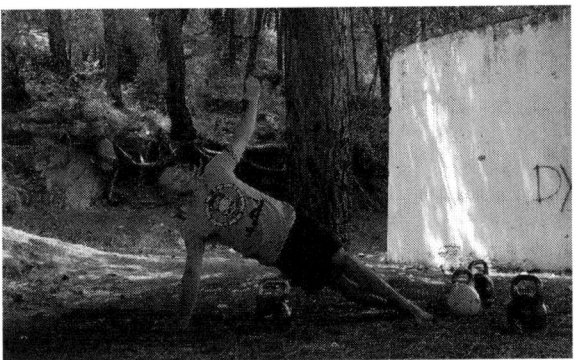

Side plank

Get our *Advanced Workout Timer* on Google Play and you can create flexible and advanced workouts like the following:

- 10-second countdown
- 5-minute warm-up
- Repeat 6 times
    - 1 minute counting up

- 30 seconds counting up
- 30 seconds countdown
- 1 minute counting up
- 30 seconds counting up
- 30 seconds countdown
* 5-minute cool-down

You need a good hand insert and know how to transition from loose to hook grip, download our free PDF on kettlebell grips and instantly take your training to the next level. Your wrist strength also plays an important part in this workout. Choose the right weight for the workout, don´t continue with a heavyweight if the elbow flexors play up. Pay attention to the kettlebell rotation implemented during the curl, this is vital to make the curl smooth.

This is a workout you can include in your training once a week but you should pay close attention to the elbow flexors and reduce weight, rest, recover, and revise if any problems in that area do occur.

If you can find a couple of seconds to rate the book on Amazon I would really appreciate it. go.cavemantraining.com/kbwc-link19

Thanks

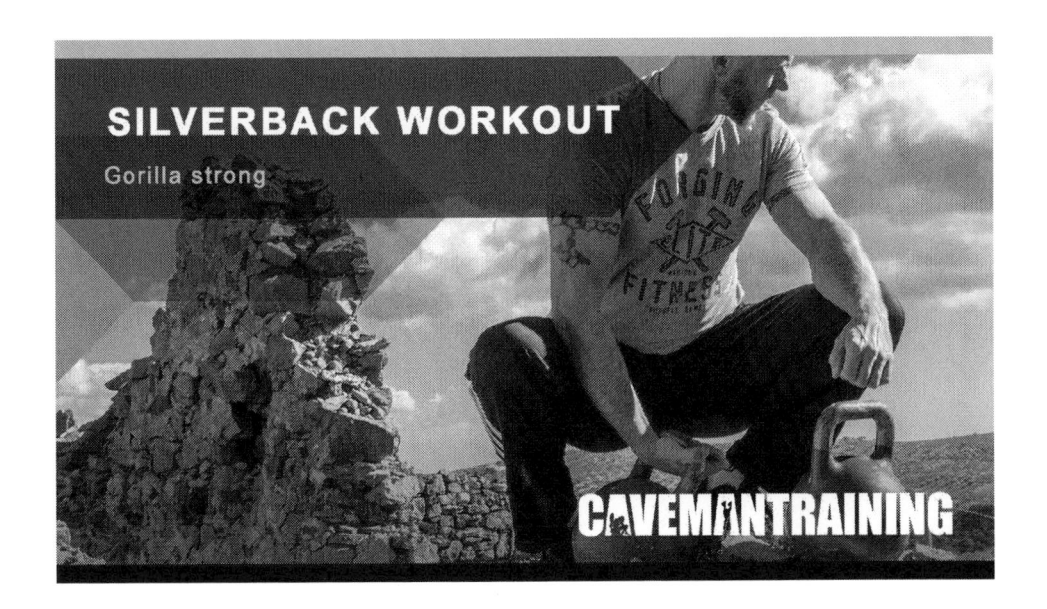

CAVEMAN KETTLEBELLS SILVERBACK WORKOUT

Level: Advanced

Weight: Medium

Kettlebell(s):

Type: Strength and light cardio

Duration: 20 minutes

Other: Full-body; short; low reps; AMRAP

▶ workout go.cavemantraining.com/kbwc-vid50

Gorilla strong.

I designed this 20-minute WOD in 2016 with low reps, medium weight, and a short time frame so that you can complete this workout going from one exercise into the next without overloading any of the muscle groups too much. It's a nice quick and easy workout to get in on those days you don't have a lot of time.

2018 and I've re-filmed this workout at one of our outdoor workout locations. Check out the video above.

The WOD consists of:

➔ 2 x bent over dead rows (wide)
➔ 2 x renegade rows
➔ 2 x overhead squat
➔ 2 x alternating hang clean and press

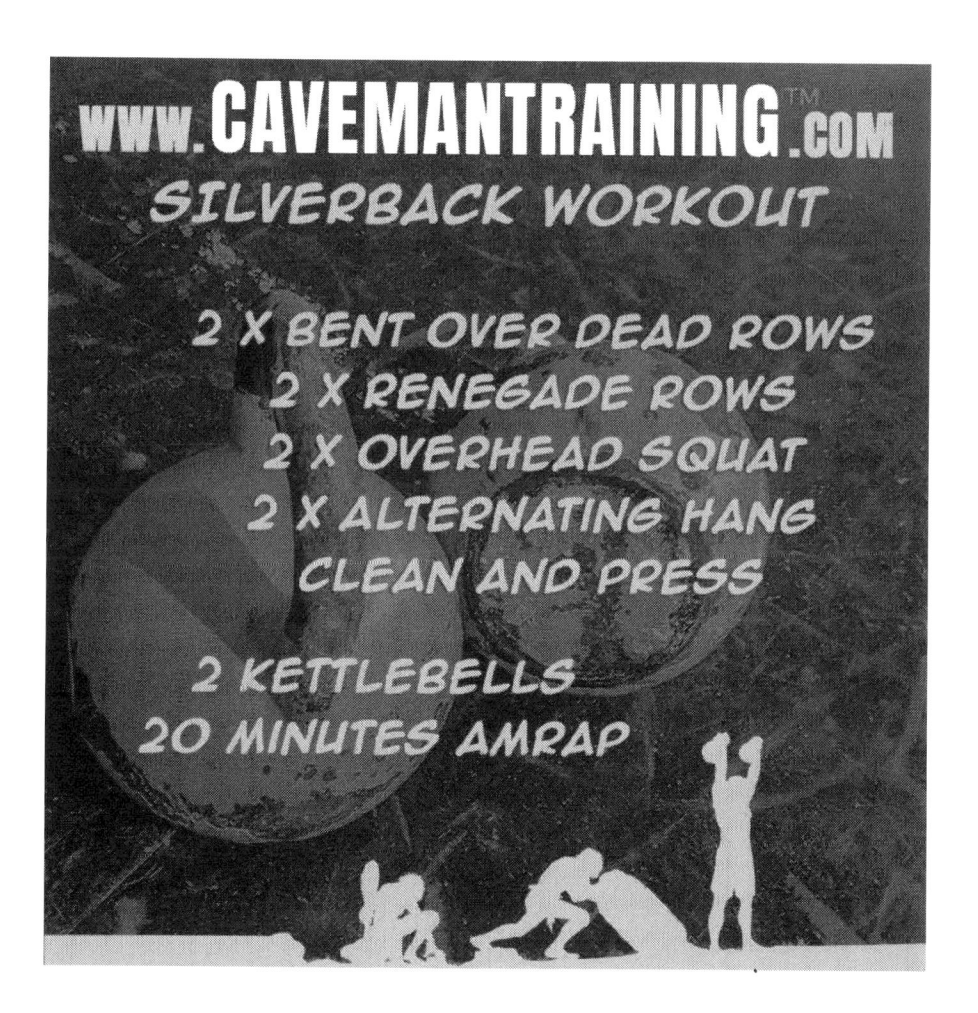

20-minute **AMRAP**

Share go.cavemantraining.com/kbwc-link11

For the rows you bent over with a hip hinge and start with the weights dead on the ground each time, row outwards squeezing the shoulder blades together, control the down phase and put the bells down dead right under your shoulders.

You can go straight into the renegade rows by kicking your feet back and landing into a plank if you placed the bells in the right place, perform a tricep push-up and row each side into the hips.

If you jump your feet back in the right position you can clean the bells straight up, then press or jerk them overhead and perform two overhead squats.

Rack your bells and let one drop straight down moving from loose grip to hook grip coming into a squat, clean the bell up from a hang position using nothing but the legs, go straight into a press and perform the same on the other side.

This is one round, mark it down on the board, you have 20 minutes to perform as many rounds as possible.

Muscles worked but not limited to:

- Triceps
- Trapezius
- Rhomboids
- Deltoids (front and back)
- Quads
- Abductors (if you squat properly, pulling your knees out)
- Latissimus dorsi (if you engage them during the plank)
- Glutes
- Core muscles (especially during the rows)

The workout step-by-step in pictures:

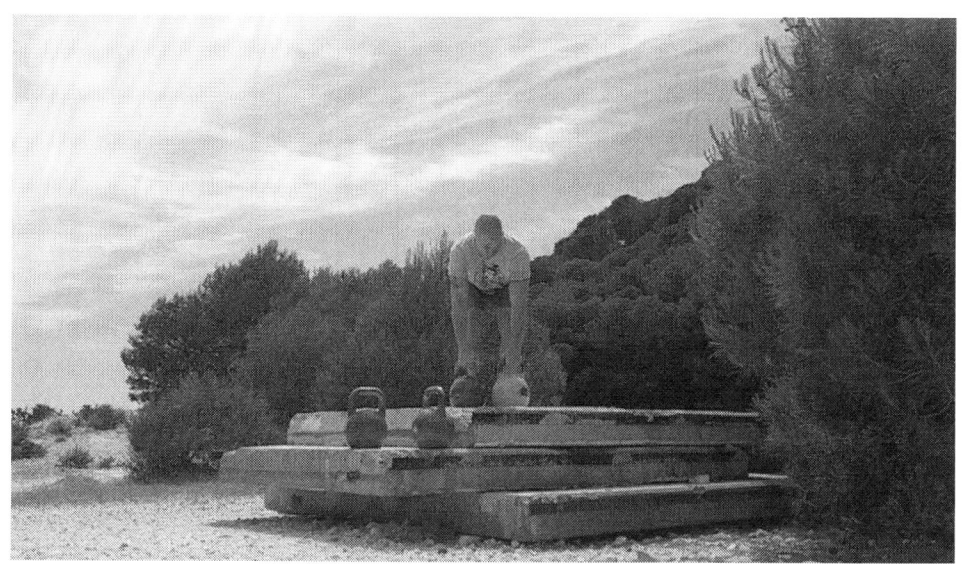

Bent over with the hip hinge.

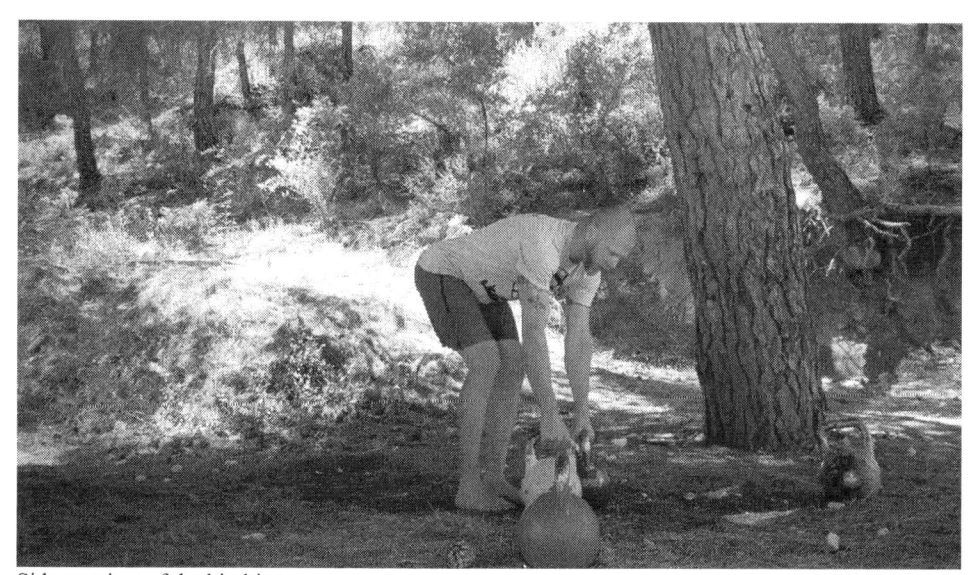

Side-on view of the hip hinge.

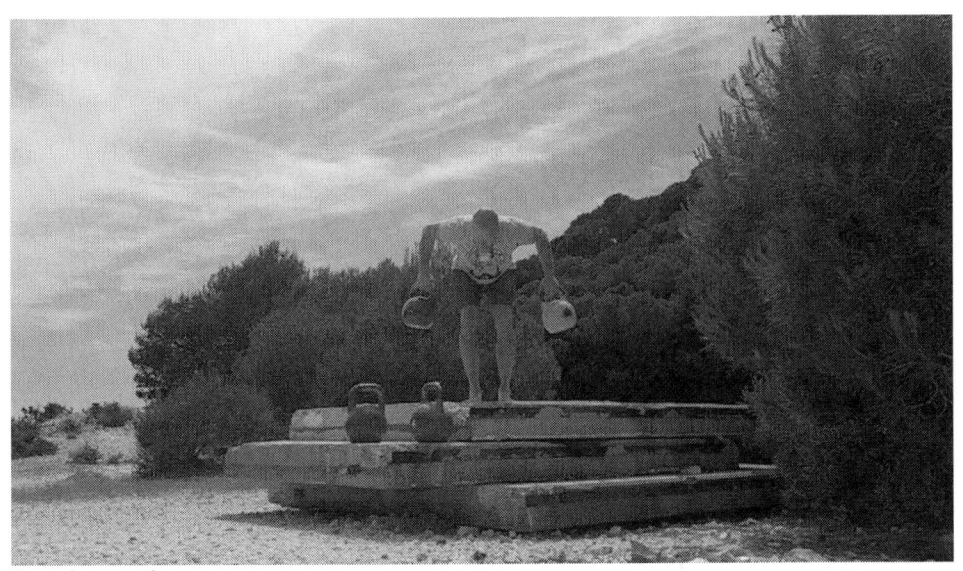

Scapula retraction

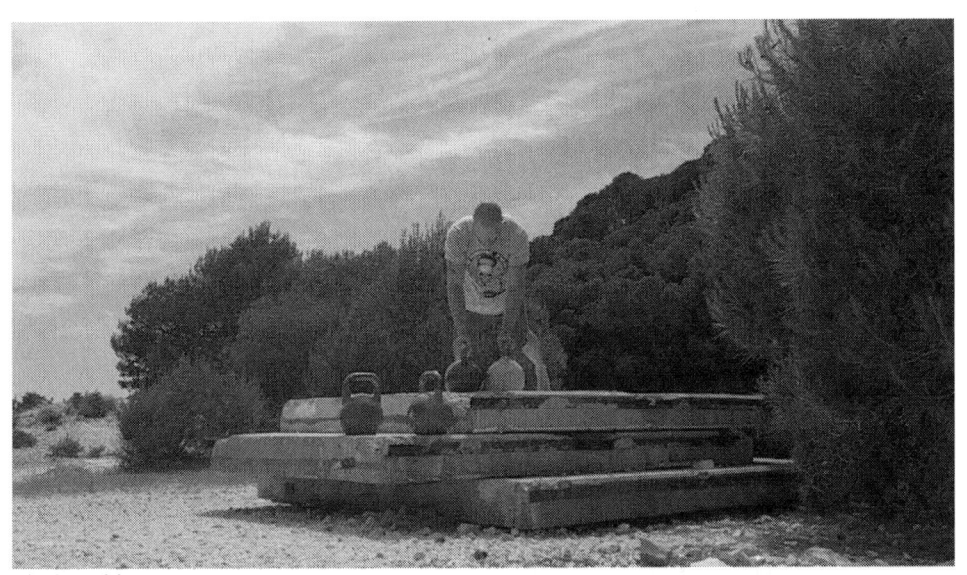

Plank position

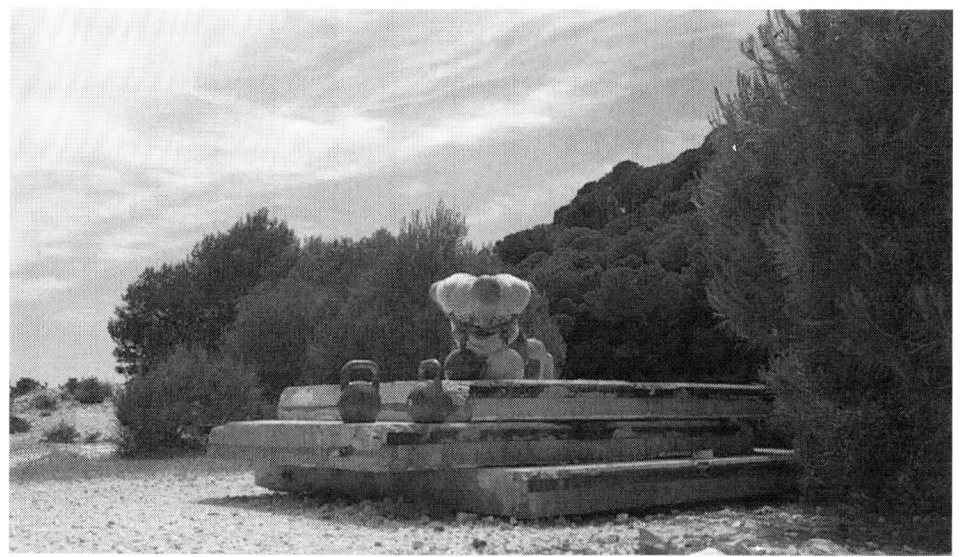

Perform a tricep push-up

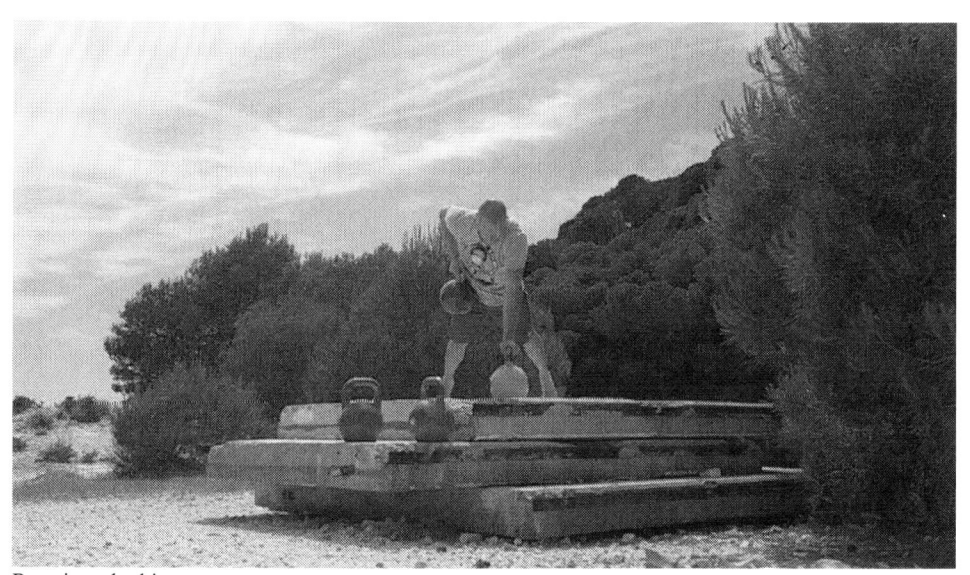

Row into the hip

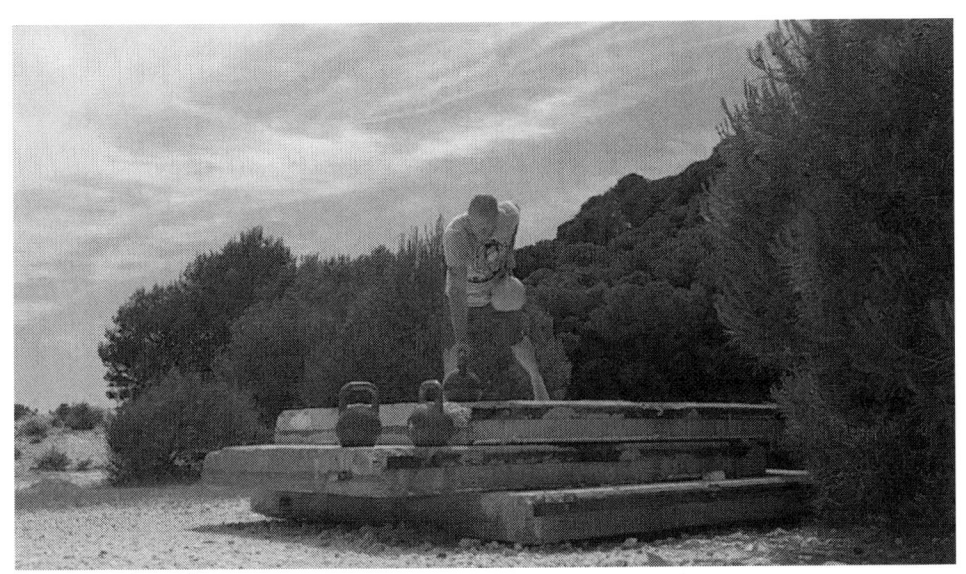

Repeat on other side

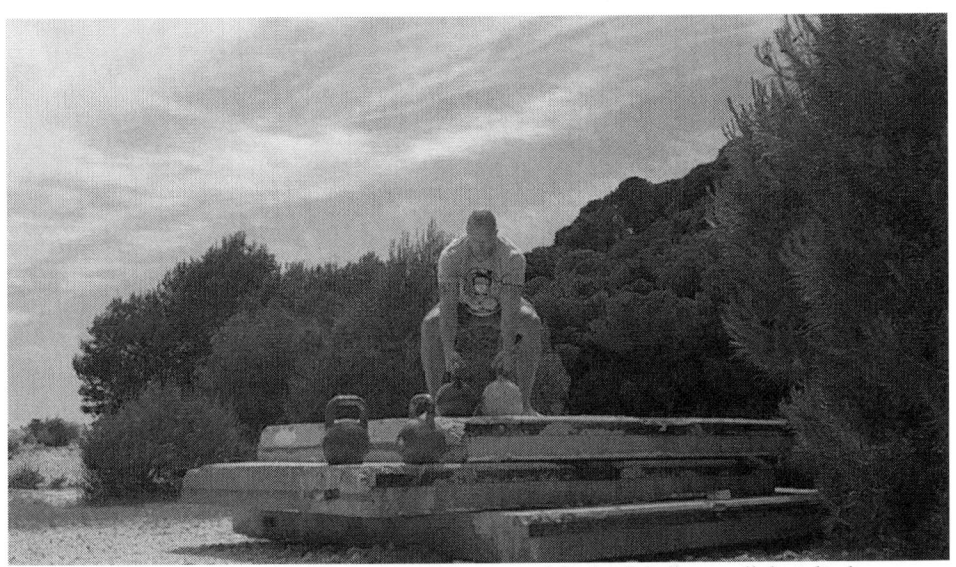

Jump the feet back in with enough space between you and the kettlebells to pull them back

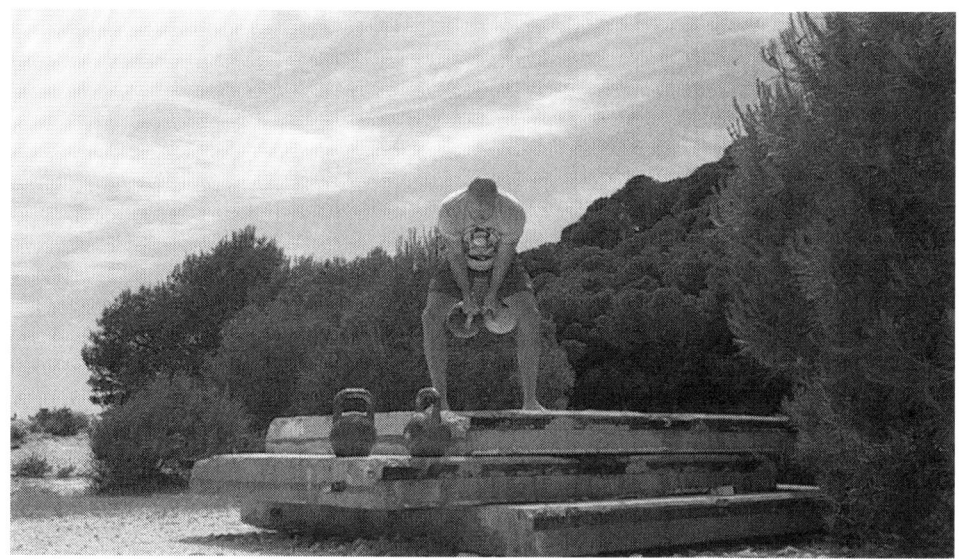

Pull the kettlebells back for the clean

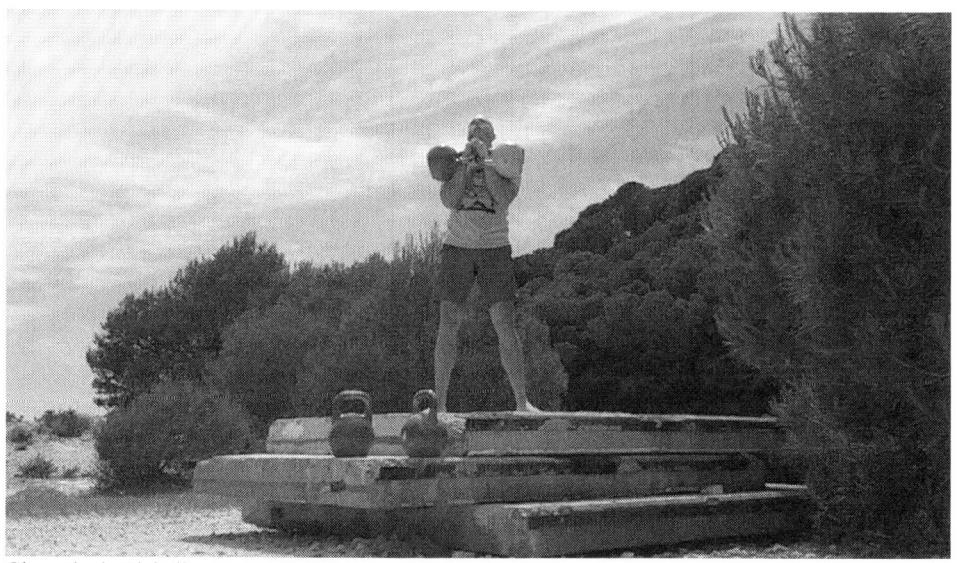

Clean the kettlebells

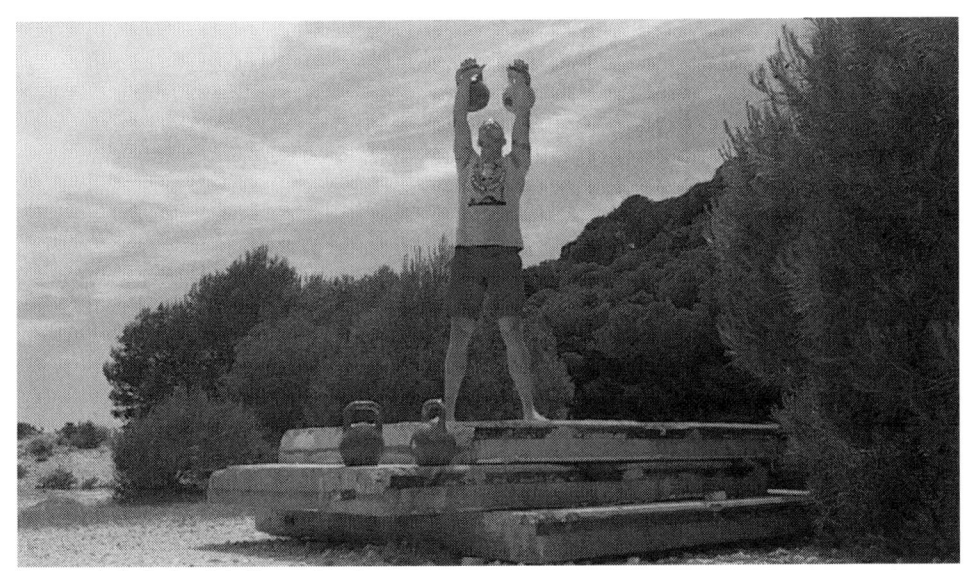

Press or jerk the kettlebells overhead

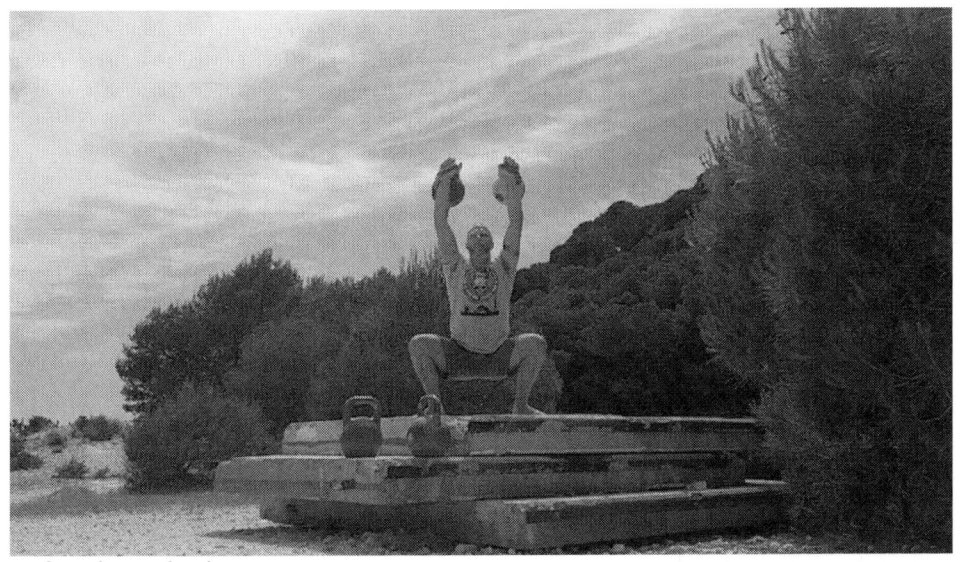

Perform the overhead squat

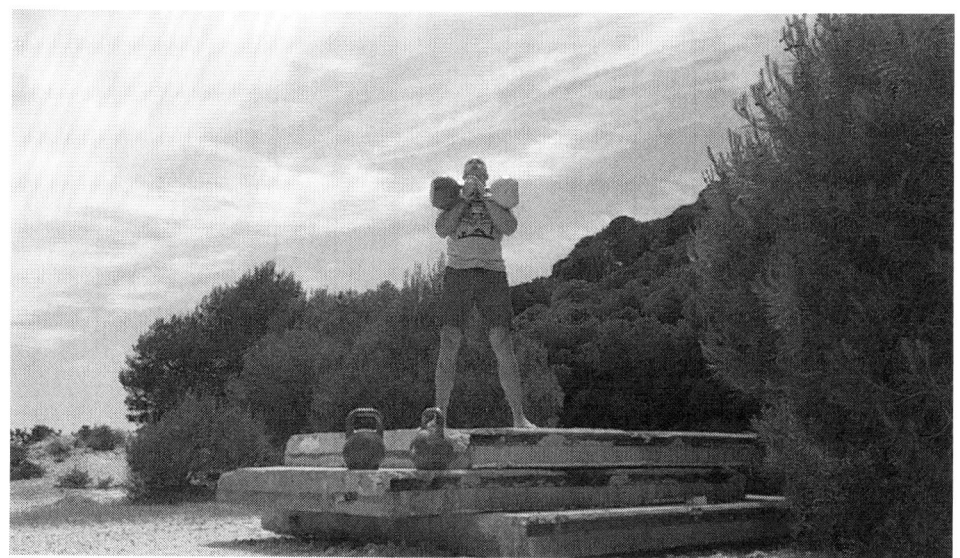

Lower both bells into racking

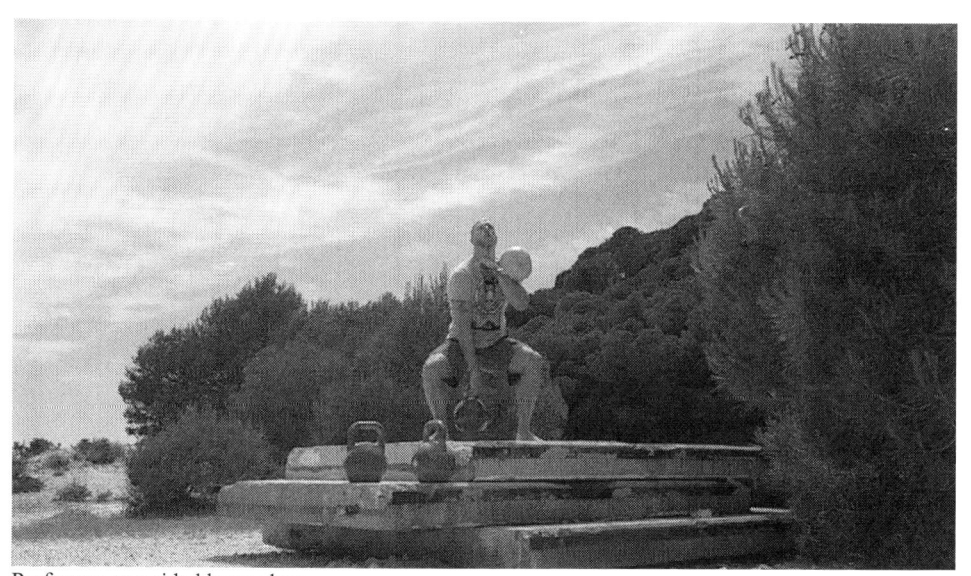

Perform a one-sided hang clean

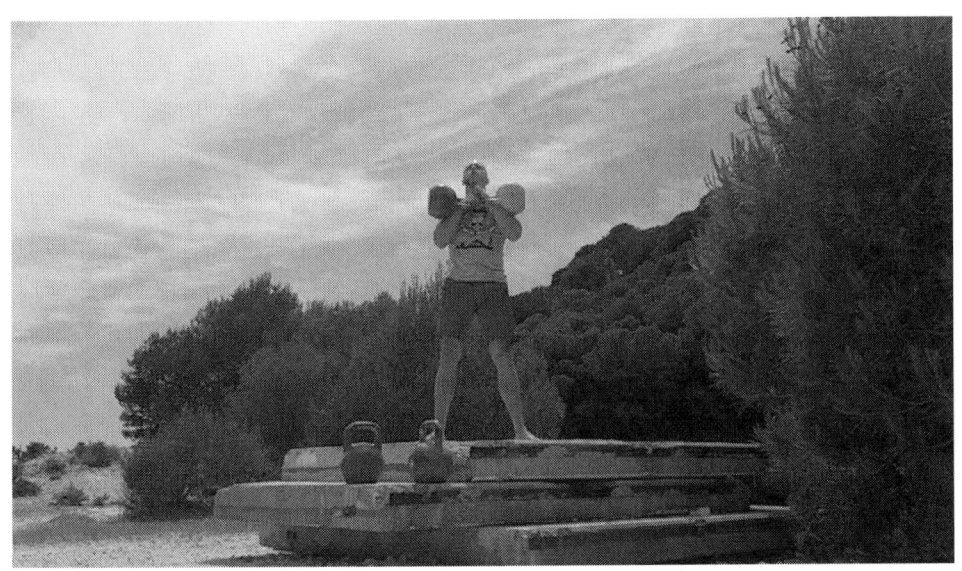

End up in racking position

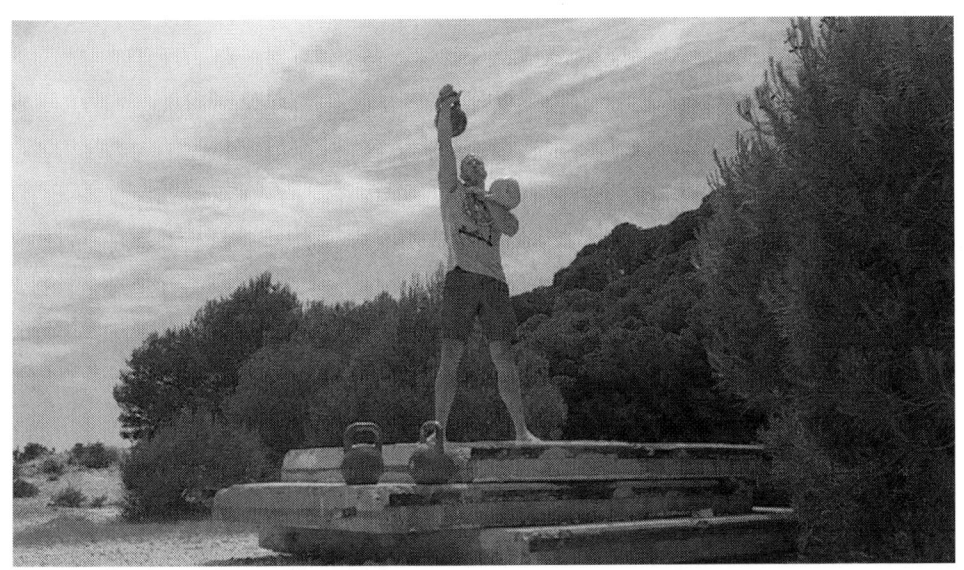

Press overhead or push press if required

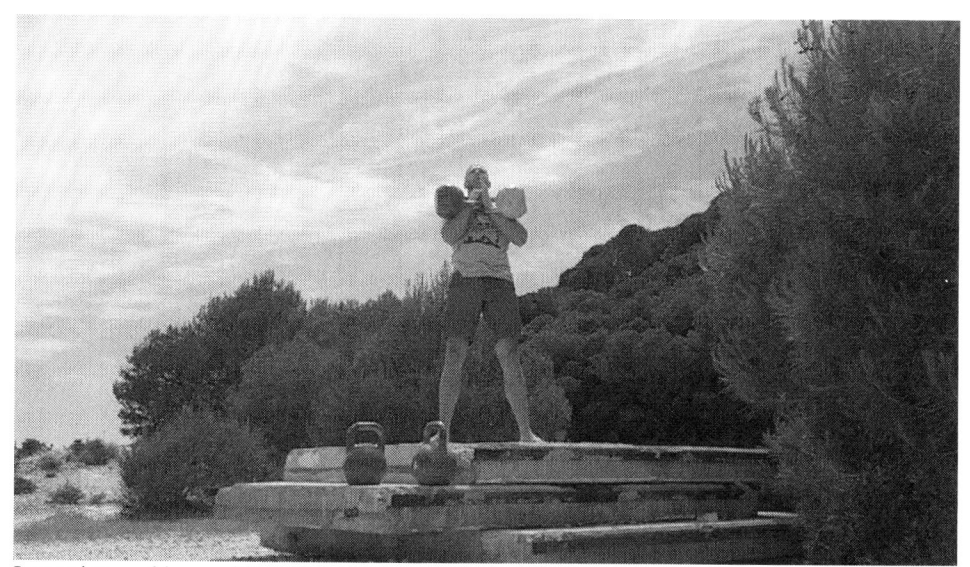

Lower into racking position

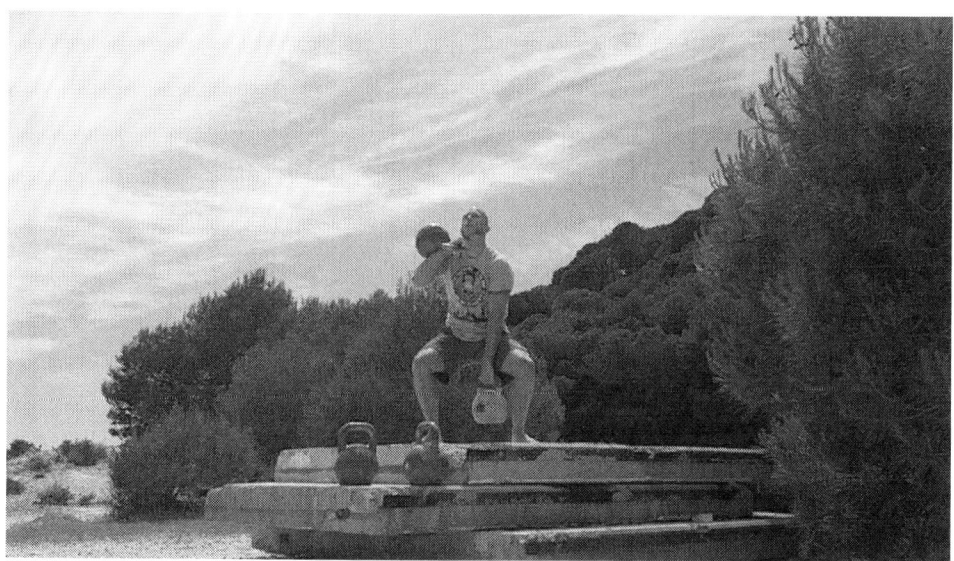

Hang clean the other side

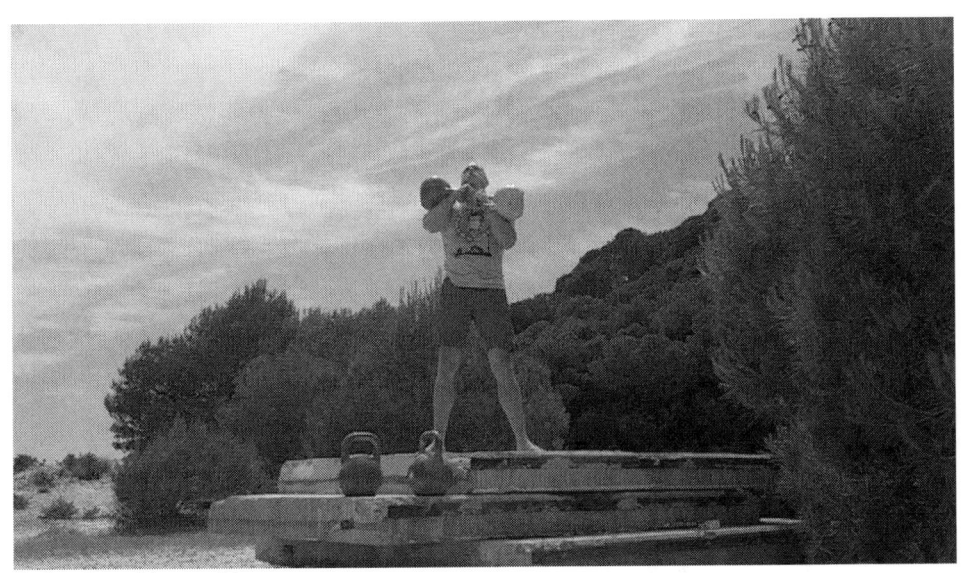

End up in racking position

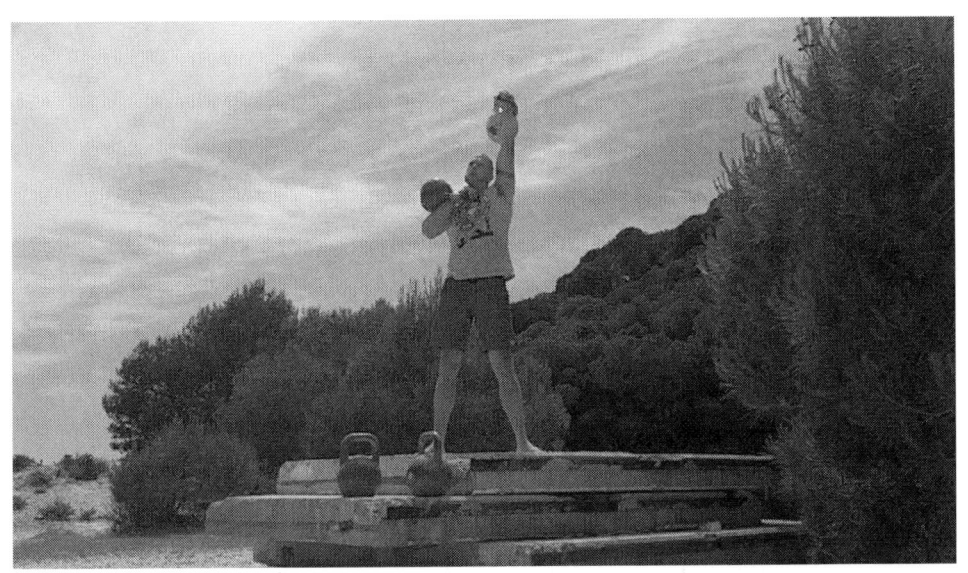

Press or push press overhead

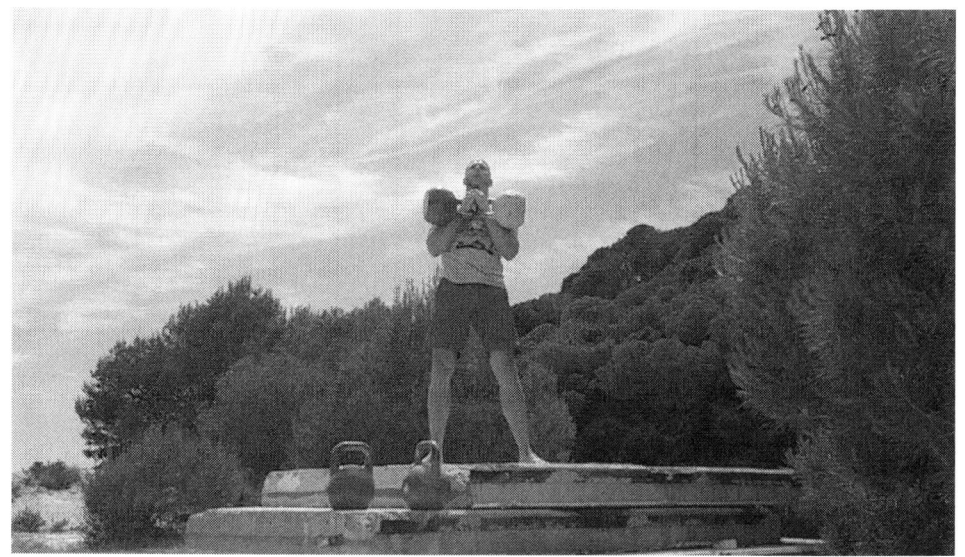

End up in racking position

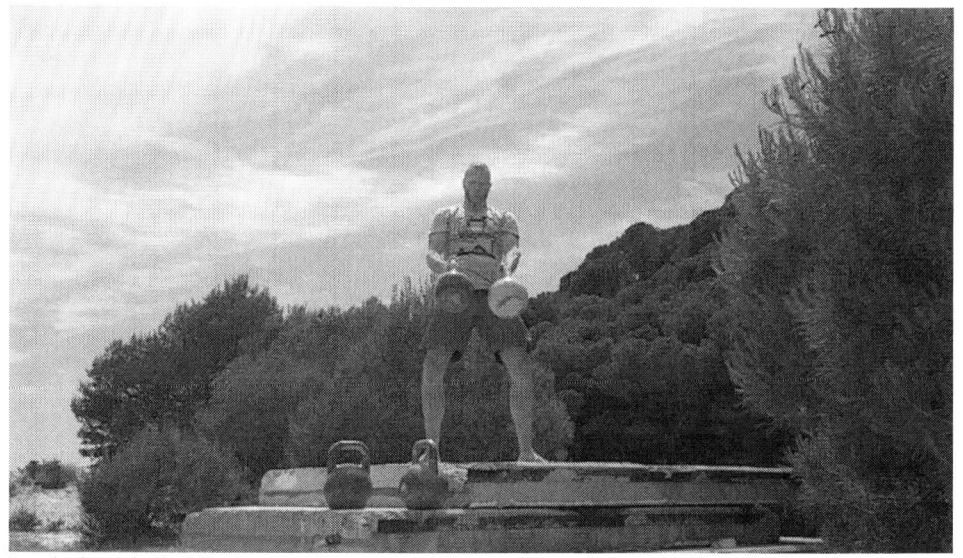

Let the kettlebells falls down while creating hip extension and transitioning to hook grip

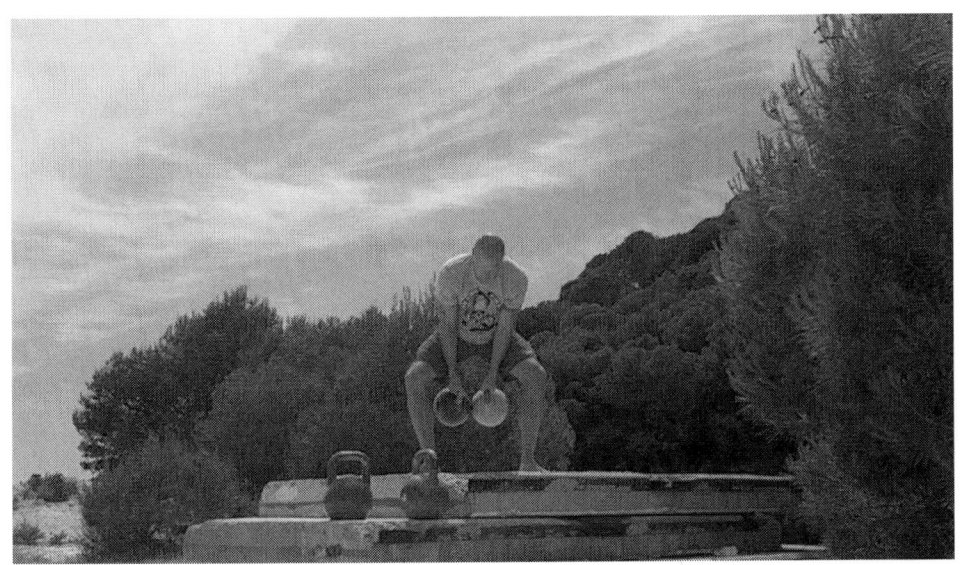

Let the bells swing back through the legs

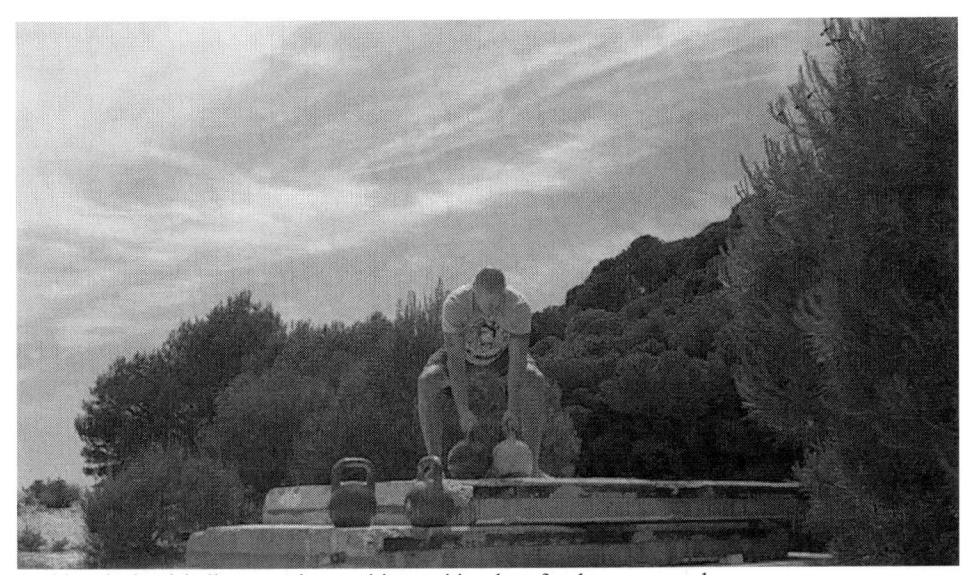

Position the kettlebells to starting position and in-place for the next round

Don't fool around with the kettlebell overhead squat! You might do barbell overhead squats, but this is a different beast all together. There is a lot more stabilization required, more direct overhead shoulder flexibility, better thoracic mobility and much more.

Check out this video for improving overhead squat mobility go.cavemantraining.com/kbwc-vid51 and the associated article here go.cavemantraining.com/kbwc-link12

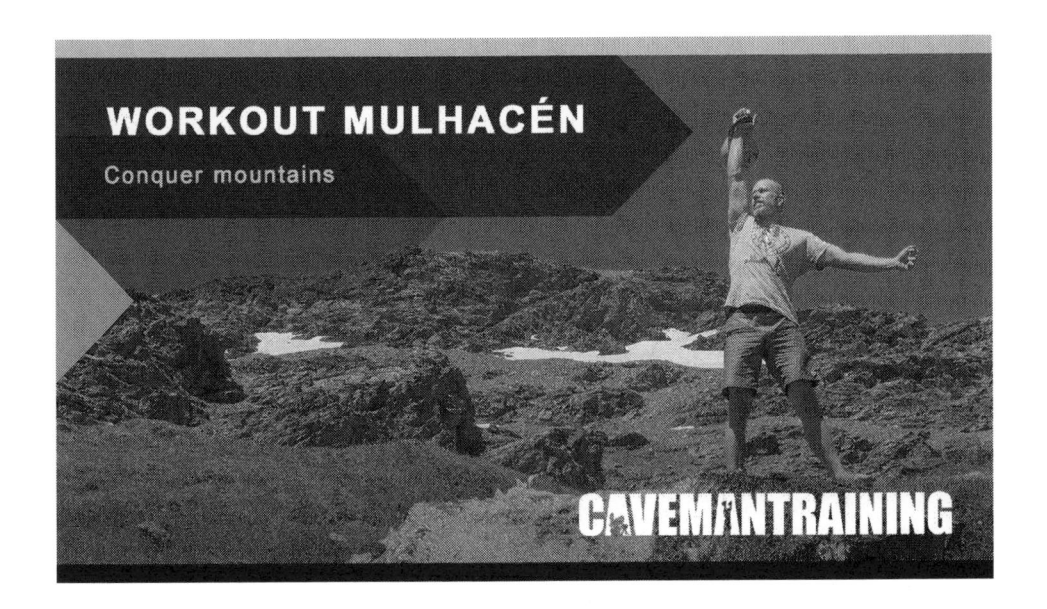

WORKOUT MULHACÉN

Level: Intermediate

Weight: Medium to heavy

Kettlebell(s):

Type: Strength and cardio

Duration: 22 to 26 minutes

Other: Full-body; FOR TIME; low reps

workout go.cavemantraining.com/kbwc-vid52

Conquer mountains.

This awesome workout is named after the mountain we've been doing a lot of our training on this year. It's the highest mountain in Spain (mainland).

The workout is as follows:

- → 3 front squats
- → 3 single arm swings
- → 3 swing high pulls
- → 3 full snatches

Performed on the left side, repeat on the right, that equals one round. Complete 5 rounds. Finish with 25 bent-over dead rows on the left, and 25 on the right. FOR TIME.

Rest 4 minutes.

Repeat the whole sequence.

Rx weight: 20kg/44lbs for male and 16kg/35.2lbs for female

MULHACÉN FOR TIME

3 FRONT SQUATS
3 SINGLE ARM SWINGS
3 SWING HIGH PULLS
3 FULL SNATCHES

PERFORMED ON THE LEFT SIDE, REPEAT ON THE RIGHT, THAT EQUALS ONE ROUND. COMPLETE 5 ROUNDS. FINISH WITH 25 BENT-OVER DEAD ROWS ON THE LEFT, AND 25 ON THE RIGHT. FOR TIME.

REST 4 MINUTES.

REPEAT THE WHOLE SEQUENCE.

RX WEIGHT: 20KG/44LBS
1 KETTLEBELL

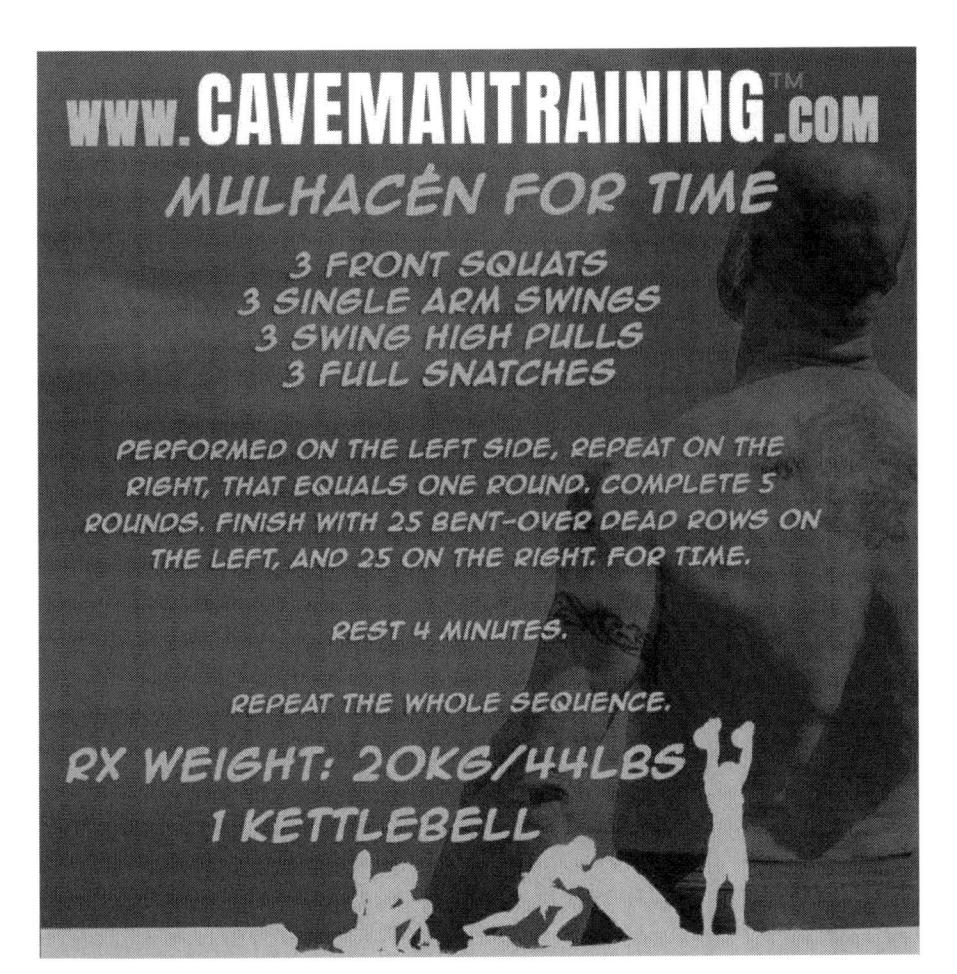

Share go.cavemantraining.com/kbwc-link13

- **Front squat:** the elbow should touch the inner thigh while the hips are below knee line.
- **Single arm swing:** the kettlebell should swing to shoulder height.
- **Swing high pull:** aim for the elbow to come in line with the shoulders.
- **Full snatch:** the kettlebell should end overhead in full lockout and drop back down into a swing.
- **Bent-over dead row:** the kettlebell should start dead under the shoulder upon each rep and the elbow should travel past the ribs.

Leave the clock running if you do this in a group format. The athlete notes their time when completing the first sequence, for example, if the time is 7:35 they rest till 11:35 and then start their second sequence noting the time they finish that.

The Kettlebell Swing High Pull

It's quite frequently that I see the kettlebell swing high pull performed incorrectly and hear of tendon issues. This is due to the pulling exercise being performed incorrectly and it turning into an elbow flexion exercise (think bicep curl), rather than a rowing/pulling exercise for the back.

When performing this exercise you should be focussing on the back muscles, the rhomboids, trapezius, and rear deltoid. Use your rear deltoid for horizontal shoulder abduction, and rhomboids plus trapezius for scapula retraction (scapula abduction). Think of this as pulling your elbow back and the forearm just follows, and think about squeezing the shoulder blades together. Avoid pulling the hand towards the shoulder which incorrectly turns this exercise into elbow flexion.

I have a few cues that I use to teach people, you can see these in the following video. These cues undoubtedly make it super clear to your athletes how to perform this exercise, what to feel, and what not to feel. go.cavemantraining.com/kbwc-vid53

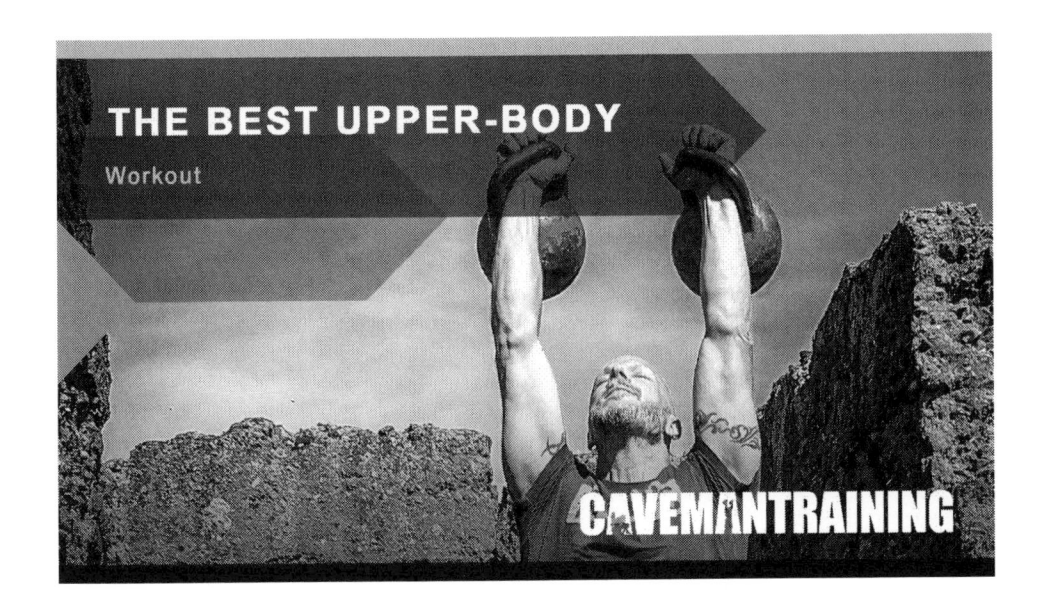

THE BEST UPPER-BODY WORKOUT

Level: Intermediate

Weight: Heavy

Kettlebell(s):

Type: Strength

Duration: 60 minutes

Other: Upper-body and back; slow

workout go.cavemantraining.com/kbwc-vid54

Strong shoulders.

If you could only do four exercises for the upper-body, then this would be the best combination for an awesome upper-body workout. This workout hits the front and rear deltoids, the lats and upper trapezius. All super important muscles for good upper-body strength.

4 Upper-body Exercises

→ Shoulder press
→ Bent-over dead row
→ Pull-up
→ Shrug

Targets:
- Anterior deltoid
- Posterior deltoid
- Lats
- Upper trapezius

Repetitions and rounds:

4 – 6 – 4 – 6 x 2 rounds @ 90%

6 – 8 – 6 – 8 x 2 rounds @ 80%

8 – 8 – 8 – 8 x 2 rounds @ 70%

Approx. 60+ minutes of work

Performed slow and controlled

Plenty of rest between exercises and rounds.

If your weight is very heavy, it's ok to clean and return the weight back to the ground with two hands.

You can put the weight down during reps, in fact, I recommend it, rather than doing one after the other and rushing it, put the weight down and take your time with each quality rep.

4 – 6 – 4 – 6 x 2 rounds @ 90% would be done as following.

4 reps of strict shoulder press at 90% of 1RM, finish one side and then do the other. Check out my book about the kettlebell press if you want the nitty-gritty on pressing a kettlebell.

6 reps of bent-over dead rows at 90% of your 1RM row, finish one side and then do the other. Because you have to hold a static hip hinge you'll not just be working your rear deltoid, but also your gluteals and back. Make sure you come out of the position if you feel the gluteals or back is giving up. Return to dead upon each rep.

4 reps of pull-ups, return to full hang upon each rep. If you can't come down in a controlled manner, make sure you rest before your next rep. An alternative to the pull-up will be the lat activation drill explained here go.cavemantraining.com/kbwc-link14

6 reps of shrugs with 90% of your 1RM. You'll only get little range out of this movement, don't force a fake range by bending to the side. Pull your shoulder up with your upper trapezius.

That's one round, repeat to make 2. Then move on doing the same exercises, the same amount of rounds (two), but increasing the reps and decreasing the weight to 80%. Same for the final 2 rounds, everything is 8 reps and the weight is 70%.

Finish off the workout with 20 tricep push-ups.

Feeling buff? Post online after you completed the workout.

FYI: I used 32kg/70lb first two rounds, then 28kg in the second set of two rounds, and 24kg/53lb in the last two rounds but stuck to the 32kg for the bent-over rows and shrugs as there was nothing heavier to start with.

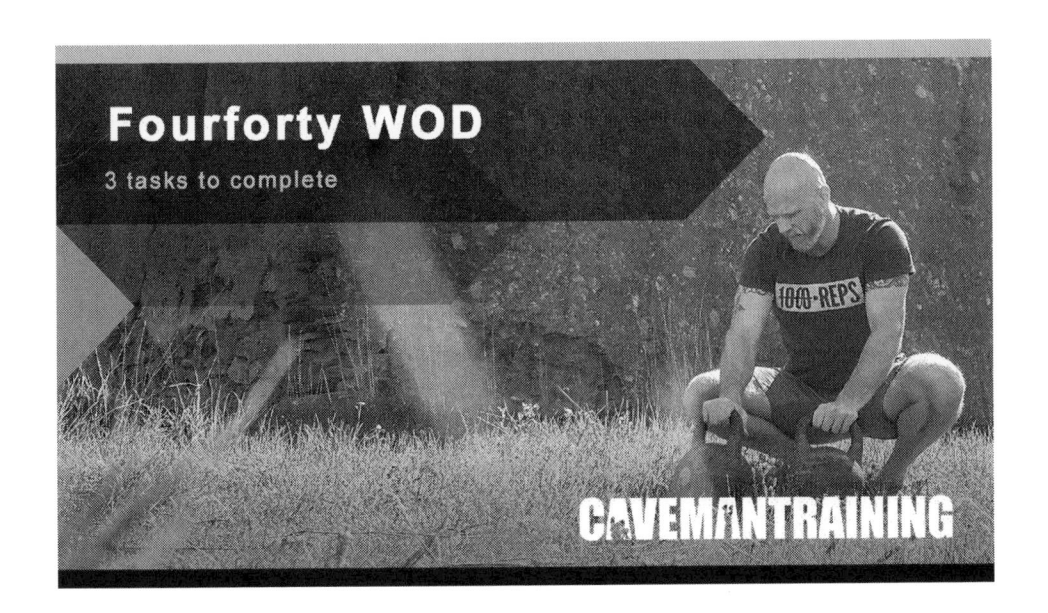

FOURFORTY WOD

Level: Beginner to intermediate

Weight: Medium

Kettlebell(s):

Type: Strength and cardio

Duration: 26 to 30 minutes

Other: Full-body; AMRAP; FOR TIME

workout go.cavemantraining.com/kbwc-vid55

Three tasks to complete.

This is Fourforty WOD. 3 tasks, 2 AMRAP, and 1 FOR TIME. It's either 4 or 40 reps. Complete and post online.

Your First Task

→ 4 squats

- → 4 crossfit burpees
- → 4 dead clean and press left
- → 4 dead clean and press right

⏱ 8 minutes AMRAP

⏳ 2 minutes rest

Your Second Task

- → 40 jump rope
- → 4 dead clean and squat left
- → 4 dead clean and squat right

⏱ 8 minutes AMRAP

⏳ 2 minutes rest

Your Third And Final Task

- → 40 squats
- → 40 alternating dead clean and press
- → 40 crossfit burpees

⏱ FOR TIME

℞ weight

♂ ℞ for a male is 16kg/35.2lbs

♀ R for a female is 12kg/26.4lbs

Watch the dead clean performed in slow-mo go.cavemantraining.com/kbwc-link15

Movement standards:

- The press is strict on the up-phase
- Hips below knee line on the squat
- Full rack and knee plus hip extension on the dead clean

Scoring: Athletes are scored over the two AMRAPs combined, and separately for the task FOR TIME. When posting, combine your rounds/reps for the first two tasks, and the time for the last task.

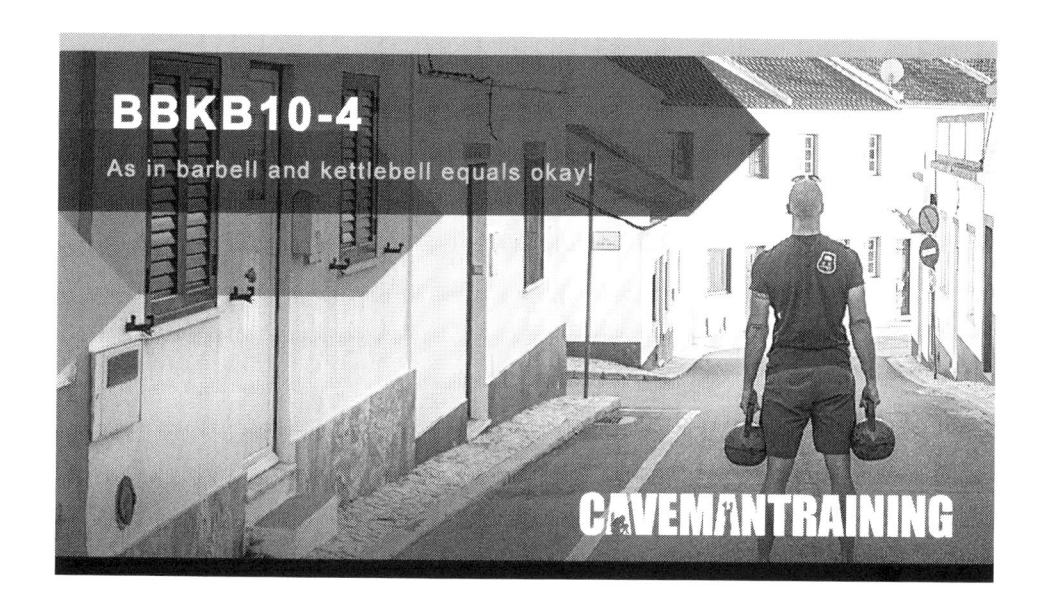

BBKB10-4

Level: Intermediate

Weight: Heavy

Kettlebell(s):

Type: Strength and cardio

Duration: 25 to 30 minutes

Other: Full-body; FOR TIME

workout go.cavemantraining.com/kbwc-vid56

BBKB10-4 as in barbell and kettlebell equals okay!

Low reps. Light barbell just to work on technique. Go heavy with the kettlebell. Seek about 80 to 90% of your max.

➜ 4 x hip hinge deadlifts (not squat style)
➜ 4 x power cleans

→ 4 x single arm swings (aim for chest height) left

→ 4 x single arm swings (aim for chest height) right

→ 4 x jerks left

→ 4 x jerks right

Repeat 2 times, add 10 tricep push-ups and that's ONE ROUND.

Complete five rounds FOR TIME.

Rx male barbell 40kg / 88lbs (light), female 30kg
Rx kettlebell 32kg / 70.5lbs (heavy), female 24kg

Find your weakness.

Scaling:
- Lower the kb weight
- Double arm swings double the reps
- Push press instead of jerks

Here is a slow-motion video of the kettlebell jerk go.cavemantraining.com/kbwc-link16

Improve your technique. Rack. Quarter squat. Knee jerk. Second dip. Elbow extension. Come up. Remember, no bouncing with the deadlift.

Movement standards:

- Single arm swing
  - Kettlebell reaches chest height
  - The bell is visible behind the legs on the back-swing
  - Hip hinge not squat movement
- Jerk
  - Full arm extension upon the second dip
  - Come into full hip and knee extension

THORAX WORKOUT
Injury proof yourself

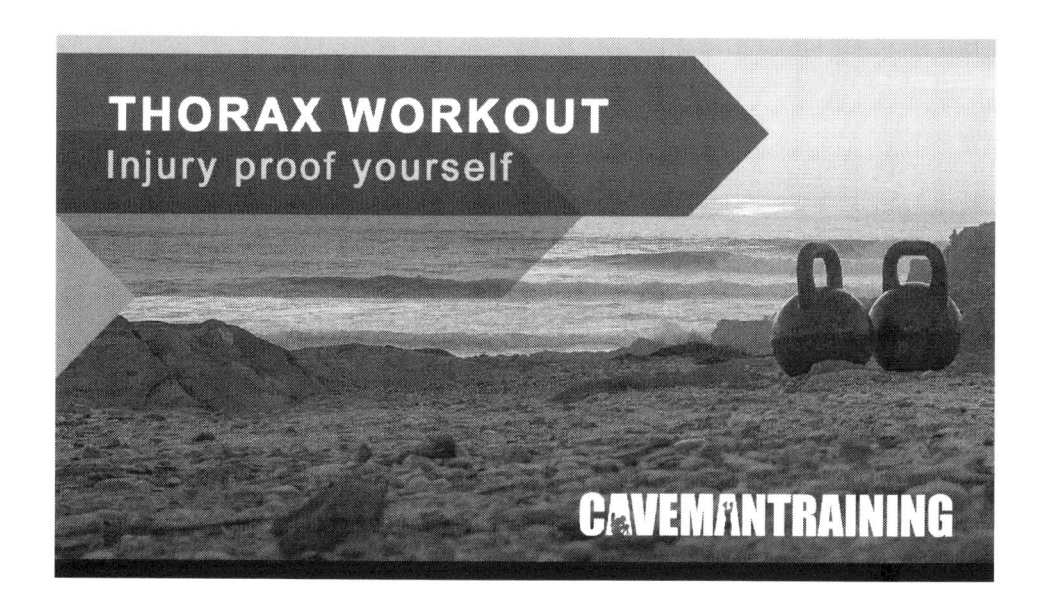

THORAX MOBILITY WORKOUT

- Level: Beginner
- Weight: Light
- Kettlebell(s):
- Type: Mobility and flexibility
- Duration: 45 to 60 minutes
- Other: Full-body but focus on the thoracic area, but not neglecting the hips, knees, and ankles

workout go.cavemantraining.com/kbwc-vid57

Injury proof yourself

I included this workout in *Kettlebell Workouts and Challenges 1.0* but I am including it in this book as well, just in case you don't have a copy of our first kettlebell workout book. The *Thorax Workout* is one of the best workouts for thoracic, scapula, and shoulder mobility. Due to the importance I believe good mobility has in your training, for injury proofing, and strength progression, I will devote a lot of time to explaining this workout.

Thoracic mobility, often overlooked. Lateral flexion, extension, and rotation of the thoracic spine, often overlooked.

Take time out to injury proof yourself. Invest in yourself.

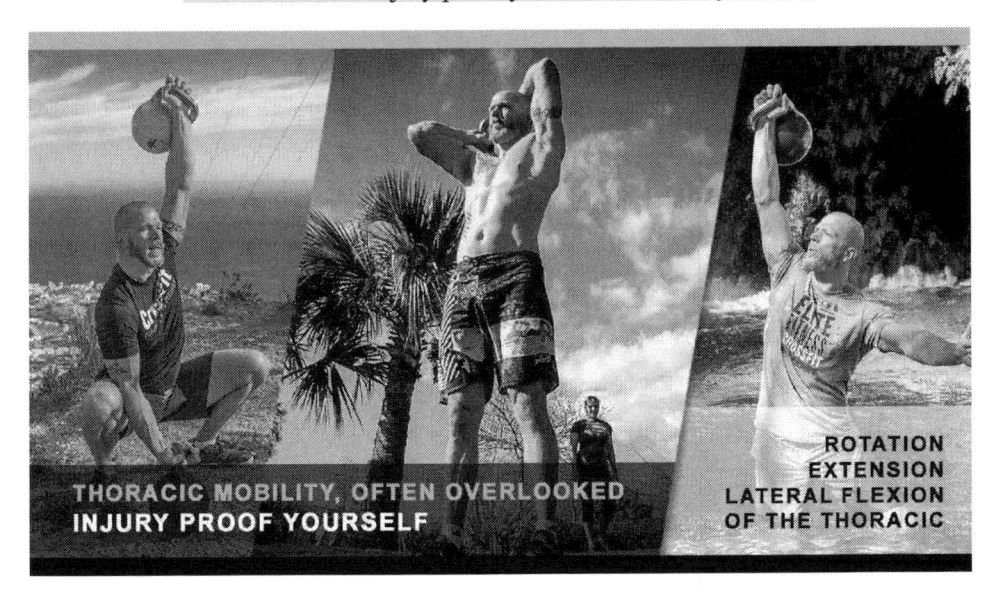

Benefits of good thoracic mobility:

- Better overhead squats
- Less chance of injury
- Lack of kyphosis – excessive curvature of the spine or hunchback
- Increased lung capacity
- Safer lumbar
- Improved posture

Bad thoracic mobility plays a huge role in a bad lower back, and shoulders.

This workout is about control, range of motion (ROM), and should be performed slowly. Form and technique first. Remember, it's about connecting with your muscles. Because this workout is all about connecting with those muscles you normally don't think about, or connect with, I will go into more details than normal. I will explain movement in simple terms, and then from a joint perspective.

This workout is one that anyone should be incorporating in their regular training – MMA fighters, BJJ fighters, kettlebell enthusiasts, and especially Crossfitters. Why did I mention especially Crossfitters? In kettlebell training, MMA, and BJJ, rotation is already included, whether you get mangled by your opponent in the twister, or throwing punches. But in CrossFit there is a distinct lack of rotation, lateral flexion, etc.

Most of you will know that bad thoracic mobility can lead to missed lifts, due to the chest being unable to open up because of stiffness in the thoracic spine, making the lift harder by pushing the weight forward. Furthermore, it makes it harder to get under the bar, minimizing power from the lower limbs (wider hand placement). Etcetera. I've designed this workout so the focus is purely on lateral thoracic flexion, rotation, extension, same for shoulders, and even included some hip work.

The thorax and back is an amazing and complex part of the body, with many muscles surrounding it. Following are illustrations to give you a better understanding of what's where. I'll cover the erector spinea, and transversospinales muscle group as a list below, just to show its complexity. From there on out they will be referred to as the erector spinae, and transversospinales muscle group.

The muscles of the back for spine extension:

Erector spinae muscle group
- Iliocastalis cervicus
- Iliocastalis thoracis
- Iliocastalis lumborum
- Longissimus capitus
- Longissimus cervicus
- Longissimus thoracis
- Spinalis cervicis
- Spinalis thoracis

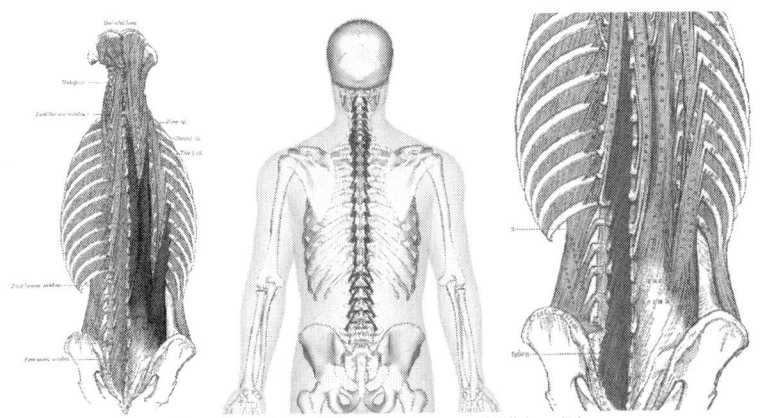

Erector spinea (R), rotatores, multifidus (L)

Transversospinales muscle group
- Rotatores breves
- Rotatores longi
- Multifidus
- Semispinalis capitus
- Interspinalis cervicis
- Interspinalis lumborum
- Intertransversarii anterioris cervicis
- Intertransversarii posterioris cervicis
- Intertransversarii medialis lumborum
- Intertransversarii laterales lumborum

Spine extension can be seen during back extensions on the GHD (Glute-ham Developer), or standing and creating extension in the spine by looking up to the sky. During this workout, when we create spinal extension we also pair it with scapula depression and adduction, which can be translated to pushing the chest out, shoulder blades down, and together.

Upper-body

Serratus anterior

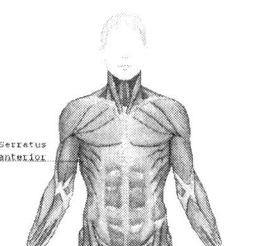

Pectoralis minor

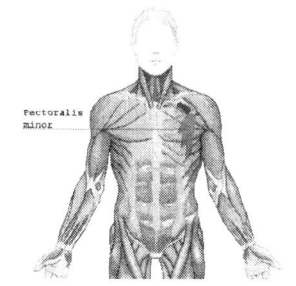

Pectoralis major

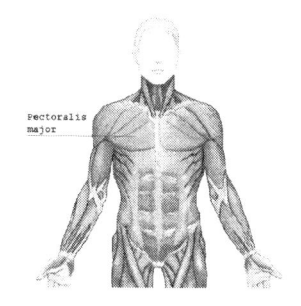

Anconeus

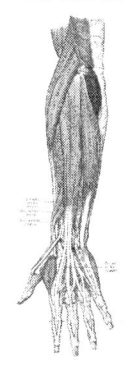

Triceps brachii

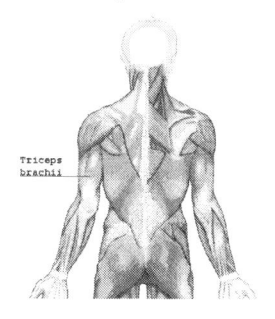

Biceps brachii

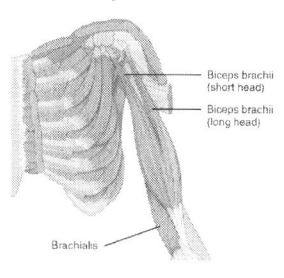

Brachialis

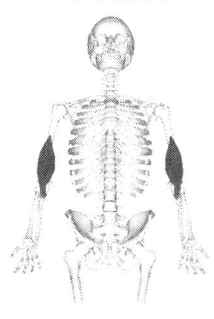

Brachioradialis

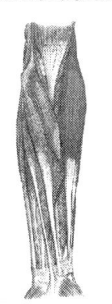

Rotatores

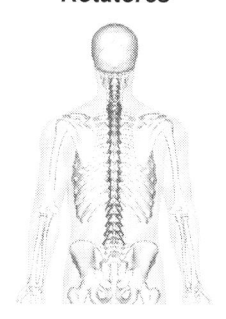

Coracobrachialis   *Teres major* 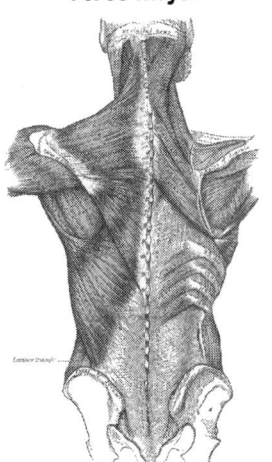   *Trapezius*

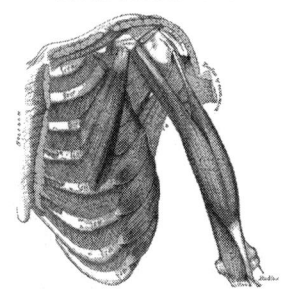

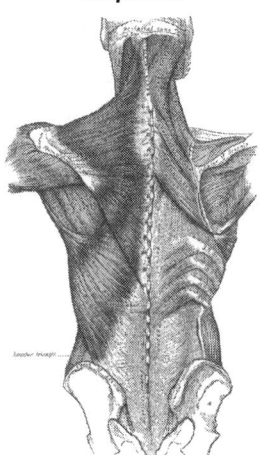

Upper, middle, and lower

Lower-body

Sartorius   *Gastrocnemius* 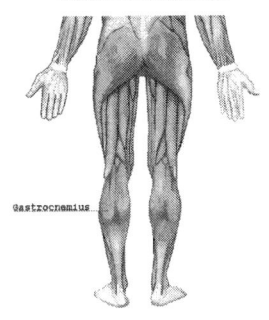   *Vastus lateralis*

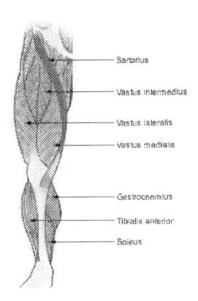

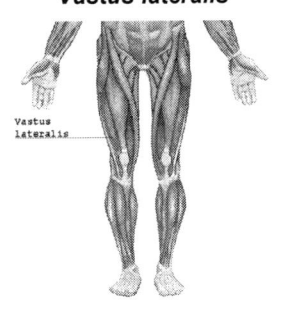

Biceps femoris

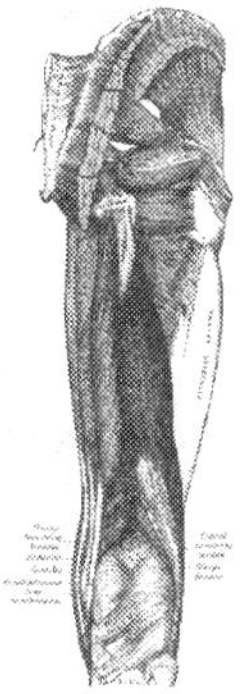

Semitendinosus

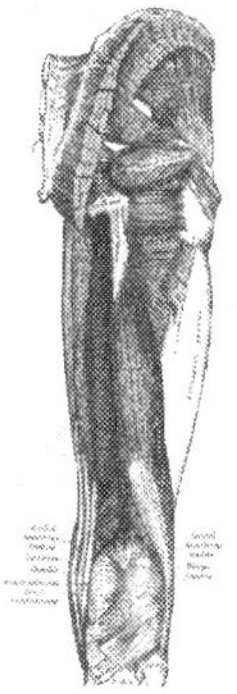

Semimembranosus

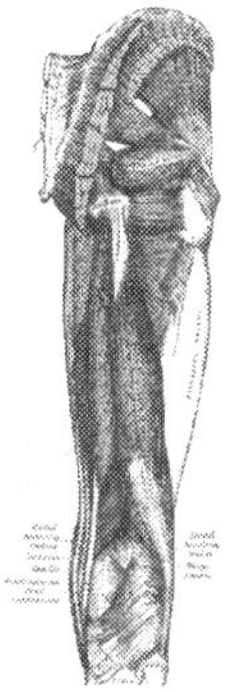

Vastus medialis, vastus intermedius

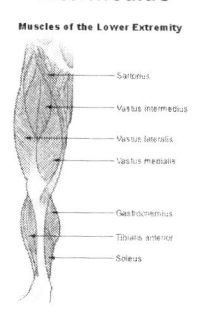

Rectus femoris

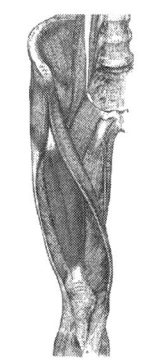

Popliteus

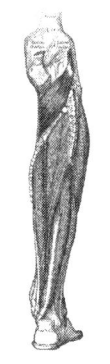

Gracilis, psoas major, illiacus, tensor fasciae latae, adductor longus, adductor brevis, pectineus

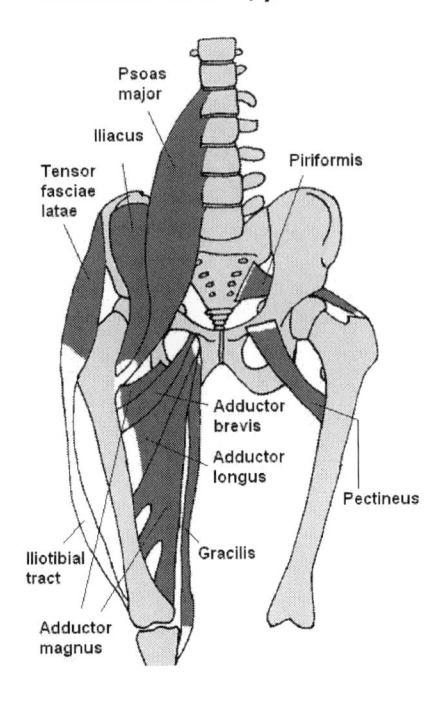

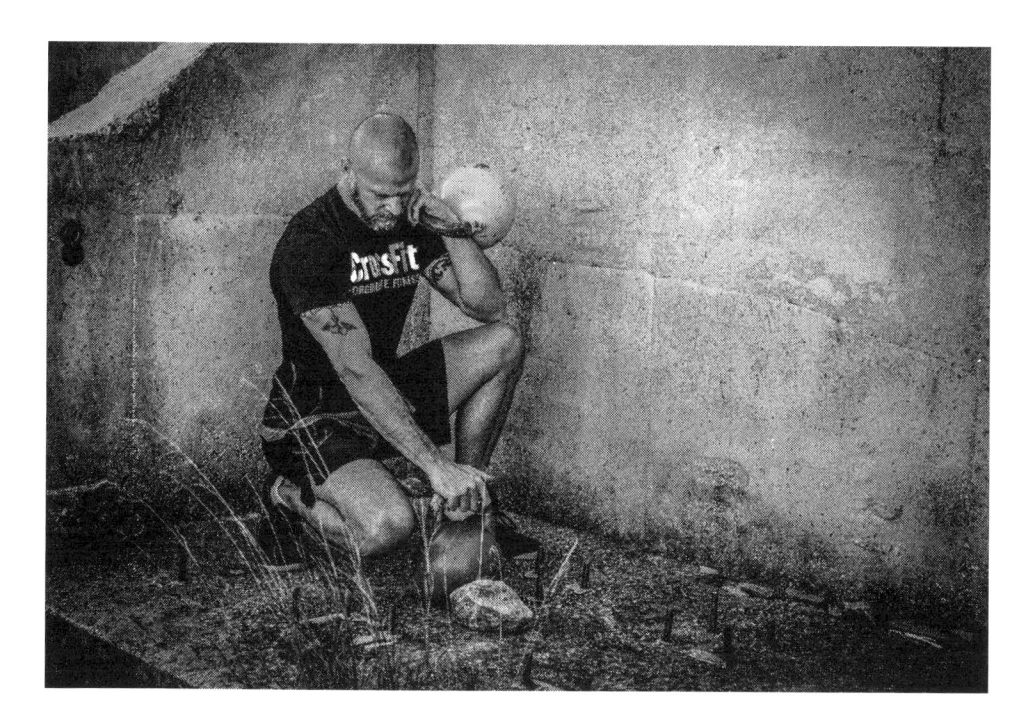

Everything done in the *Thorax Workout* is to be performed in a slow and controlled fashion, with maximum muscle engagement of the appropriate muscle groups. Don't think about weight, nor reps. This is all about creating max range of motion. It's about movement and connecting with your body.

The weight to use for this workout should be light, or about 35 to 40% of your 1RM press. Aim for 4 to 6 rounds. Each round takes about 5 minutes to complete, with some added rest in between. You should include this workout at least once a week, but 2 to 3 times would be optimal if you're not including any other similar work.

If you're just starting out, it's important to progress safely. What might not feel or look like a huge range, could very well be the right and appropriate range for your abilities at this moment in time. Rushing, pushing, and wanting to progress too quickly will result in injury.

The best way to get the most out of this workout is by watching the video first, then reading this document, and then performing the workout while watching the video. Don't expect to soak up all the information in one go. Don't get frustrated if you don't get the moves right away. It takes some time. Invest in it.

The *Thorax Workout* consists of the following exercises and reps:

→ 8 alternating halo reverse lunge and twist

→ 4 squat dead curl

→ 4 hang and lateral thoracic flexion L / R

→ 4 squat dead curl

→ 4 overhead and lateral thoracic flexion L / R

→ 4 squat dead curl

→ 4 kneeling bent press L / R

→ 4 squat dead curl

→ 4 pull-over scap opener

→ 4 squat dead curl

→ 4 spiral press L/ R

If at this stage you're not familiar with all the variations of kettlebell grips, download the kettlebell grip PDF from *Cavemantraining* at www.cavemantraining.com/shop/ebook/kettlebell-grip-ebook/

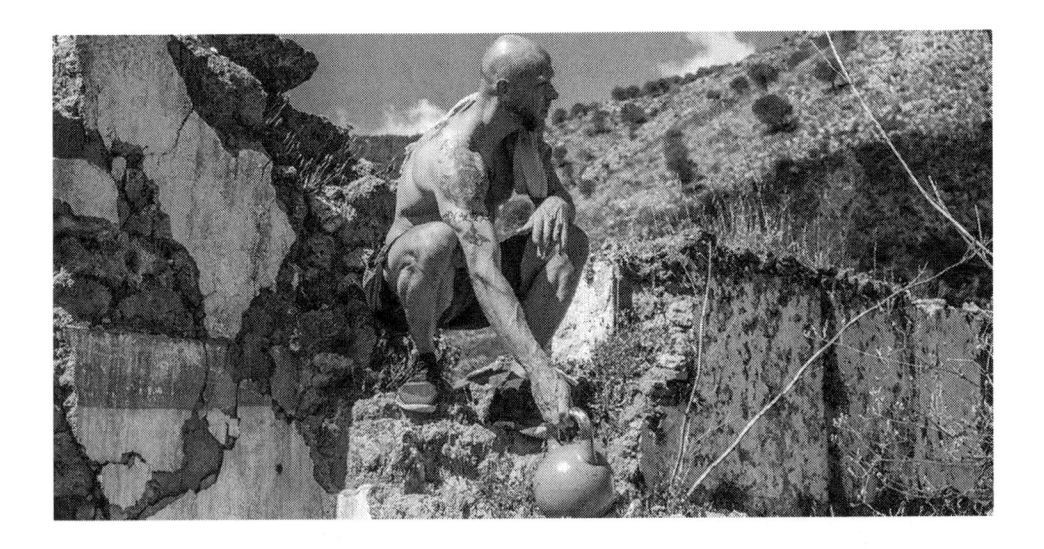

Squat dead curl

The curl is added to load and unload the bottom of the squat, not to tax the elbow flexors. This exercise is to work the ankles, knees, hips and thoracic area. To perform:

- ➔ Grab a kettlebell by the horns with the base facing down
- ➔ Bring the kettlebell into racking position
- ➔ Create **knee flexion** through contraction of the biceps femoris, semitendinosus, semimembranosus, gracilis, sartorius, gastrocnemius, and popliteus
- ➔ Create **hip abduction** through contraction of the gluteus medius, gluteus minimus, and sartorius
- ➔ Create **hip flexion** through contraction of the psoas major, illiacus, tensor fasciae latae, sartorius, and rectus femoris
- ➔ Create **ankle dorsiflexion** through contraction of the tibialis anterior, extensor digitorum longus, and extensor hallucis longus
- ➔ Come into a deep squat
- ➔ Stop about 3% before max squat depth
- ➔ Keep the glutes contracted
- ➔ Keep pressing the heels into the ground
- ➔ Connect the elbows with the inside of the thighs near the knee
- ➔ Push the elbows out to open up the hips
- ➔ Push the chest out (thoracic extension)
- ➔ Create **scapula depression** through contraction of the lower trapezius, serratus anterior, and pectoralis minor (shoulder blades down)
- ➔ Create **scapula adduction** through contraction of the trapezius, and rhomboids (shoulder blades towards each other)
- ➔ Slowly lower the kettlebell with an eccentric curl
- ➔ Maintain some elbow flexion, slowly lower by creating **elbow extension** through contraction of the triceps brachii, and anconeus
- ➔ The weight is dead on the ground
- ➔ Curl the kettlebell to the chest

- → Create **elbow flexion** through contraction of the biceps brachii, brachialis, and brachioradialis
- → Transition from horn to open palm grip
- → Position the forearms and elbows under the bell if you want to avoid tension on the elbow flexors
- → Come back up into neutral standing position
- → Create **knee extension** through contraction of the rectus femoris, vastus lateralis, vastus medialis, and vastus intermedius
- → Create **hip adduction** through contraction of the adductor longus, adductor brevis, pectineus, and gracilis
- → Create **hip extension** thought contraction of the gluteus maximus, biceps femoris (long head), semitendinosus, semimembranosus, and adductor magnus
- → Create **ankle plantarflexion** through contraction of the gastrocnemius, soleus, tibialis posterior, flexor digitorum longus, flexor hallucis longus, and plantaris
- → Press the heels into the ground
- → Contract the glutes
- → Come into full hip and knee extension
- → Repeat

Related videos:

▶ http://bit.ly/kb-wk-vid17

▶ Squat dead curl http://bit.ly/kb-wk-vid18

▶ Alternating Sots press http://bit.ly/kb-wk-vid19
http://bit.ly/kb-wk-vid20 http://bit.ly/kb-wk-vid21

▶ Squat, dead curl, and press http://bit.ly/kb-wk-vid22

Halo reverse lunge and twist

This exercise is great because there is so much involved, so much benefit, including the use of the gluteus minimus and medius. To perform:

- Hold a kettlebell with an upside down horn grip
- Perform a halo
- Pack the chest to create a firm base to move from
- Squeeze the glutes and lock out the knees
- Bring the kettlebell next to one ear
- Bring the kettlebell behind the head
- Lats and triceps should be fully engaged when the kettlebell is behind the head
- Bring the kettlebell next to the other ear
- Your arms should be making a boxed shape around the head
- Bring the kettlebell in-front of the chest
- Create a ribbon like pattern
- Keep the movement flowing without pausing
- Move the kettlebell towards the obliques while still going in the same direction
- Lunge back with the leg away from the bell
- The leg remaining planted is the leg now close to the kettlebell
- Bring the kettlebell all the way next to the hip
- Create thoracic rotation to get the bell next to the hip
- Do not use the arms to get the bell where it needs to end up
- Look at the bell to create a more natural rotation
- Bring the kettlebell back in the same pattern you used to get it there
- Come back out of the reverse lunge
- Halo around the other side
- Repeat the ribbon pattern
- Lunge back on the other side
- Repeat

Halo reverse lunge and twist:

http://bit.ly/kb-wk-vid23

http://bit.ly/kb-wk-vid24

Hang, scapula depression and lateral thoracic flexion

This exercise focuses on the thoracic and scapula. To perform:

- ➔ Let one kettlebell hang to the side
- ➔ Align the shoulders
- ➔ Lift the hanging kettlebell through scapula depression and lateral flexion on the opposite side
- ➔ Create **scapula depression** through contraction of lower trapezius, serratus anterior, and pectoralis minor
- ➔ Pull the shoulder down and to the side
- ➔ Create **lateral thoracic flexion** through contraction of quadratus limborum, erector spinae, obliques, and latissimus dorsi
- ➔ The head and neck can move along to the side
- ➔ Range will be minimal
- ➔ Release contraction
- ➔ Align the shoulders by slight contraction on the hanging side
- ➔ Repeat
- ➔ There is no shoulder raise through upper trapezius contraction

Hang, scapula depression and lateral thoracic flexion:
http://bit.ly/kb-wk-vid25

Overhead, scapula depression and lateral thoracic flexion

To perform:

- ➔ Bring a kettlebell overhead
- ➔ Create **shoulder flexion** through contraction of the anterior deltoid, pectoralis major, biceps brachii, coracobrachialis, serratus anterior
- ➔ Create **elbow extension** through contraction of the triceps brachii, and anconeus
- ➔ The shoulder flexion and elbow extension will remain isometric from here on

- → Align the shoulders
- → Your goal is to raise the overhead kettlebell through lateral flexion at the opposite side
- → Create **scapula depression** through contraction of lower trapezius, serratus anterior, and pectoralis minor
- → Pull the shoulder down and to the side
- → Create **lateral thoracic flexion** through contraction of quadratus limborum, erector spinae, obliques, and latissimus dorsi
- → The head and neck can move along to the side
- → Range will be minimal
- → Release contraction
- → Align the shoulders by slight contraction on the overhead side
- → There is no shoulder raise through upper trapezius contraction

Kneeling bent press

To perform:

- → Rack a kettlebell
- → There should be minimal pressing involved throughout this movement
- → Pressing should only happen at the end if there is any required at all
- → Reverse lunge and kneel with opposing side of the racked kettlebell
- → Remain in kneeling position throughout the movements
- → Thoracic rotation and hip hinging happens at the same time
- → Create **thoracic rotation** through contraction of internal and external obliques, rotatores breves and longi, and multifidus
- → Flex the hip extensors, slowly release while creating hip flexion
- → Create **hip flexion** through contraction of psoas major, iliacus, tensor fasciae latae, sartorius, recturs femoris
- → Pull the elbow down with the lat throughout the rotation

- ➔ Create **shoulder adduction** through contraction of latissimus dorsi, pectoralis major, teres major, coracobrachialis
- ➔ Keep the forearm vertical through extension and flexion of the elbow
- ➔ Look at the bell
- ➔ The non working hand can touch the ground
- ➔ Continue and come under the kettlebell
- ➔ Come up once full elbow extension is reached
- ➔ Press the knee into the ground
- ➔ Contract the obliques on opposite side
- ➔ Focus on the shoulder rotation as you come up
- ➔ Come into full lockout position
- ➔ Lower and rack the kettlebell
- ➔ Repeat

Kneeling bent press:
http://bit.ly/kb-wk-vid26

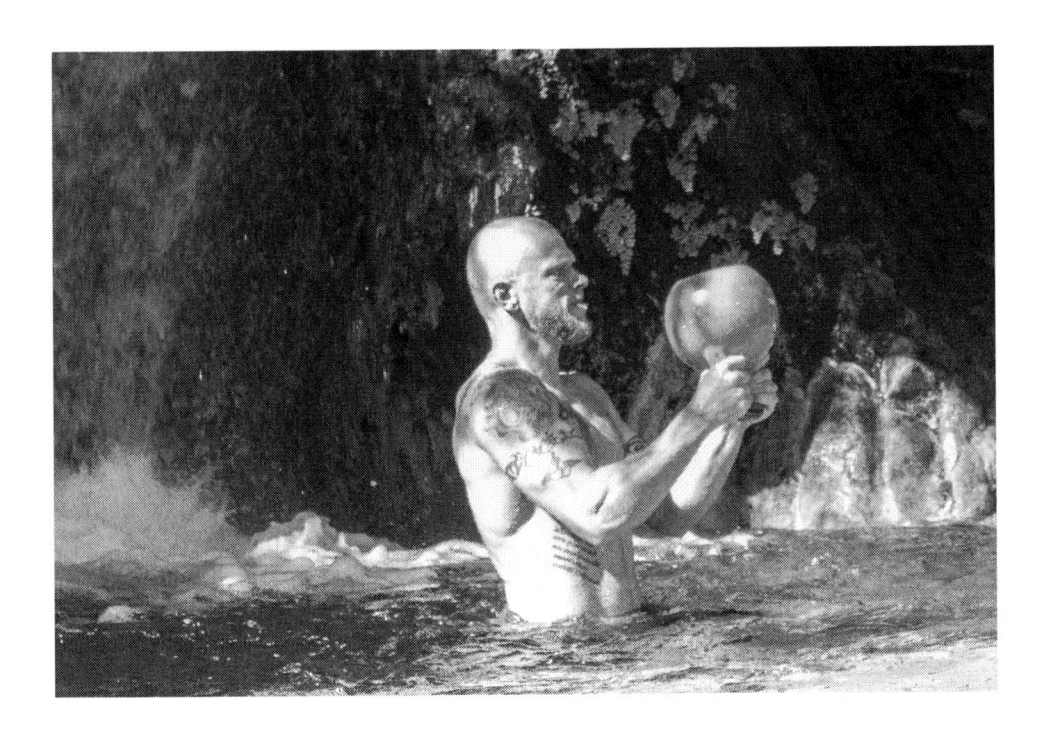

Pull-over and scap opener

To perform:

- → Hold a kettlebell with an upside down horn grip
- → Elbows close to the ribs
- → Don't let the elbows flare out during the movement
- → Bring the kettlebell over and behind the head
- → Create **shoulder flexion** through contraction of the anterior deltoid, pectoralis major, biceps brachii, coracobrachialis, serratus anterior
- → Create **scapula depression** through contraction of the lower trapezius, serratus anterior, and pectoralis minor (shoulder blades down)
- → Let the bell hang and feel the pull
- → Don't let the kettlebell touch on the other side
- → Push the chest out through thoracic extension
- → Create spinal extension
- → Pull the lats down to protect the shoulders

- → Feel the stretch in the triceps
- → Slowly open up and let the elbows come out
- → Create **scapula adduction** through contraction of the trapezius, and rhomboids (shoulder blades towards each other)
- → The bell can now touch
- → Bring the elbows back in
- → Tighten the grip on the horns
- → Engage the triceps and lats to bring the kettlebell up and over
- → Bring the kettlebell back to starting position
- → Repeat

Related videos:

Kettlebell pull-over into scap opener http://bit.ly/kb-wk-vid27

Standing pull-over http://bit.ly/kb-wk-vid28

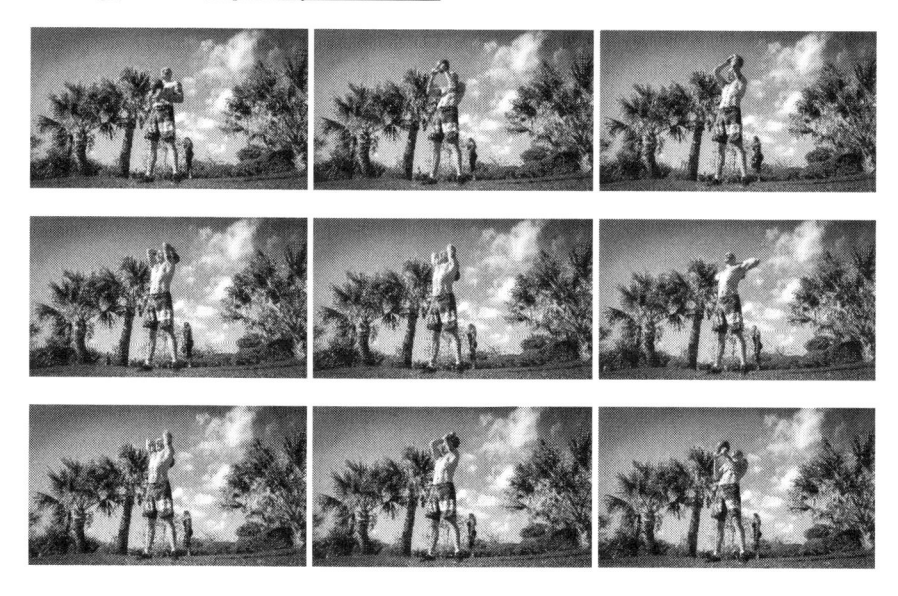

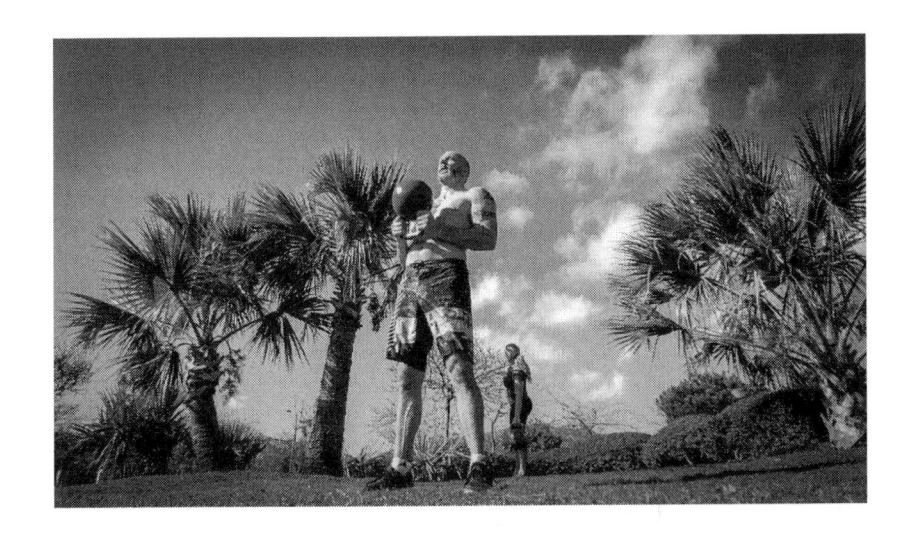

Spiral press

To perform:

→ Rack a kettlebell
→ Hold the opposite arm out (shoulder abduction)
→ Rotate into opposite side of the bell
→ Create **thoracic rotation** through contraction of internal and external obliques, rotatores breves and longi, and multifidus
→ Rotation should start at the top of the thoracic and follow through
→ Create max safe range
→ Create controlled rotation in the opposite direction
→ At the same time start to press
→ Follow through with the press in a spiral motion
→ Move into max safe range
→ Look at the kettlebell
→ Bring the kettlebell back into racking through the same path
→ Repeat
→ Knees should not hurt

Spiral press:
http://bit.ly/kb-wk-vid29
http://bit.ly/kb-wk-vid30

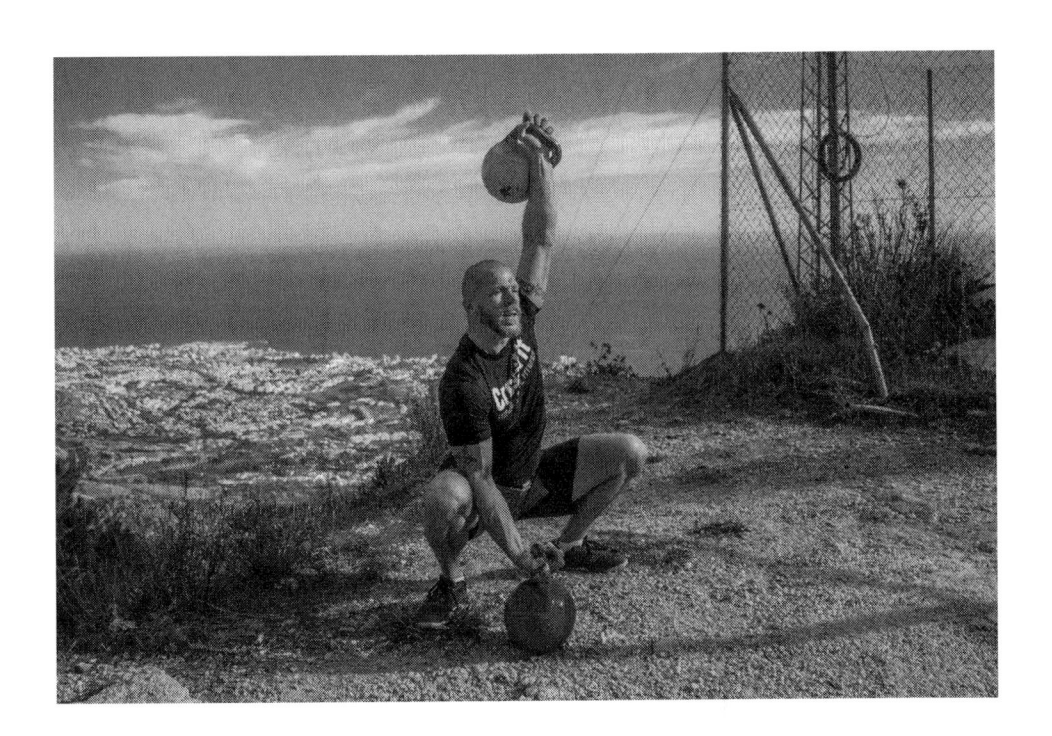

Other mobility related videos:

▶ Best mobility exercise routine http://bit.ly/kb-wk-vid31
▶ Kettlebell and movement flow for mobility http://bit.ly/kb-wk-vid32
▶ Caveman ROM flow: 20 minutes of mobility http://bit.ly/kb-wk-vid33
▶ Shoulder mobility and stability: kettlebell windmill http://bit.ly/kb-wk-vid34
▶ 32 minutes of mobility and body maintenance http://bit.ly/kb-wk-vid35
▶ Overhead shoulder mobility and strength training http://bit.ly/kb-wk-vid36
▶ Shoulder mobility: tea cup exercise http://bit.ly/kb-wk-vid37
▶ Thoracic and shoulder mobility http://bit.ly/kb-wk-vid38
▶ OH lunge and twist for thoracic mobility http://bit.ly/kb-wk-vid39
▶ Shoulder warm up + mobility: arms in and out http://bit.ly/kb-wk-vid40

For questions, join our discussion group and post
www.facebook.com/groups/unconventional.training/

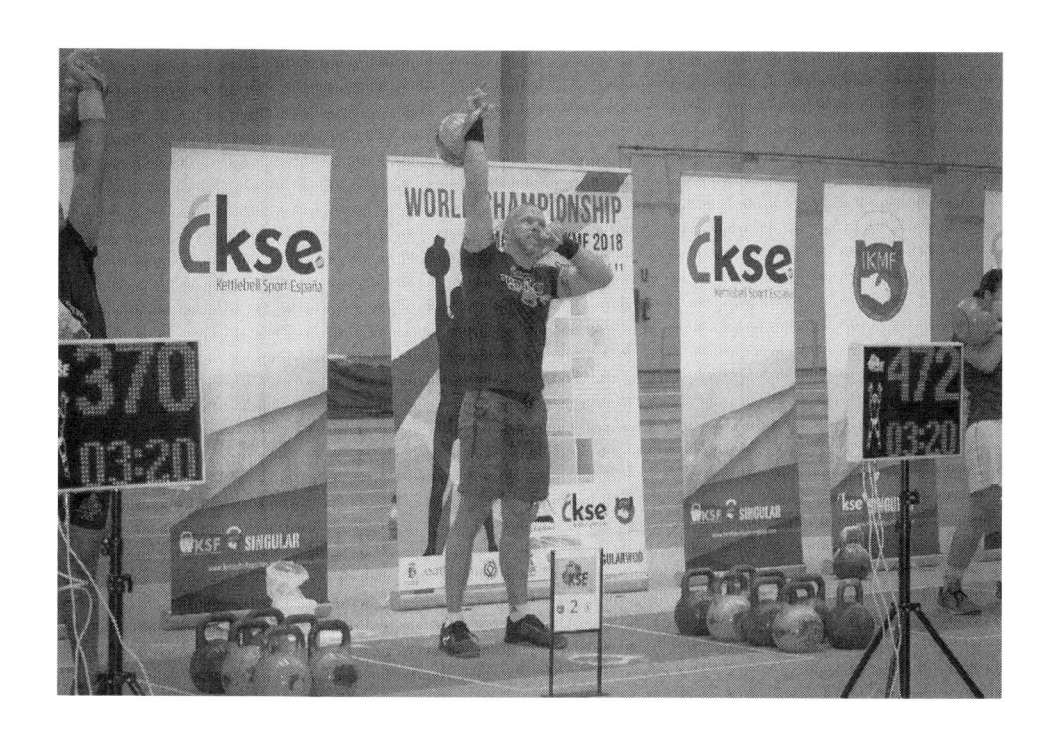

Easter egg
20% discount on our online course, use coupon code: **QCQUV1722X**
www.cavemantraining.com/shop/training-course/kettlebell-fundamentals-trainer-l3-0/

T-shirt kettlebell skull
www.cavemantraining.com/shop/t-shirts/short-sleeve-soft-t-shirt-kettlebell-skull-girya/

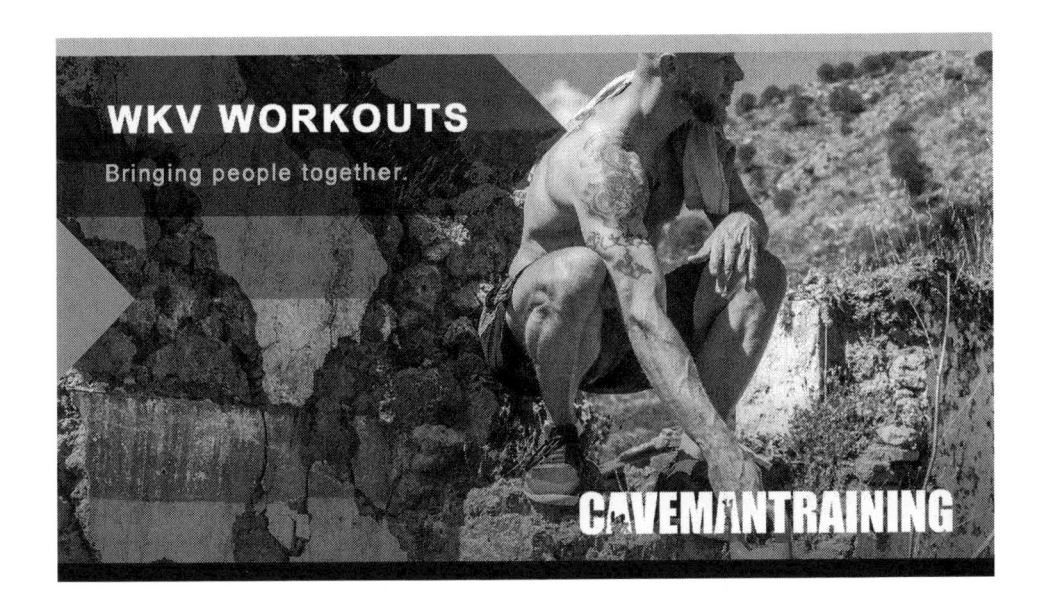

WORLD KETTLEBELL VIDEO WORKOUTS

Level: Beginner to advanced

Weight: Light to heavy

Kettlebell(s): 🔔 to 🔔🔔

Type: Mix

Duration: Mix

Other: Full-body

Brining people together from across the world.

These are the world kettlebell video workouts, a Cavemantraining project to spread the word of kettlebells and show that our workouts can be done by anyone and every body. Each workout has beginner, intermediate, and advanced.

The beginner workout progresses to intermediated, and intermediate to advanced. More details on the project can be found here go.cavemantraining.com/kbwc-link17

WKV1

This full body kettlebell workout is for beginners, intermediate, and advanced. The workout can be done with one kettlebell and two hands, one kettlebell and one hand, or two kettlebells.

What is a full body workout?

You can create a full body workout by going through the muscle groups one by one and work them in isolation, or you can work with compound movements that involve multiple muscle groups with one exercise. Both have their own benefits. This workout focusses on the following compound exercises:

- Kettlebell swing
- Kettlebell front squat
- Kettlebell overhead press
- Kettlebell overhead reverse lunge

Kettlebell swing muscles used

To give you an idea of what a compound exercise involves in regards to muscles, I'm going to use the kettlebell swing as an example.

Forearm:

- Flexor digitorum superficialis
- Flexor digitorum profundus
- Flexor digit minimi brevis
- Lumbricals

Back:

- Rhomboideus minor
- Rhomboideus major
- Lower trapezius
- Levator scapulae
- Latissimus dorsi
- Iliocostalis
- Longissimus
- Spinalis

Upper legs:

- Bicep femoris (long head)
- Semitendinosus
- Semimembranosus
- Adductor magnus
- Gracilis
- Sartorius
- Gluteus maximus

Lower legs:

- Gastrocnemius
- Soleus
- Popliteus

This is keeping it simple, there are many more muscles used.

Beginner

workout go.cavemantraining.com/kbwc-vid58

Dead start and holding on to the kettlebell with two hands throughout the workout.

→ 5 x double arm swings

→ 5 x front squat

→ 5 x Press

→ 3 / 3 x Reverse lunge and twist

(or just hold the kettlebell without twist)

2 rounds followed by 1-minute of rest and repeat 6 times, or 1 round followed by 30 seconds rest and repeat 12 times.

Detailed instructions here go.cavemantraining.com/kbwc-vid59

Intermediate

▶ workout go.cavemantraining.com/kbwc-vid60

Dead start

- ➔ 5 x swing
- ➔ 5 x Squat
- ➔ 5 x Press
- ➔ 5 x Overhead reverse lunge
- ➔ (alternative racked reverse lunge)

Switch or dead start and do the other side, both sides equal one round

2 rounds followed by 30 seconds of rest and repeat 12 times

Detailed instructions here go.cavemantraining.com/kbwc-vid61

Advanced

▶ workout go.cavemantraining.com/kbwc-vid62

Double bell

Dead start

- ➔ 5 x swings
- ➔ 5 x squat
- ➔ 5 x press
- ➔ 3 / 3 x overhead reverse lunge

Complete 12 rounds

Detailed instructions here go.cavemantraining.com/kbwc-vid63

WKV2

Yes, you might have recognized it from a workout earlier on, this is the Gorilla Blackback workout, but here you can progress to the advanced workout.

The second world kettlebell video workout is the Gorilla Blackback workout and has been designed as three progressional level, beginners, intermediate, and advanced. This workout is V2 of the famous and awesome Silverback Workout, if you've been following *Cavemantraining* for a while, you'll know this from 2016 and the remake in 2018.

Beginner

▶ workout go.cavemantraining.com/kbwc-vid64

1 kettlebell

- ➔ 4/4 x Rows (wide staggered stance elbow on knee)
- ➔ 4/4 x Assisted Hang Cleans (double hand switch)
- ➔ 4 x Double-arm Curls
- ➔ 4 x Alternating Deadlift

Each round is followed by 30 seconds of rest

Complete 8 to 10 rounds

Detailed instructions here go.cavemantraining.com/kbwc-vid66

Intermediate

▶ workout go.cavemantraining.com/kbwc-vid65

1 kettlebell

- ➔ 4 x Alternating Gorilla Rows
- ➔ 4 x Alternating Hang Cleans
- ➔ 4/4 x Gorilla Curls (wide staggered stance elbow on knee)
- ➔ 4 x Burpee Deadlift

Every two rounds 30 to 60 seconds rest

Complete 10 to 12 rounds

Detailed instructions here go.cavemantraining.com/kbwc-vid67

Advanced

workout go.cavemantraining.com/kbwc-vid68

2 kettlebells

- → 4 x Gorilla Rows
- → 4 x Gorilla Cleans
- → 4 x Gorilla Curls
- → 4 x Renegade Rows Deadlift

20 minutes AMRAP

Detailed instructions here go.cavemantraining.com/kbwc-vid69

WKV3

This is the third and final WKV for this book, WKV4 is already out and I'm working on WKV5, so do make sure you come and join all the social channels to find out when the details for that are released, and join in.

Beginner

workout go.cavemantraining.com/kbwc-vid70

Transition: Deadlift to a neutral stance
→ 6 x hang lift (double-arm squat style)
Transition: Double-arm dead clean
→ 3 x presses L
Transition: Double hand switch and clean
→ 3 x presses R
Transition: Double-arm backswing drop to dead in position for dead swing start
→ 4 x swing double-arm
Transition: Open hand horn clean
→ 4 x squat thumb through horn grip

2 rounds and 1-minute rest.

Repeat 4 times.

Detailed instructions here go.cavemantraining.com/kbwc-vid71

Intermediate

workout go.cavemantraining.com/kbwc-vid72

This is an intermediate kettlebell workout using 1 kettlebell.

- → 3 x squat dead lift L
- → 3 x squat dead lift R

  Transition: Dead clean the other kettlebell

- → 3 x strict presses L

  Transition: Swing switch

- → 3 x strict presses R

  Transition: Single arm drop to dead in position for dead swing

- → 4 x dead swing double-arm

  Transition: Open hand horn grip clean

- → 4 x squat open hand horn grip

  Transition: Drop to dead

Detailed instructions here go.cavemantraining.com/kbwc-vid73

Advanced

workout go.cavemantraining.com/kbwc-vid74

This is an advanced kettlebell workout with 2 kettlebells.

Transition: Dead clean and press one kettlebell

- → 3 x Overhead deadlift L

  Transition: Drop 1kb to dead and dead clean to press the other

- → 3 x Overhead deadlift R

  Transition: 1 kb hang clean to bring both in racking

➔ 6 x alternating presses

Transition: Drop both to dead in position for the dead swing clean

➔ 4 x dead swing clean and squat

Transition: Drop to dead

8 minutes AMRAP

3 minutes rest

Repeat

Scoring is rounds plus reps for unfinished rounds. If you do 7 rounds and 5 reps, that would be 7.5, if you do 6 rounds plus 11 reps in your second task, it's 6.11, you add the two up which comes to 13.16.

Detailed instructions here go.cavemantraining.com/kbwc-vid75

Kettlebell Challenges

A challenge is great to test your abilities. It also gives you something to work towards, i.e. you might complete a challenge in 35 minutes, next time strive to shave one minute off; you might do 7 rounds, next time strive to do 8. Give these challenges a go and post on our *Facebook* when completed, no matter your time, your weight, number of reps, or number of rounds. Just post.

300 Clean and Jerk Challenge

The 300 clean and jerk challenge is a mental game. This is one you will need to work up to over time. You can start with aiming for 30 unbroken, then 50, 60, and so on. You can switch when you want, you can rest when you want, but you can't put the weight down. So, you need to learn how to rack well.

▶ go.cavemantraining.com/kbwc-vid76

This book has covered the swing clean which is what happens every-time before a jerk, but I will cover a bit more about the jerk.

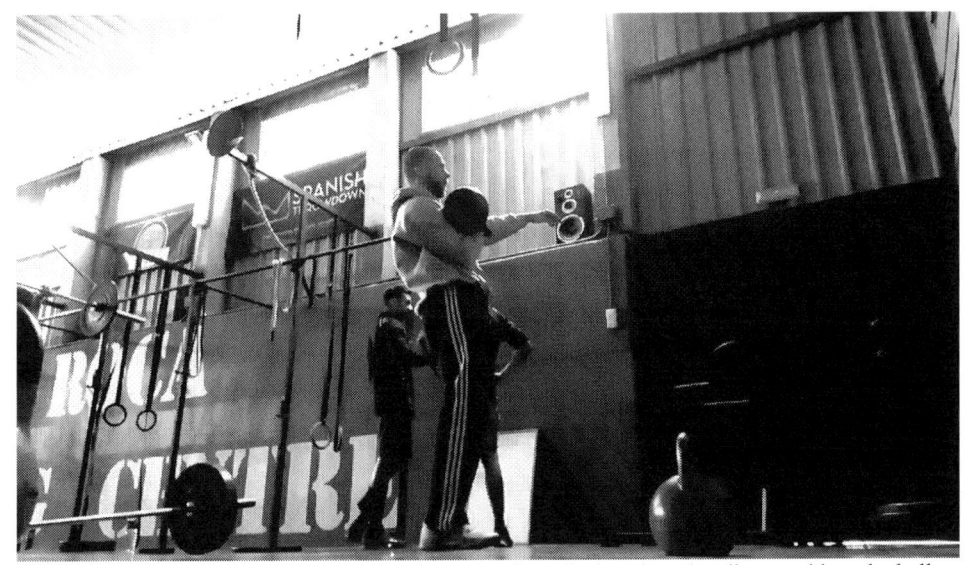

Start position in a good rack to transfer the power from the legs into the elbow and into the bell.

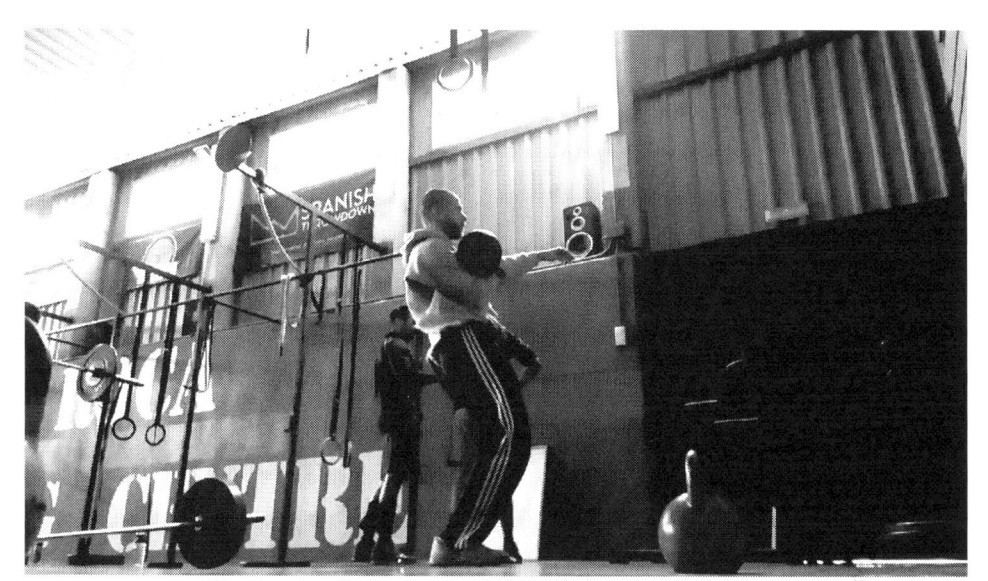

Keeping the elbow connected while the knees come forward.

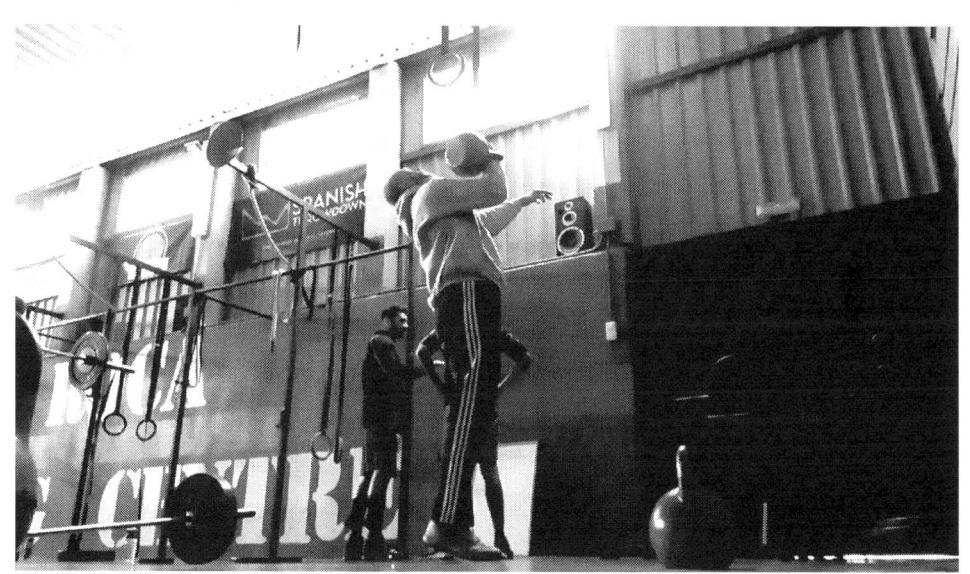

Pulling the knees back and launching the weight with the power from the legs.

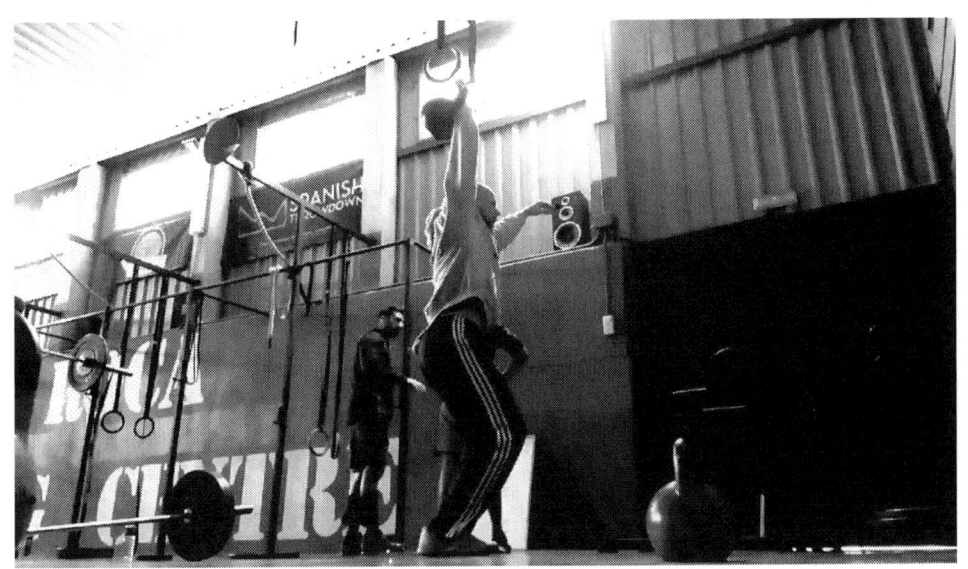

Coming under the weight and fully extending the arm before coming up.

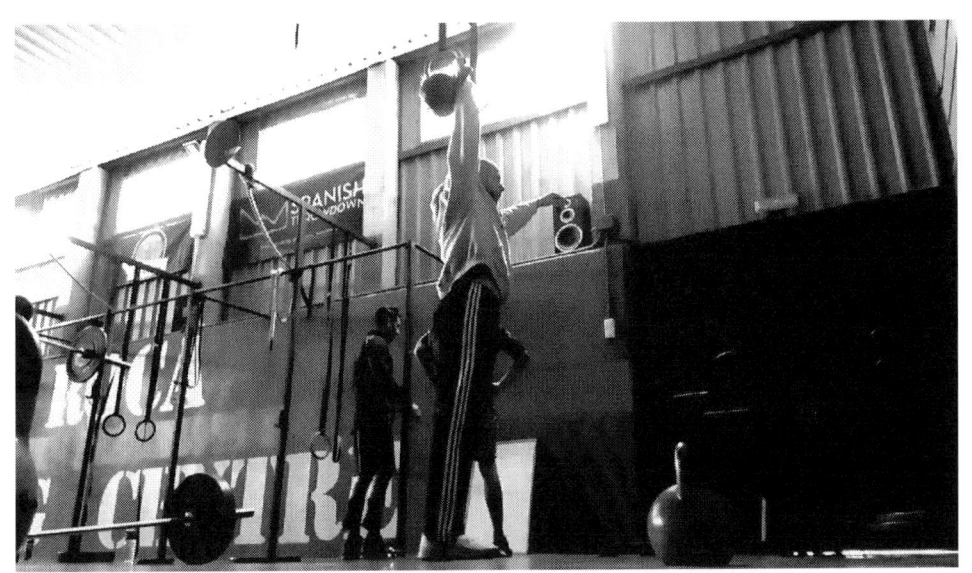

Standing up and keep the weight overhead for a split second. Then:

- Drop into rack
- Drop into backswing
- Swing back up
- Clean
- Rack
- Repeat

11-Day Sots Press Challenge by Cavemantraining

The Sots press challenges is very advanced and you need to have good mobility and strength before thinking about attempting this challenge. Stop the challenge if anything hurts or even feels like it's going to hurt. It's 11 days long.

▶ go.cavemantraining.com/kbwc-vid77

11 days to spend on your mobility and strength. The sequence is double kettlebell Sots press with the first alternating rep being straight up and the second alternating rep with thoracic rotation.

Pick a lightweight to start with. Use just bodyweight if you're still working on your overhead flexibility. Double the reps by 4 if you're working with just bodyweight. From bodyweight you should progress to the Sots press with rotation.

CONTROL. FOCUS. RANGE.

Better posture. Better overhead squat.

Day 1

Perform 1 round of the sequence.

Post and hashtag #cavemantraining #sotspresschallenge

Day 2

Perform 2 rounds of the sequence.

Day 3

Perform 3 rounds of the sequence.

Day 4

Perform 4 rounds of the sequence.

Day 5

Perform 5 rounds of the sequence.

Day 6

Perform 6 rounds of the sequence.

Day 7

Perform 7 rounds of the sequence.

Day 8

Perform 8 rounds of the sequence.

Day 9

Perform 9 rounds of the sequence.

Day 10

Perform 10 rounds of the sequence.

Day 11

Perform 11 rounds of the sequence.

If you've been doing bodyweight reps up till now then today is the day you'll try one weighted Sots press on both sides with rotation. If you're able to do it then you've achieved your goal and completed the challenge. Well done.

Film, post and hashtag #cavemantraining #sotspresschallenge.

You can break the set up, come out of position and rest. Safety first. Remember, a safe weight is the right weight.

For clarity, one round of the sequence is Sots press on one side and the other, Sots press with thoracic rotation on one side and the other. The sequence is 4 reps in total. On day one you would have done 4 reps in total, which is 1 round of the sequence. On day two you would have done 8 reps in total, which is 2 rounds of the sequence, and so on.

Increase the weight if you perform the challenge again.

To test if you can perform the Sots you can try squatting overhead in-front of a wall which will also prep you for the Sots press go.cavemantraining.com/kbwc-vid78

Sots Press Tutorial

The Sots press is an amazing exercise and I like the alternating Sots press in particular because it has several exercises into one, squat, curl, and press. All of these things require progression, great precision and flawless technique. Proper hand insertion. Rotating at the right time. Creating tension in the right areas and maintain that. And so on.

If you're performing the Sots press with one kettlebell you can choose to rotate at the thoracic spine, rotation will make the press easier and there is nothing wrong with using this for progression to the neutrally aligned press, plus your objective might be to work the thoracic. Thoracic rotation is an area most athletes neglect. In this tutorial I'll cover both the version with rotation and without.

Before you attempt this exercise you will need to be able to squat deep properly, being able to keep the torso upright and heels on the ground.

This kettlebell exercise is great for so many things, but here are some:

- Shoulder stability
- Range of motion
- Working on creating and maintaining tension throughout the body
- Squat depth
- Stability

"One of the most incredible kettlebell exercises you can do for strength, flexibility, and mobility in one. Every CrossFit box should incorporate this exercise in their mobility sessions." ~ Taco Fleur

Links:
- Facebook post www.facebook.com/Cavemantraining.Magazine/videos/1108791549255719/
- Article www.cavemantraining.com/caveman-kettlebells/incredible-sots-press/
- Video go.cavemantraining.com/kbwc-vid79
- Challenge www.cavemantraining.com/challenge/11-day-sots-press-challenge/

Learn all the kettlebell fundamentals from one book, lay a proper foundation to become a kettlebell PRO whether enthusiast or trainer. http://www.cavemantraining.com/shop/ebook/kettlebell-training-fundamentals-ebook/

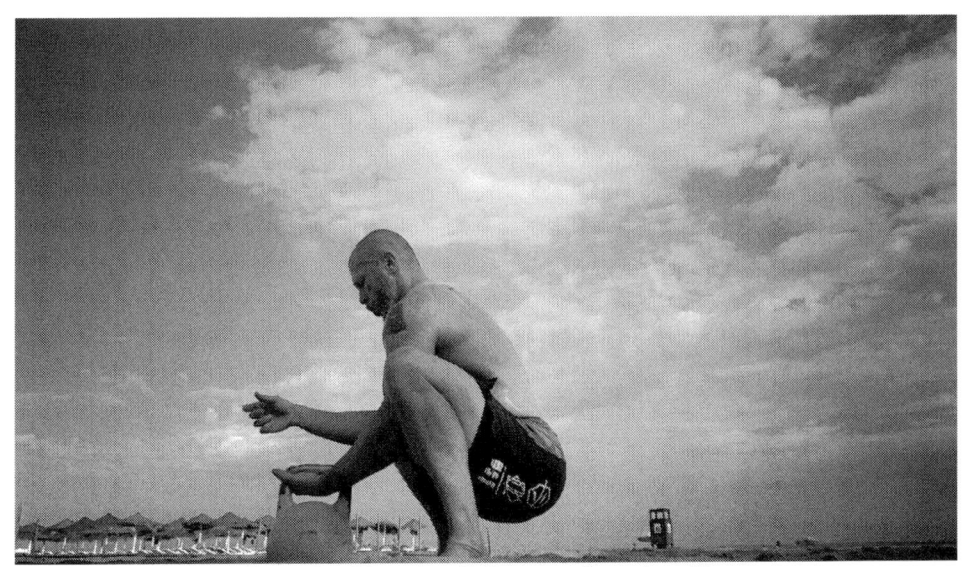

Proper hand insertion. Refer to our free grip guide.

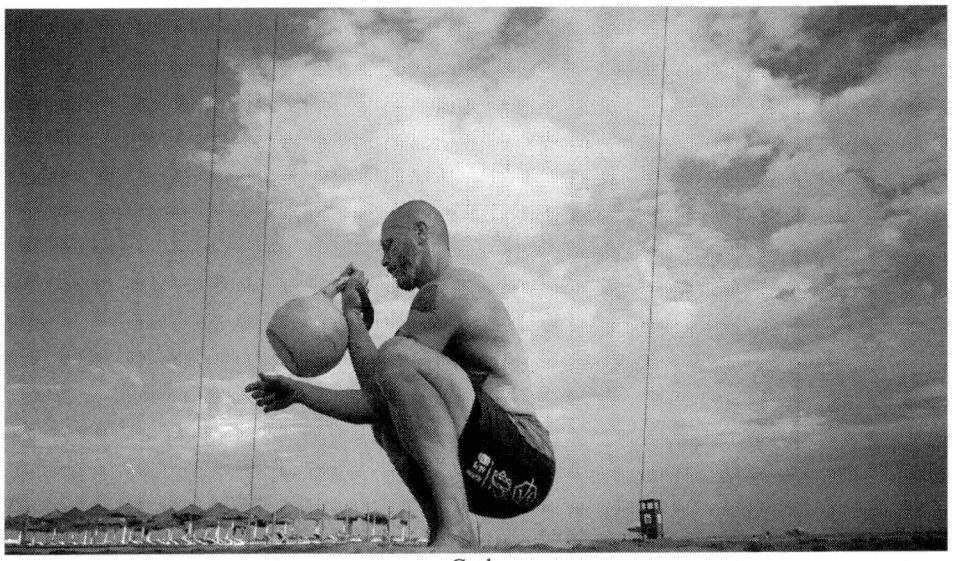

Curl.

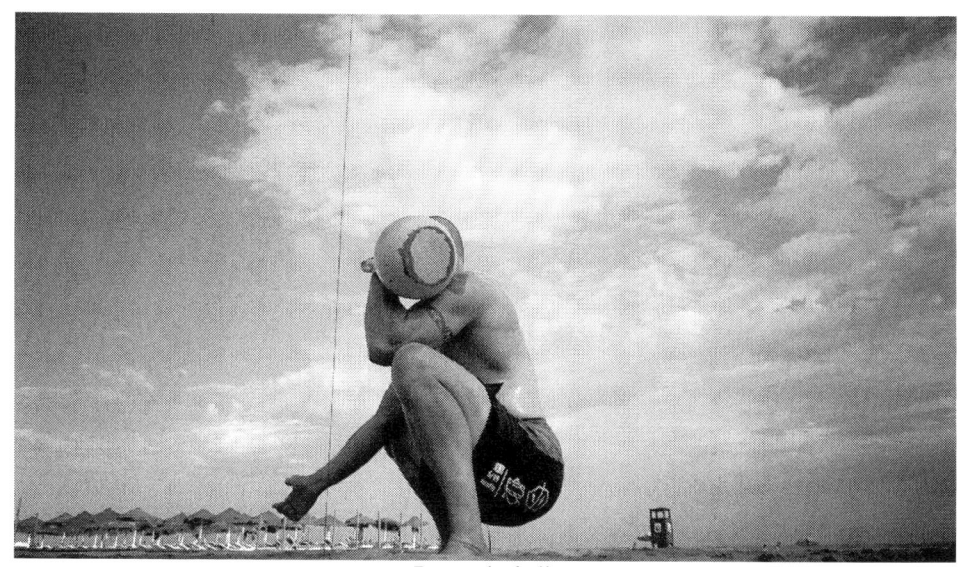

Rotate the bell.

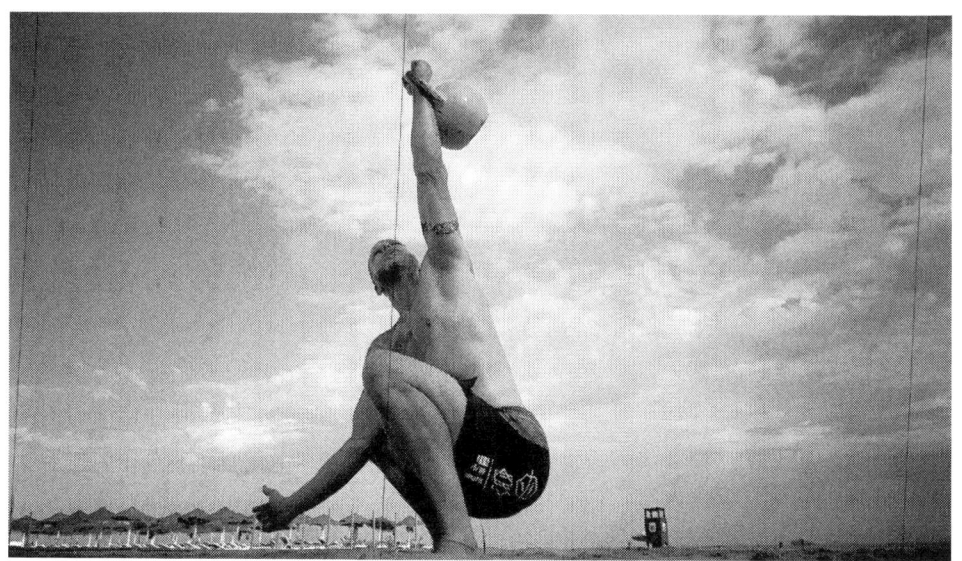

Press and lock out.

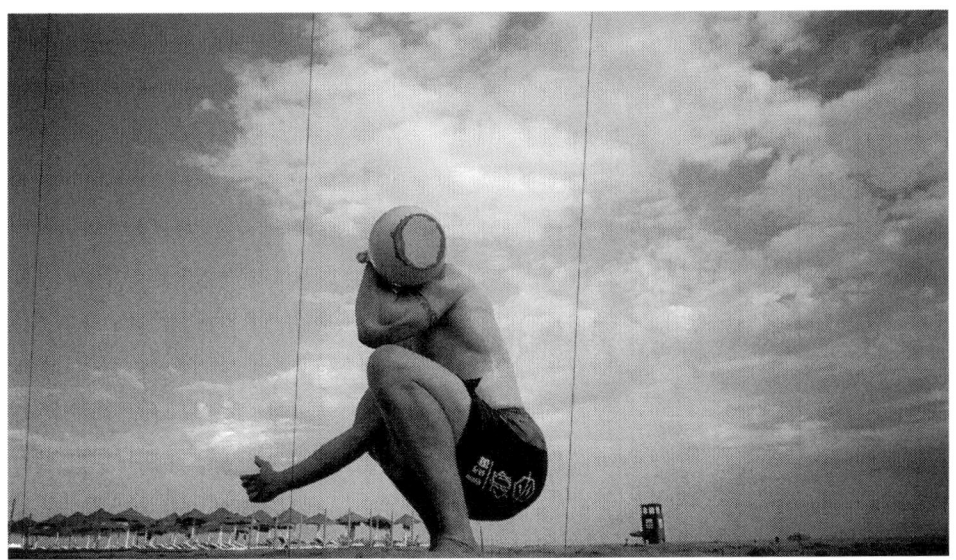

Lower into a shallow rack.

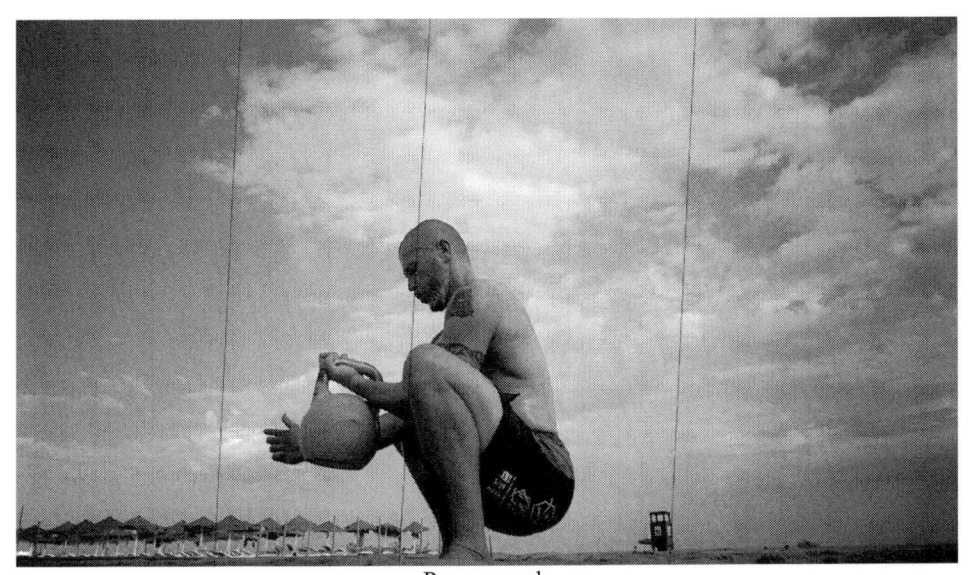

Reverse curl.

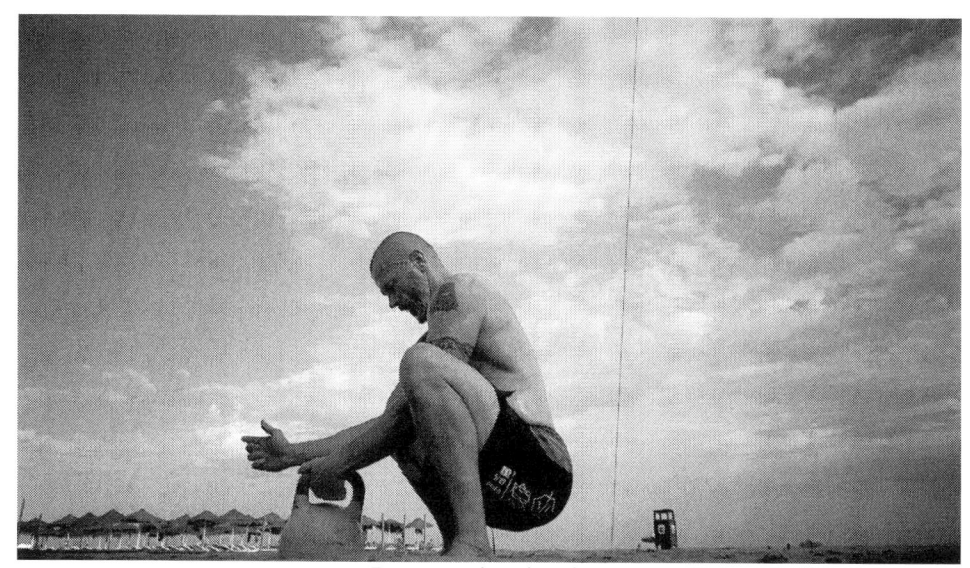

Repeat on the other side.

The advantage of working with one kettlebell is that you can use the other arm to open up the legs. It's quite common for the knees to cave in and pushing against that knee will give you additional support to open up. Don't keep relying on that support though and work your way up to being able to pull those knees apart and keeping them in place with the strength in your legs.

Hundreds of kettlebell videos on our website
KETTLEBELL.VIDEO
Check it out

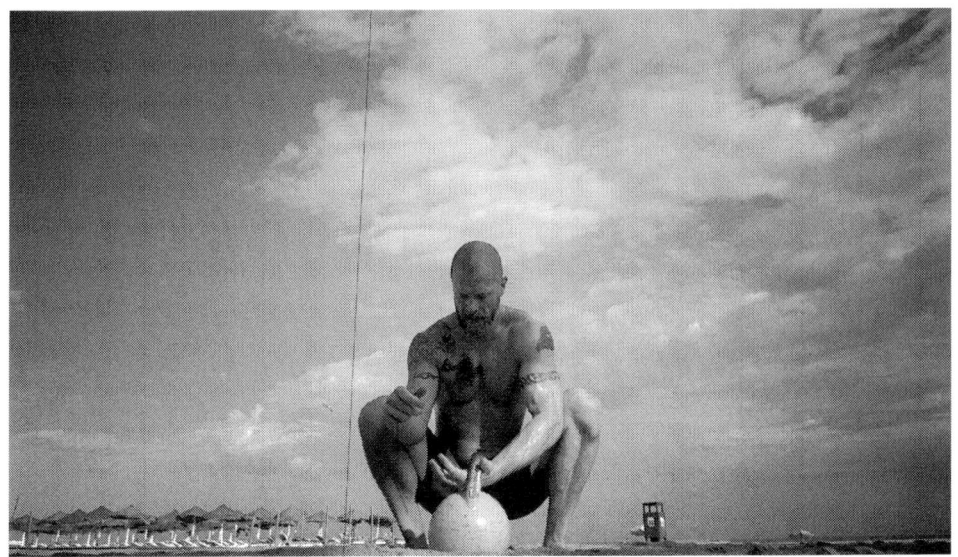

Kettlebell placed in the middle.

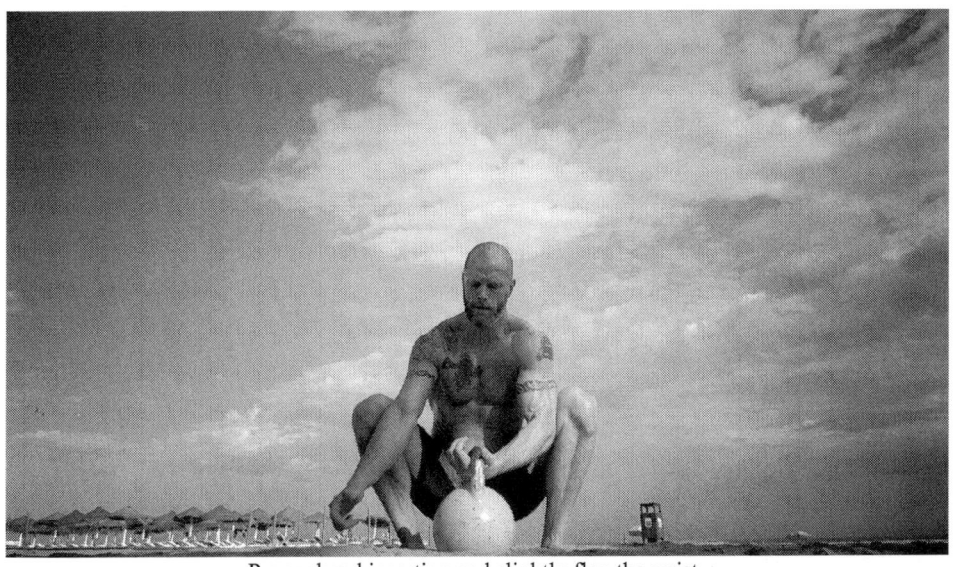

Proper hand insertion and slightly flex the wrist.

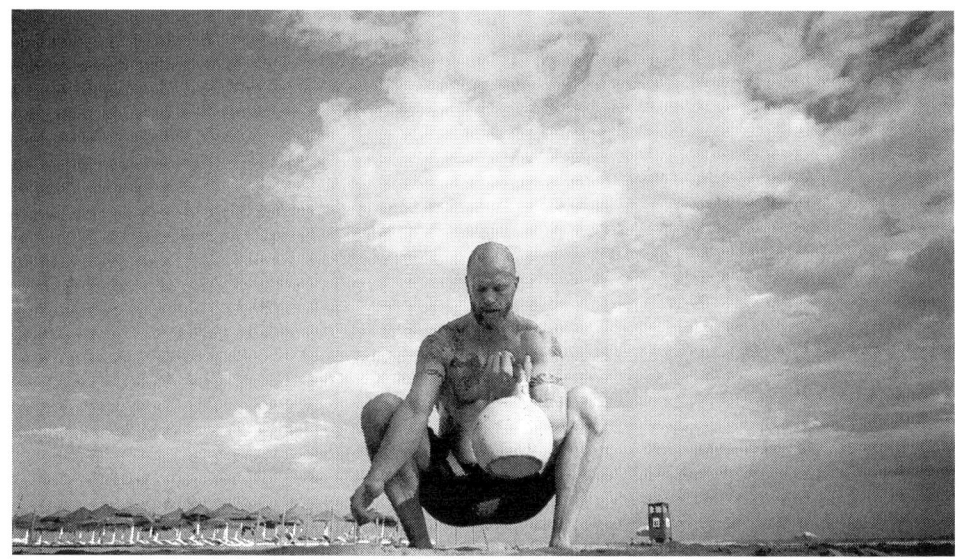

Elbow against the inside of the leg to open up.

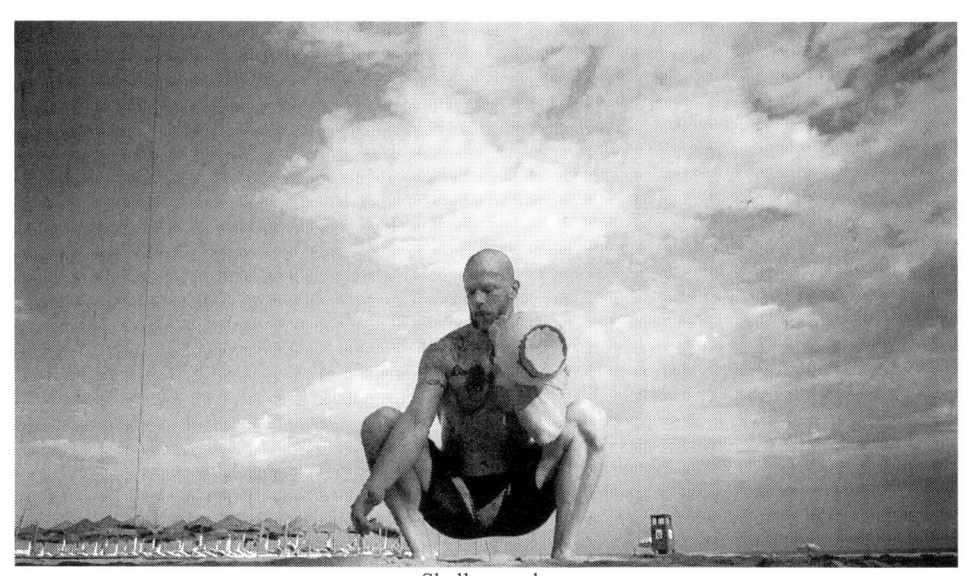

Shallow rack.

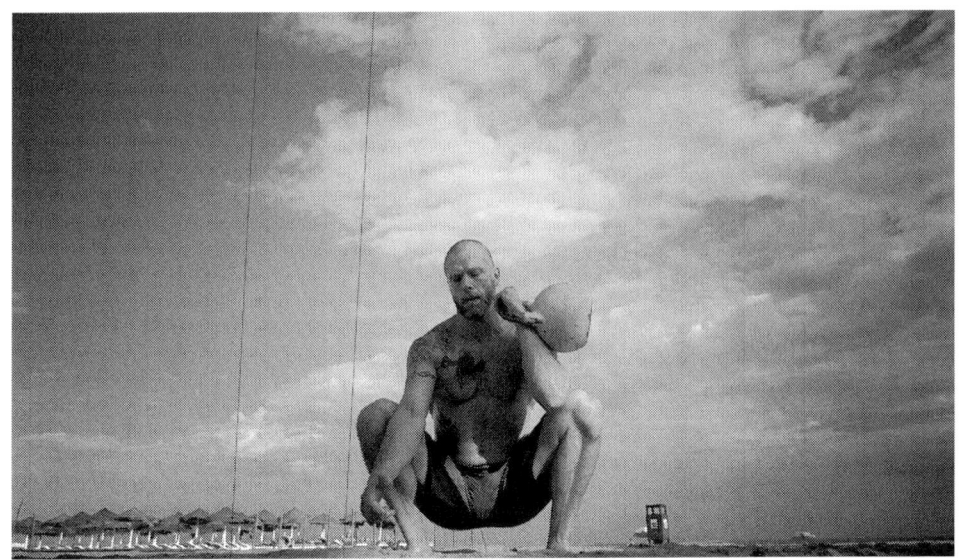

Laterally rotate the weight.

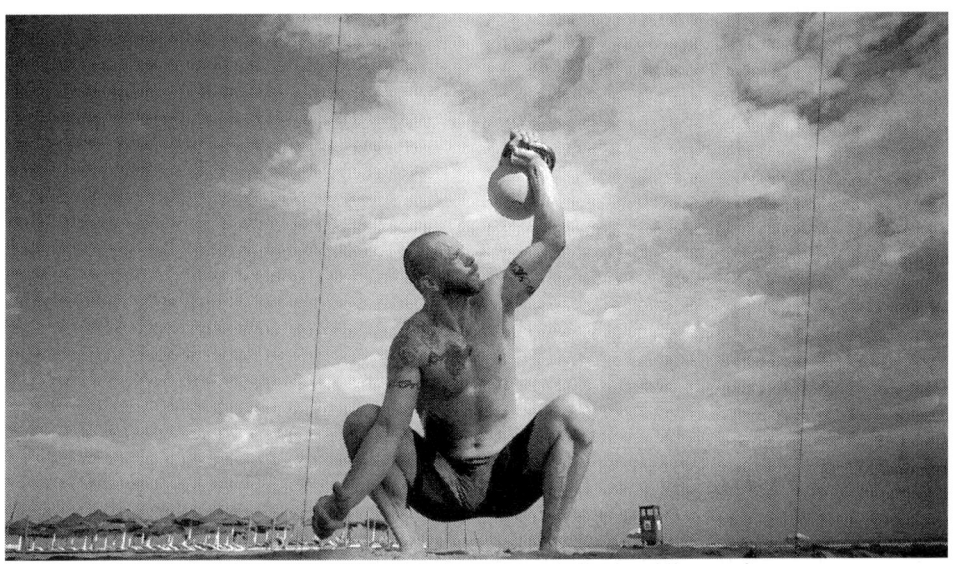

Create and maintain tension throughout the body while pressing.

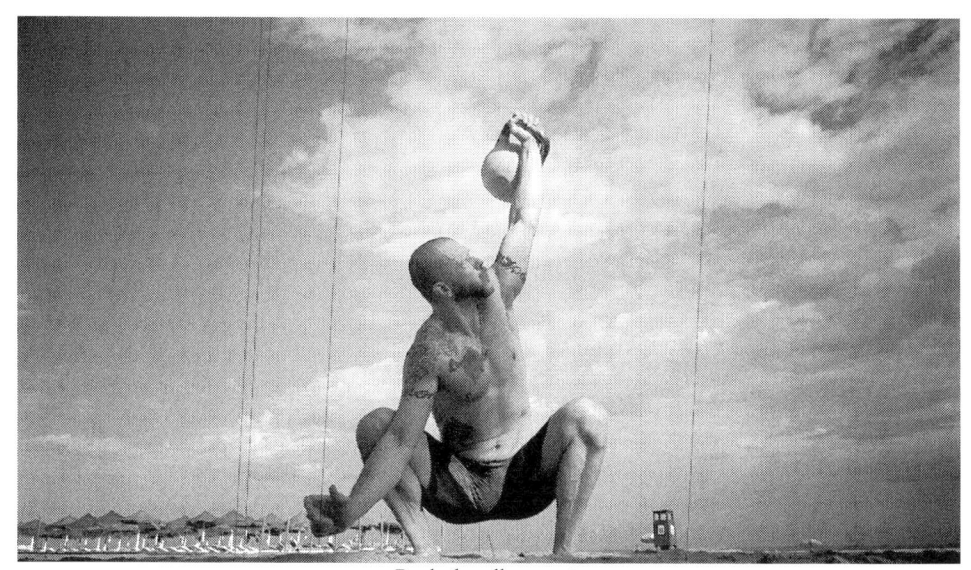

Push the elbow out.

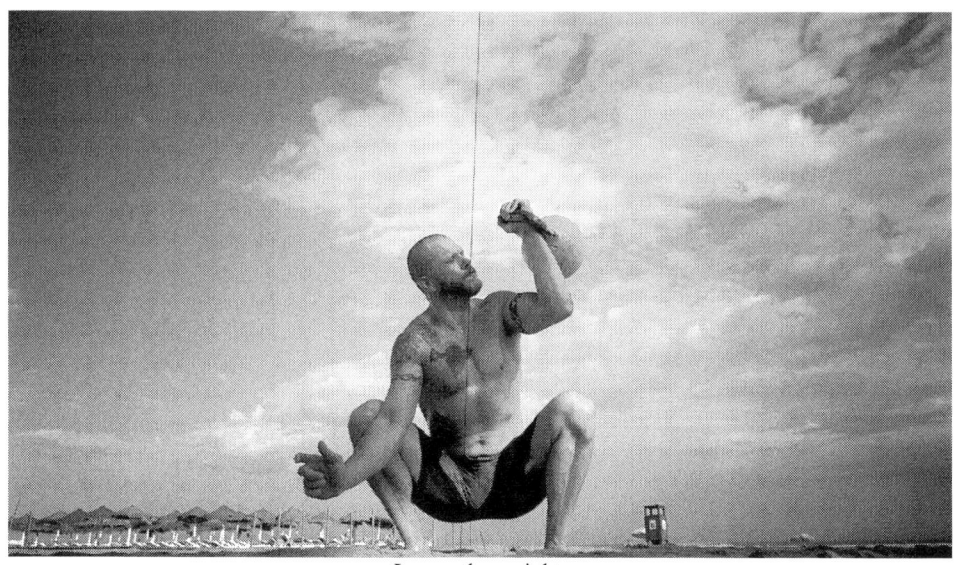

Lower the weight.

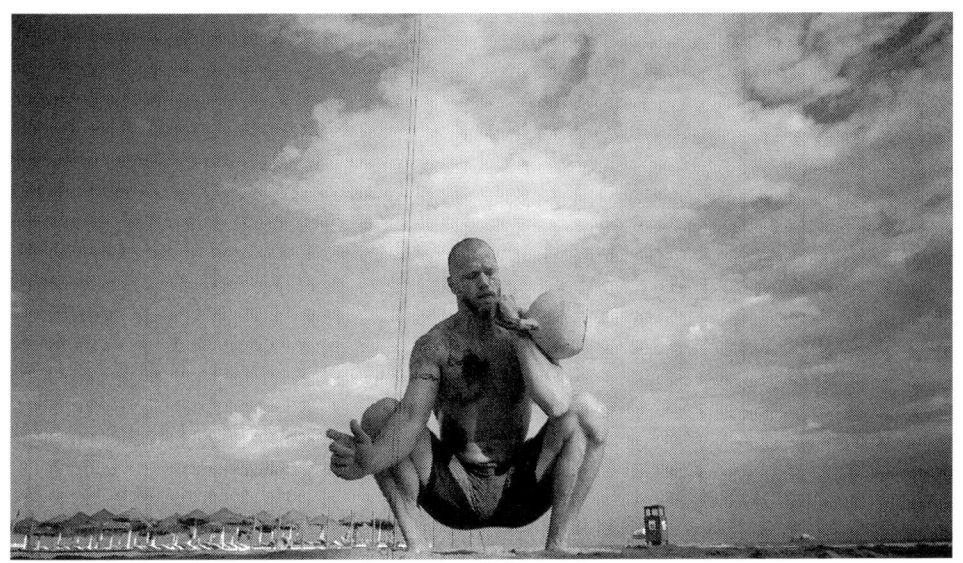

Return to a shallow rack.

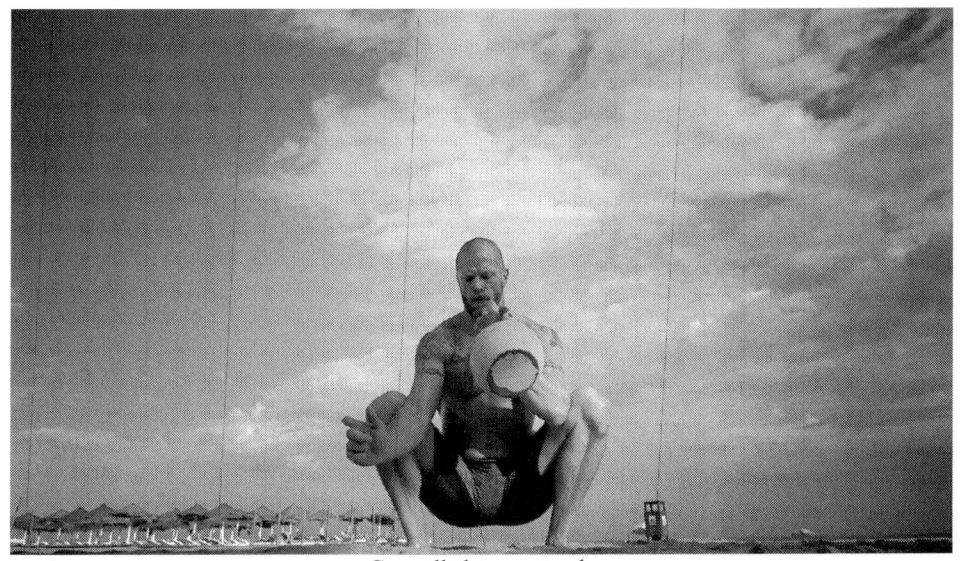

Controlled reverse curl.

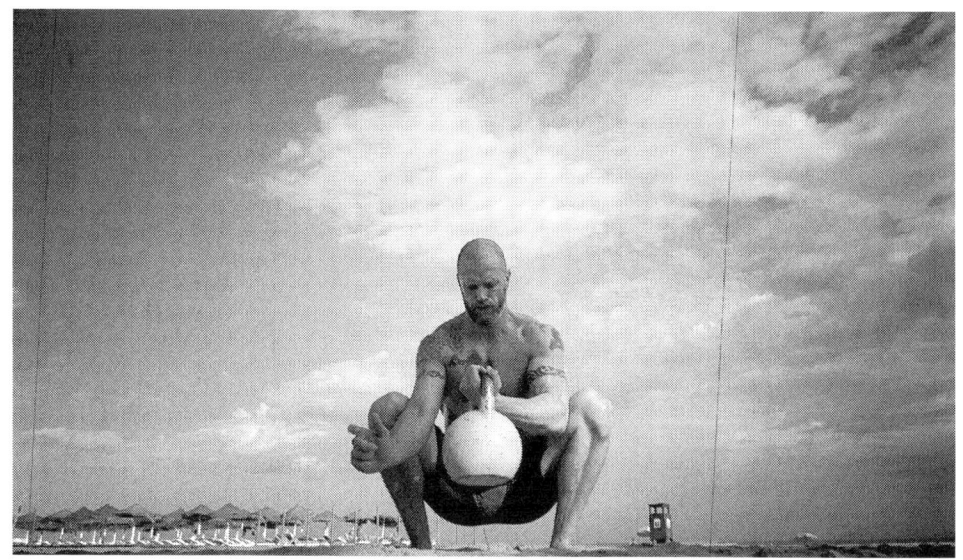

Flex the wrist slightly.

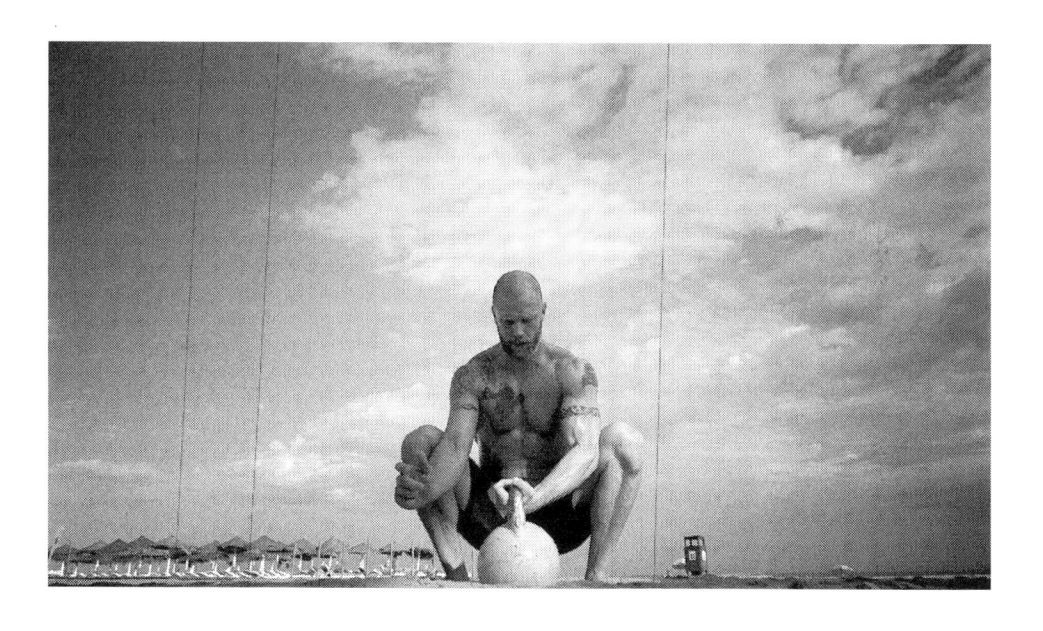

Double Kettlebell Alternating Sots Press Tutorial

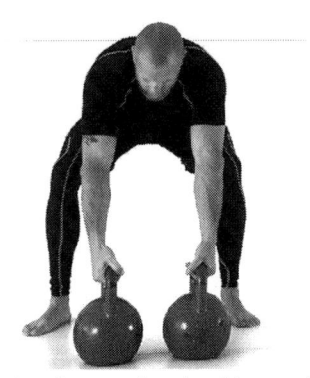

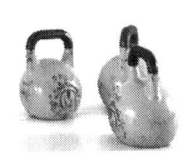

The previous example was that of the Sots press with rotation and alternating which required a curl in between and is a good progression to the alternating Sots press with double kettlebell which is what's used in the challenge. This example of the Sots press is with two kettlebells and is <u>without</u> thoracic rotation.

Position the kettlebells just far enough to be able to pull them back but no overextend.

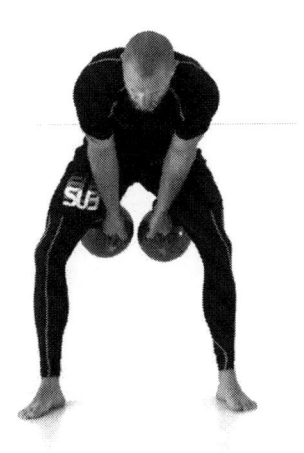

Pull the kettlebells through the legs.

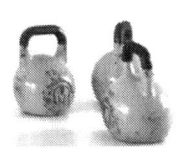

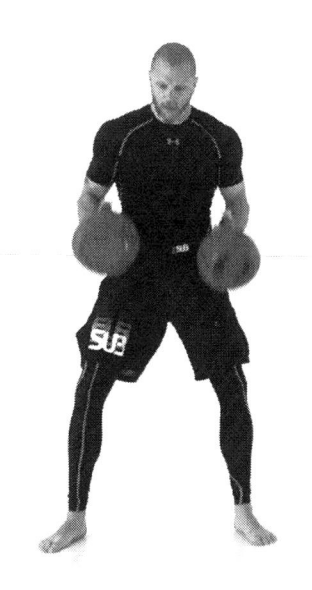

Clean the kettlebells.

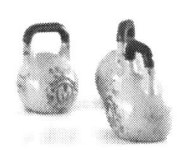

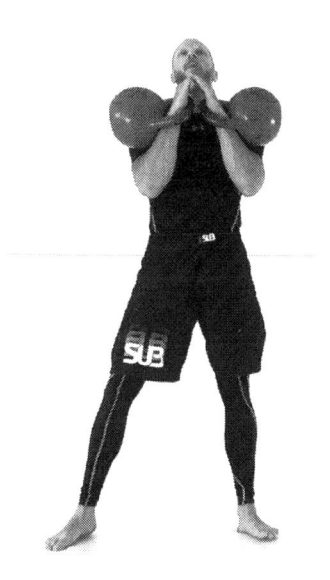

Come into proper racking position.

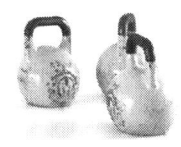

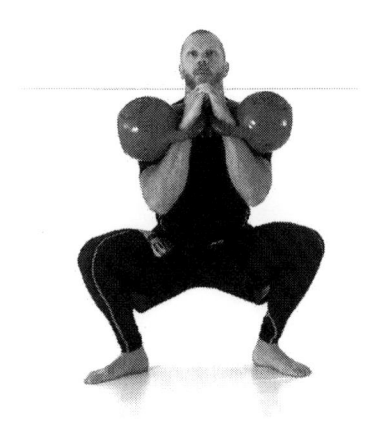

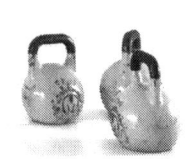

Squat deep but don't hang or sit relaxed into the squat.

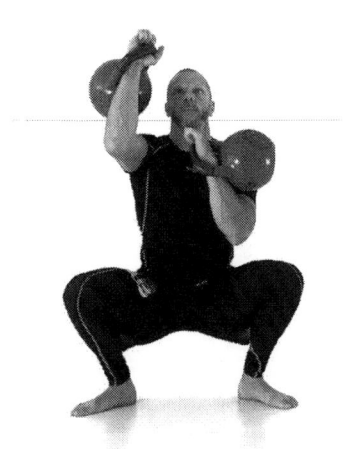

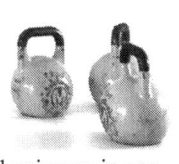

Create tension and press into the ground before pressing. Keep the kettlebell going up in one straight line, not to the side.

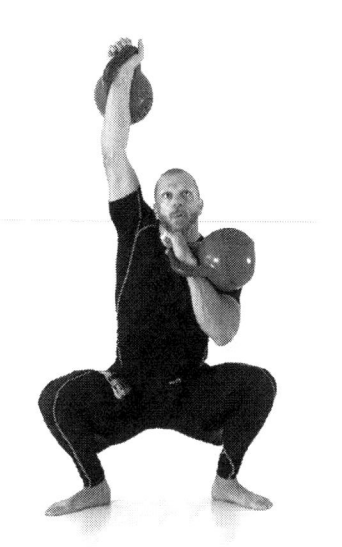

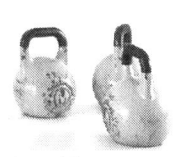

Take your time and spend some time at the top to work on the overhead position.

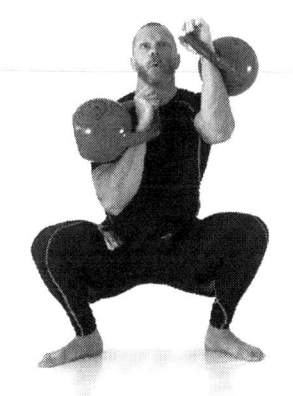

Repeat on the other side.

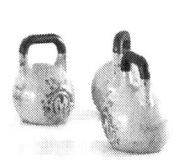

Maintain a good rack during the press.

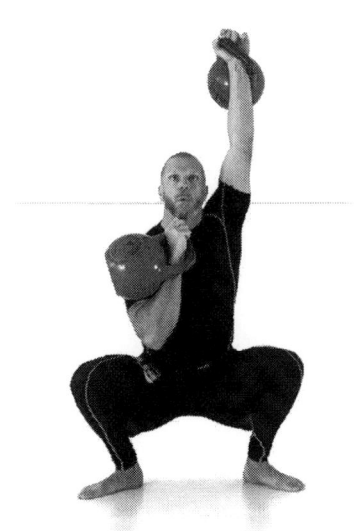

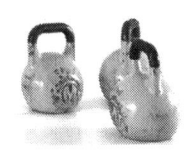

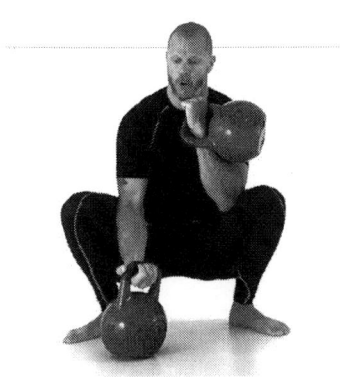

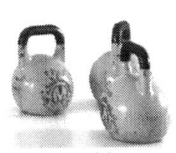

If you're having issues balancing you can use one of the kettlebells as an anchor to provide some stability during the press.

11-DAY SOTS PRESS CHALLENGE

INCREASE MOBILITY
INCREASE STRENGTH

#SOTSPRESSCHALLENGE
#CAVEMANTRAINING

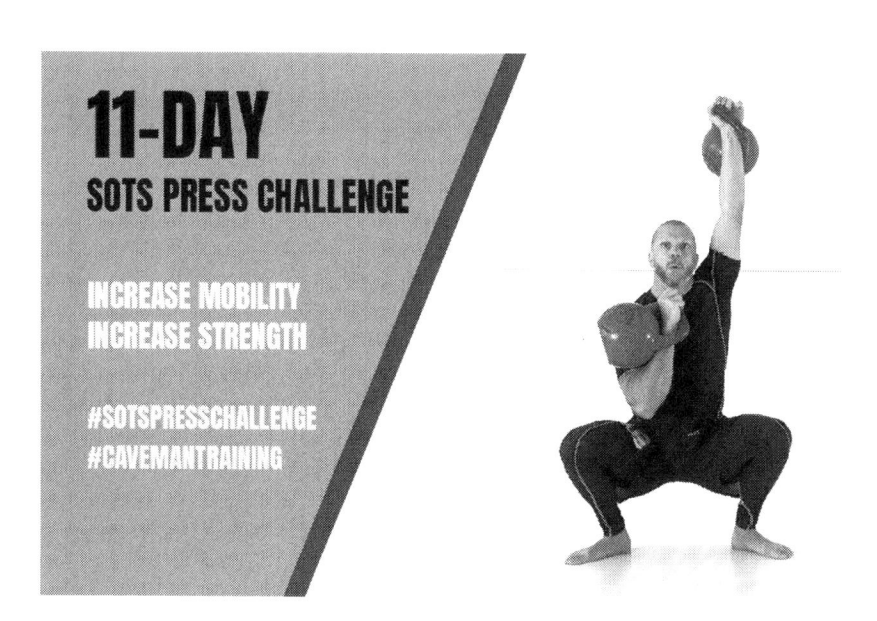

Join the 11-day Sots press challenge to increase your mobility and strength.

11 days to spend on your mobility and strength. The combo is double kettlebell Sots press with the first alternating rep being straight up and the second alternating rep with thoracic rotation.

Pick a lightweight to start with. Use just bodyweight if you're still working on your overhead flexibility. Double the reps by 4 if you're working with just bodyweight. From bodyweight you should progress to the Sots press with rotation.

CONTROL. FOCUS. RANGE.

Better posture. Better overhead squat.

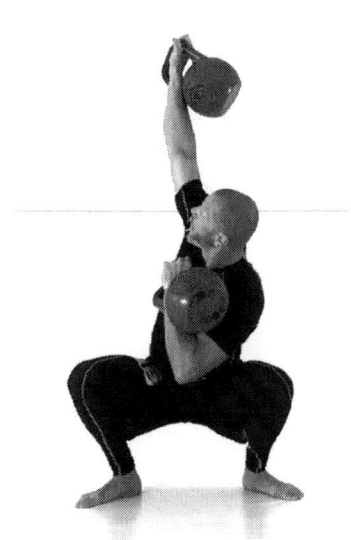

Sots press with thoracic rotation.

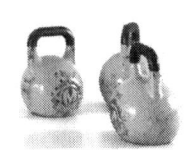

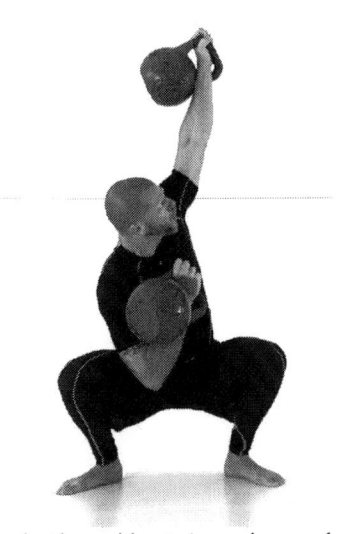

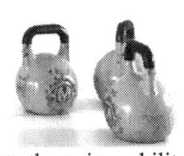

With thoracic rotation is easier than without. Assuming you have some moderate thoracic mobility.

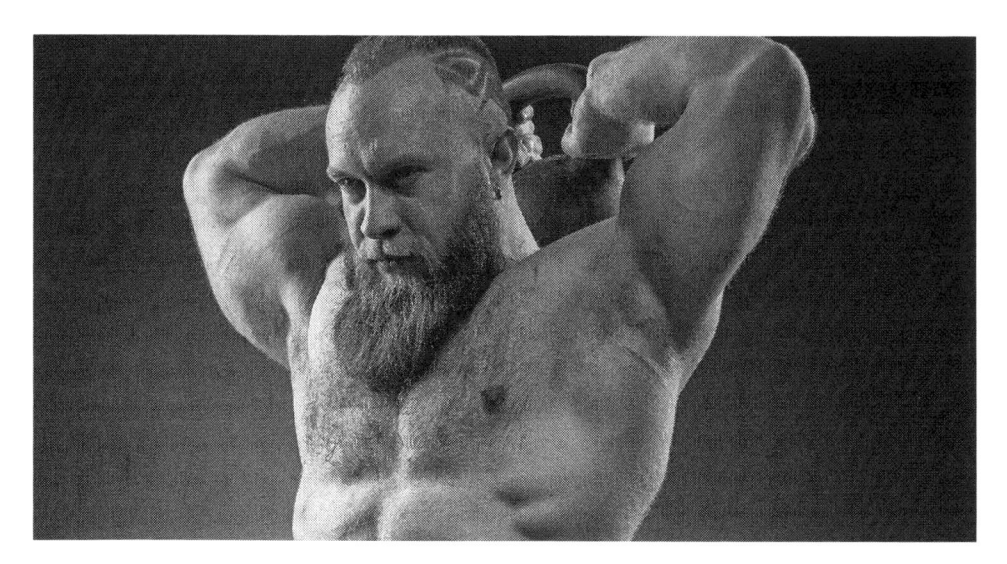

The HULK Test

Level: Intermediate to Advanced

Weight: Medium

Kettlebell(s):

Type: Strength, cardio, and explosiveness

Duration: 20 to 40 minutes depending on whether working solo or with a buddy

I sneaked this challenge in from the Kettlebell Workouts and Challenges 1.0, simply because it's such a good one. Enjoy!

Targets:

- **Shoulder**
    - Front
        - Deltoid anterior
    - Top
        - Trapezius superior
- **Chest**
    - Pectoralis major
- **Upper-arm**
    - Front
        - Biceps brachii
    - Inside
        - Coracobrachialis
    - Back

- ○ Triceps brachii
- ○ Anconeus
- **Scapula**
  - ○ Serratus anterior
- **Hips / pelvis**
  - ○ Psoas major
  - ○ Iliacus
- **Upper-leg**
  - ○ Front
    - ○ Tensor fasciae latae
    - ○ Sartorius
    - ○ Rectur femorus
    - ○ Vastus lateralis
    - ○ Vastus medialis
    - ○ Vastus intermedius
  - ○ Back
    - ○ Biceps femoris (long head)
    - ○ Semitendinosus (hamstring)
    - ○ Semimembranosus (hamstring)
    - ○ Adductor magnus
  - ○ Inside
    - ○ Gracilis
    - ○ Sartorius
- **Lower-leg**
  - ○ Back
    - ○ Gastrocnemius
    - ○ Popliteus
    - ○ Soleus
    - ○ Tibialis posterior
    - ○ Flexor digitorum longus
    - ○ Flexor hallucis longus
    - ○ Plantaris
  - ○ Outside
    - ○ Fibularis (peroneus) longus
  - ○ Front
    - ○ Tibalis anterior
    - ○ Extensor digitorum longus
    - ○ Extensor hallucis longus
- **Buttocks**
  - ○ Gluteus maximus

This beast of a workout can be used as a test or simply as a workout. You decide. You can do this on your own, or you can work with a partner. It's a lot more fun with a partner.

The HULK Test
Can you smash it!?

The test is as follows:

- 1 minute of strict presses with double kettlebells
- 2 minutes of half snatch into squat with double kettlebells
- 1 or 5 minutes rest

5 rounds AMRAP

If you're working with a partner, it's 1 minute rest after you've performed your task, and then you're counting or no repping for your partner. In effect you still have 5 minutes rest.

The HULK Test

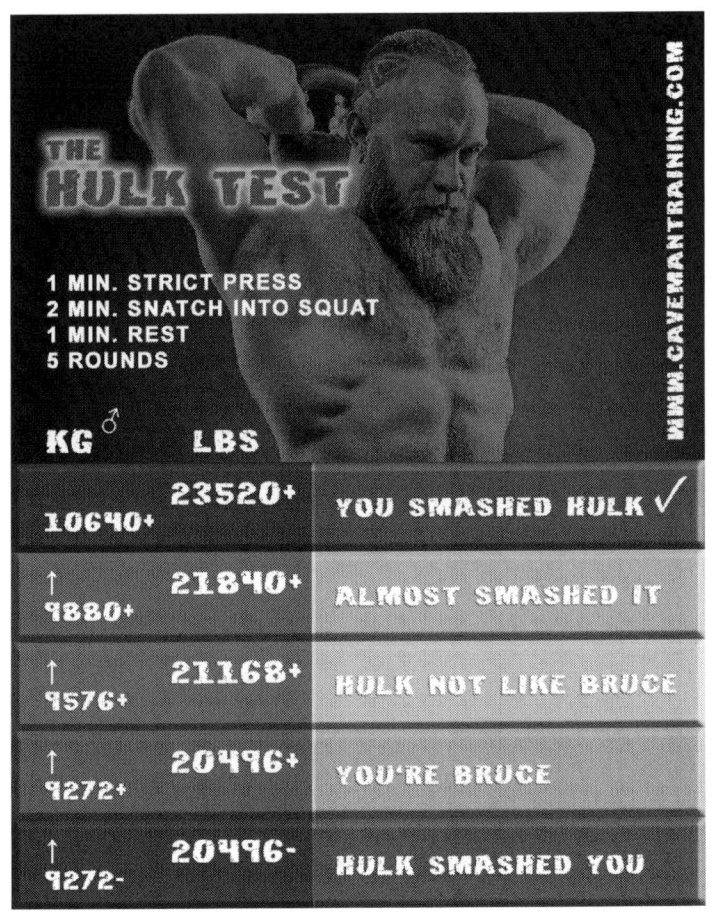

1 MIN. STRICT PRESS
2 MIN. SNATCH INTO SQUAT
1 MIN. REST
5 ROUNDS

KG ♂	LBS	
10640+	23520+	YOU SMASHED HULK ✓
↑ 9880+	21840+	ALMOST SMASHED IT
↑ 9576+	21168+	HULK NOT LIKE BRUCE
↑ 9272+	20496+	YOU'RE BRUCE
↑ 9272-	20496-	HULK SMASHED YOU

The HULK Test scorecard.

Weight

The weight for your strict press is approx. 70% of your 1RM strict press. If you can press a 32kg/70.4lbs for one time, then this is your 1RM. The easiest way to calculate your weight for this workout is by taking your 1RM, 32kg/70.4lbs / 100 = 0.32 x 70 = 22kg/48.5lbs. Hence you should be working with two 22kg/48.5lbs kettlebells.

The weight for your snatch and squat is of medium weight, approx 50% of your strict press, i.e. two 16kg/35.2lbs kettlebells.

Rx weights

If you want to Rx it:

- *Rx* for strict press
  - ♂ 2 x 20kg/44lbs for male
  - ♀ 2 x 16kg/35.2lbs for female

- *Rx* for snatch and squat
  - ♂ 2 x 16kg/35.2lbs for male
  - ♀ 2 x 12kg/26.4lbs for female

Scoring

To calculate your score, add up the total weight of your strict press plus the weight used for the snatch and squat, and times that by the total reps at the end. If you dropped down in weight during the test (no harm in that, stay safe), then your lowest weight is used for this calculation. There is no going up in weight during the workout. Use the scoring card at the top of this document to check whether you smashed it. Remember to write down the reps for yourself or partner at the end of each round.

My score was:

22kg + 22kg for strict press equals 44kg (97lbs)
16kg + 16kg for snatches and squat equals 32kg (70lbs)
Total of 76kg times 134 equals 10184
Hence, my score is 10184

The scoring card above shows the results for male. The following is the scoring card for a female Rx.

Kg	Lbs	
7560+	16660+	You smashed hulk
7020+	15470+	Almost smashed it
6804+	14994+	Hulk not like Bruce
6588+	14518+	You're Bruce
6588-	14518-	Hulk smashed you

Time

If you do this alone, the timing works as follows:

- 0 to 1 minute strict press
- 1 to 3 minutes half snatch and squat
- 3 to 4 minutes rest
- 4 to 5 minutes strict press
- 5 to 7 minutes half snatch and squat

- 🏋 7 to 8 minutes rest
- 8 to 9 minutes strict press
- 9 to 11 minutes half snatch and squat
- 🏋 11 to 12 minutes rest
- 12 to 13 minutes strict press
- 13 to 15 minutes half snatch and squat
- 🏋 15 to 16 minutes rest
- 16 to 17 minutes strict press
- 17 to 19 minutes half snatch and squat
- 🚩 **Done**

If you do this with a partner, the timing works as follows:

- 0 to 1 minute strict press
- 1 to 3 minutes half snatch and squat
- 3 to 4 minutes rest SWITCH
- 4 to 5 minutes strict press
- 5 to 7 minutes half snatch and squat
- 7 to 8 minutes rest SWITCH
- 8 to 9 minutes strict press
- 9 to 11 minutes half snatch and squat
- 11 to 12 minutes rest SWITCH
- 12 to 13 minutes strict press
- 13 to 15 minutes half snatch and squat
- 15 to 16 minutes rest SWITCH
- 16 to 17 minutes strict press
- 17 to 19 minutes half snatch and squat
- 19 to 20 minutes rest SWITCH
- 20 to 21 minutes strict press

- 21 to 23 minutes half snatch and squat
- 23 to 24 minutes rest SWITCH
- 24 to 25 minutes strict press
- 25 to 27 minutes half snatch and squat
- 27 to 28 minutes rest SWITCH
- 28 to 29 minutes strict press
- 29 to 31 minutes half snatch and squat
- 31 to 32 minutes rest SWITCH
- 32 to 33 minutes strict press
- 33 to 35 minutes half snatch and squat
- 35 to 36 minutes rest SWITCH
- 36 to 37 minutes strict press
- 37 to 39 minutes half snatch and squat
- 🏳 **DONE**

Movement Standards

Strict press:

- Full lockout of the knees and hips
- Press starts from the rack each rep
- No momentum used from the legs or torso
- Full overhead lockout
- Hands end up above the shoulders with elbows locked out
- Drop the kettlebells into racking position
- Repeat

Half Snatch into Squat:

- You can start dead or from rack
- Base of the kettlebell should be behind the legs upon the back swing
- One continuous explosive movement to overhead

- Full lockout overhead
- Drop into racking position
- Keep the kettlebells racked
- Squat down till hips reach below the knees
- Heels remaining on the ground
- Coming back up into full knee and hip extension
- Repeat

Scaling

There is no scaling for *The HULK Test*; you either Hulk it or you don't...

Kettlebell Half Snatch

The kettlebell half snatch is performed right before the squat. **Here's how it's done:**

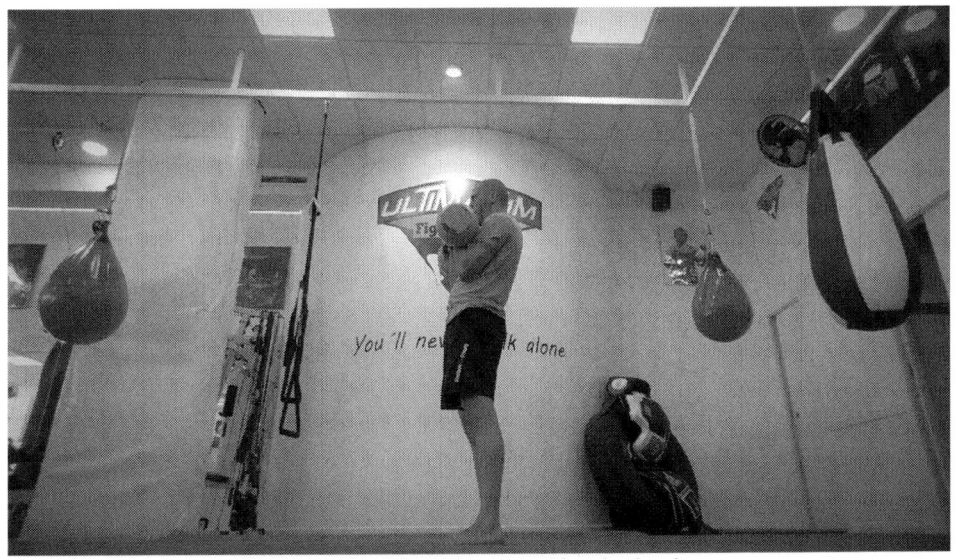

Rack your kettlebells, or start with a dead swing.

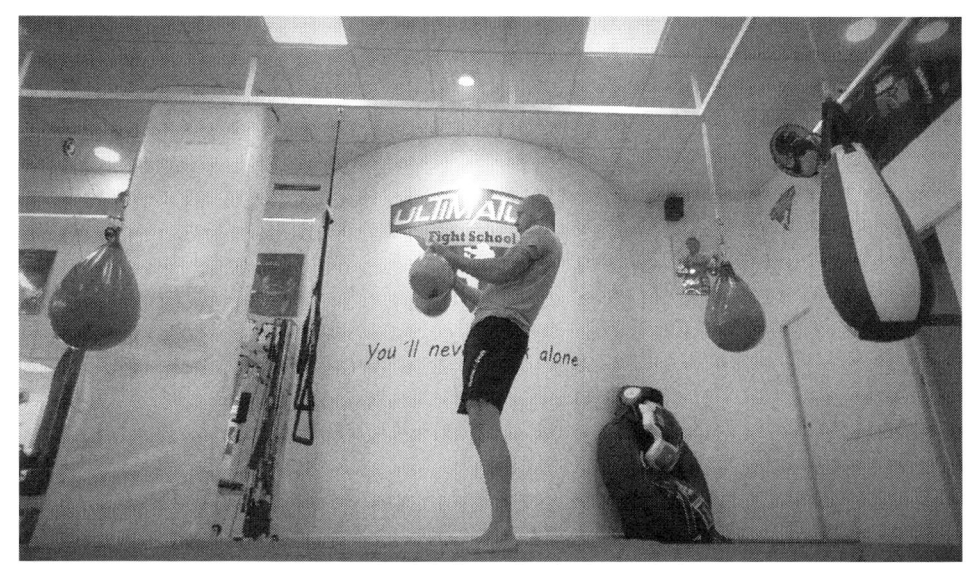

Drop your kettlebells. Bell to body proximity.

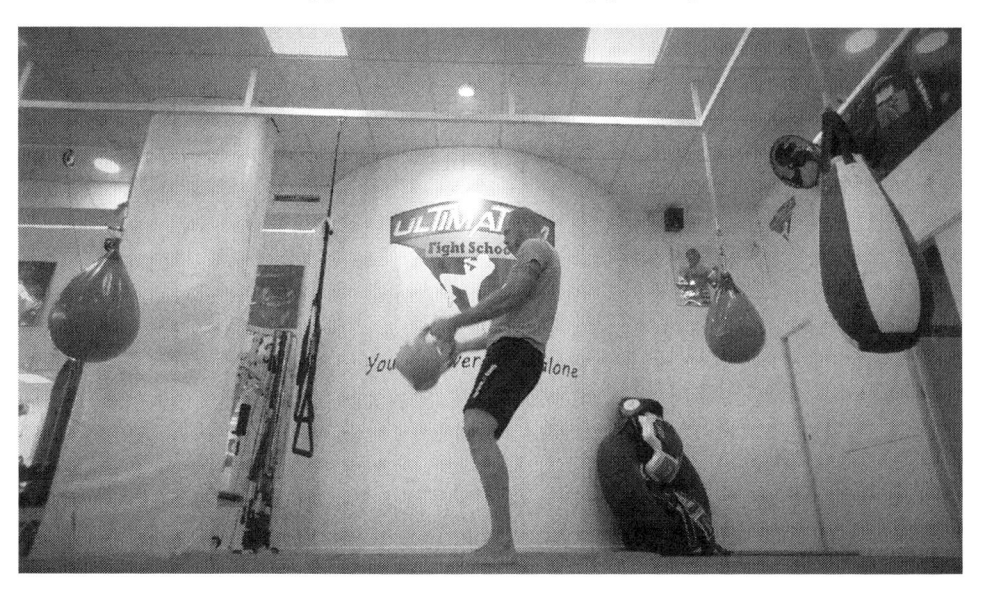

Pull out into hook grip and start the back swing.

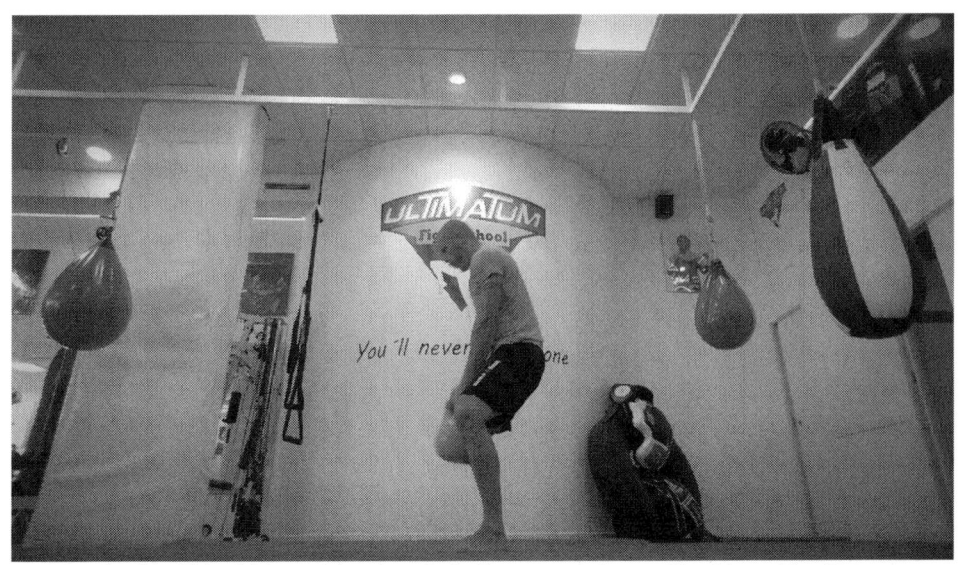

You should still be fairly upright when the bells pass your knees. Shoulder ankle alignment.

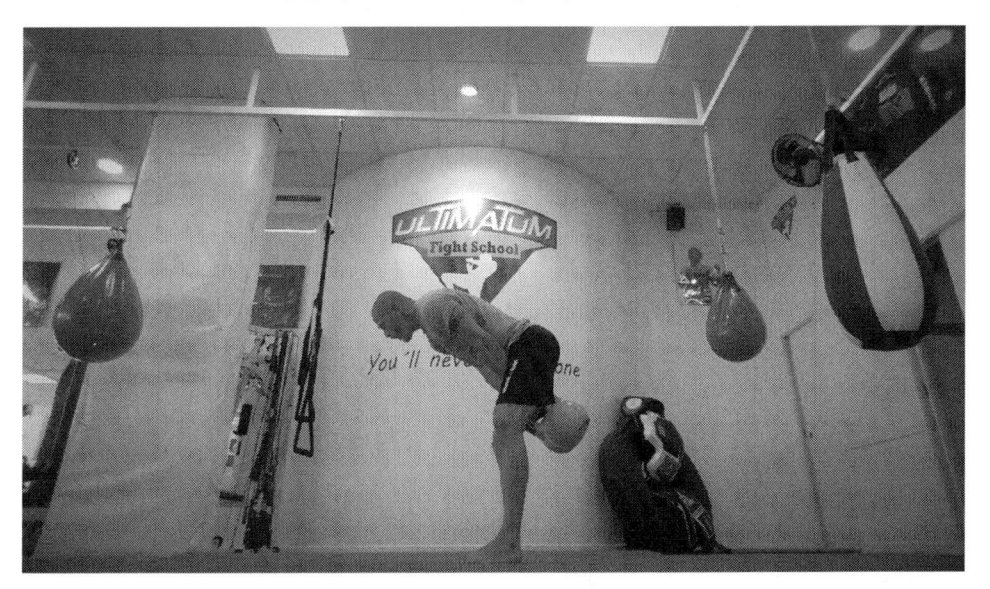

Back swing, neutral head alignment.

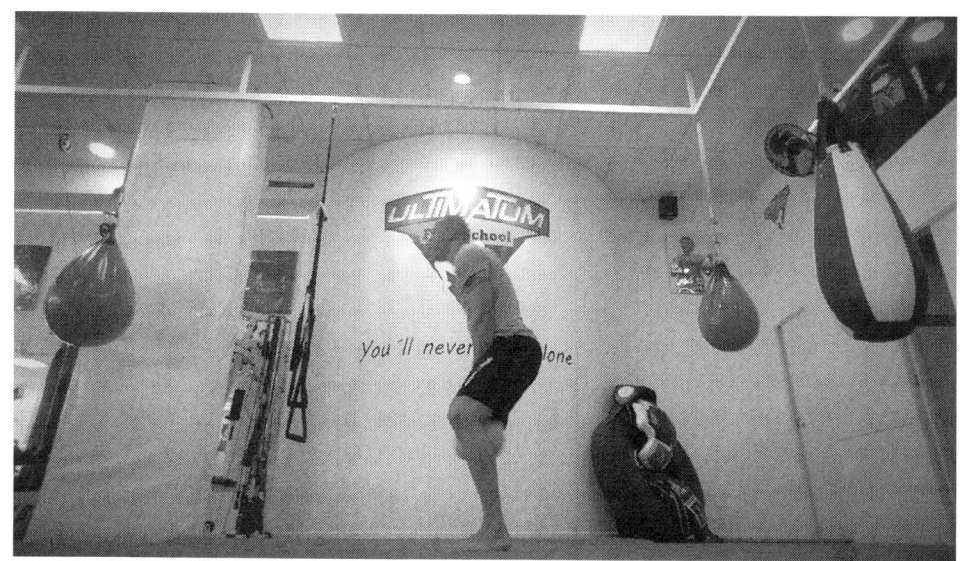

Up swing.

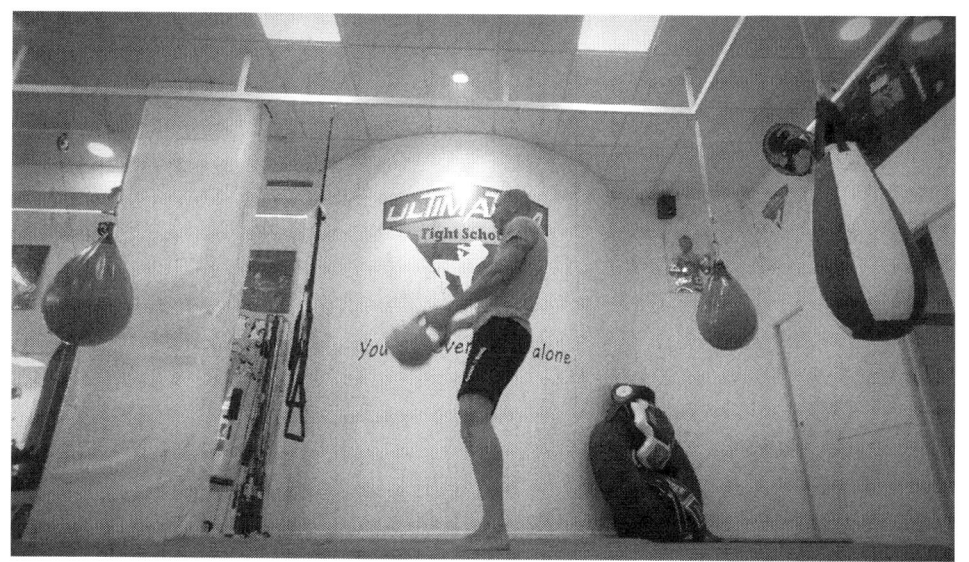

Pull.

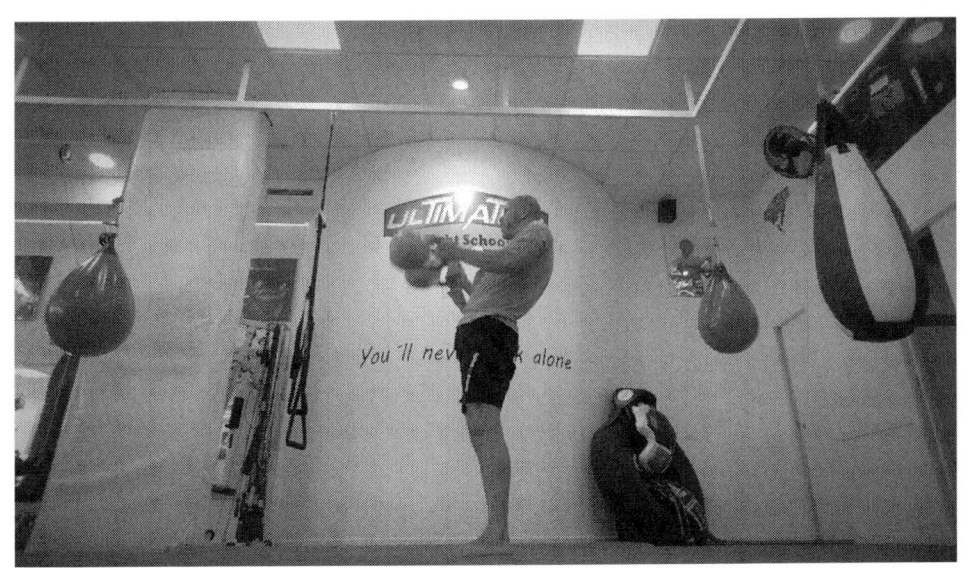

Bell to body proximity.

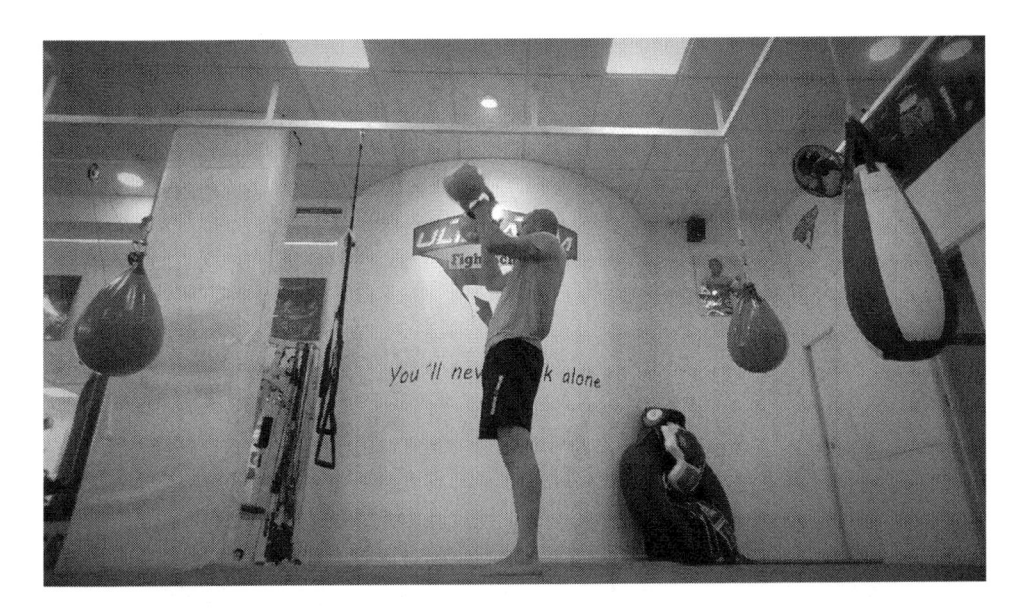

Open up.

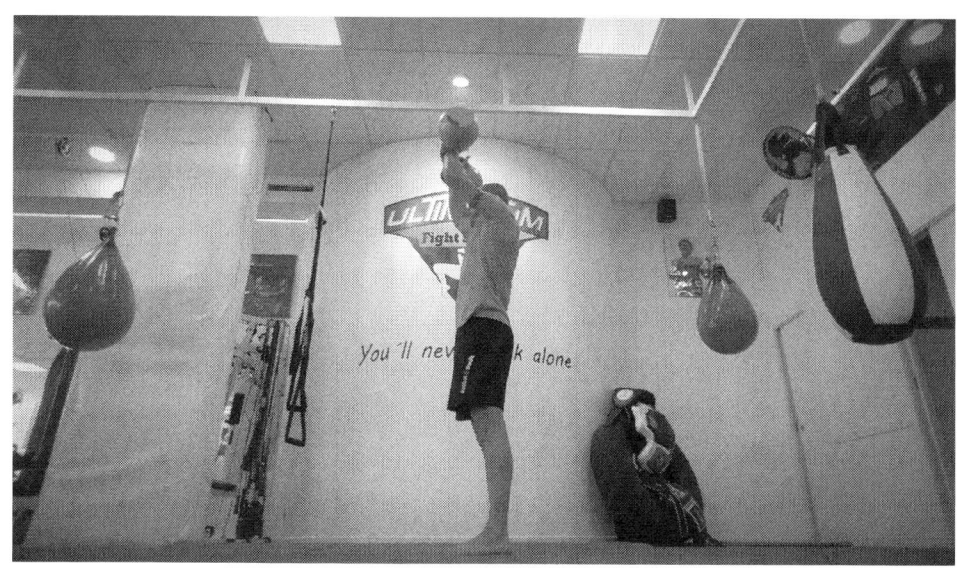

Corkscrew and hand insert.

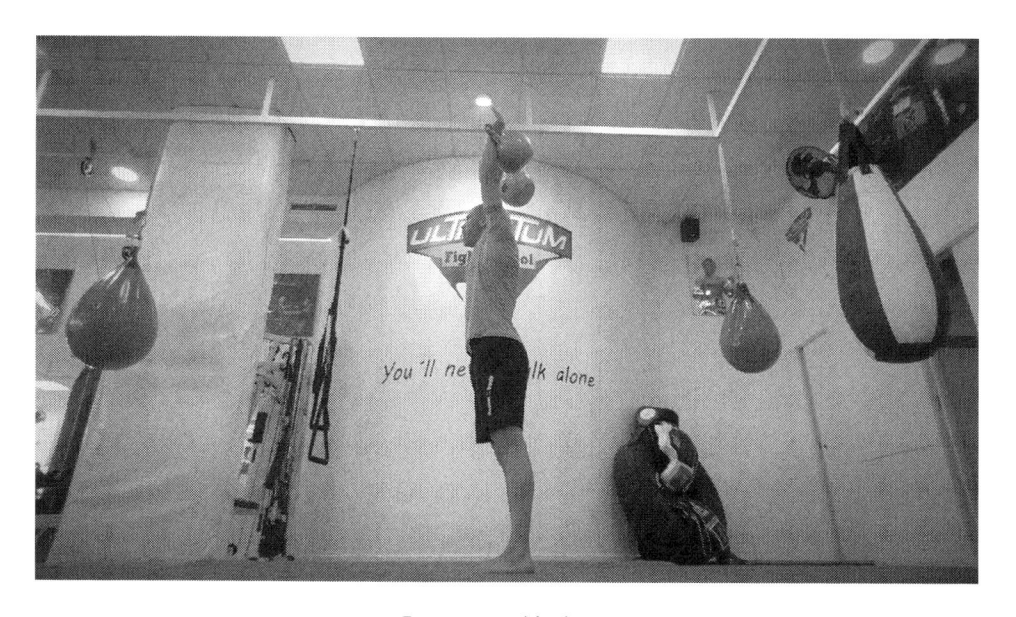

Press out and lockout.

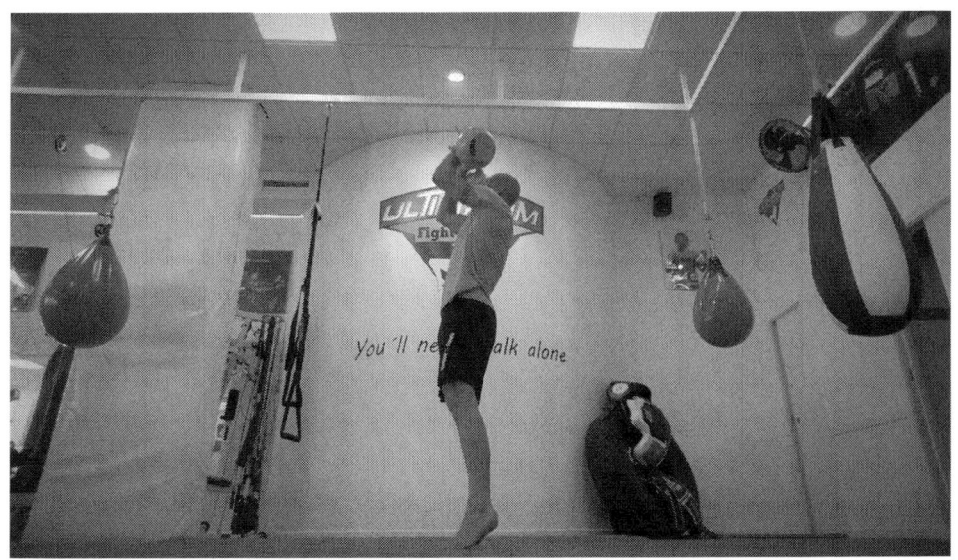

Drop and catch.

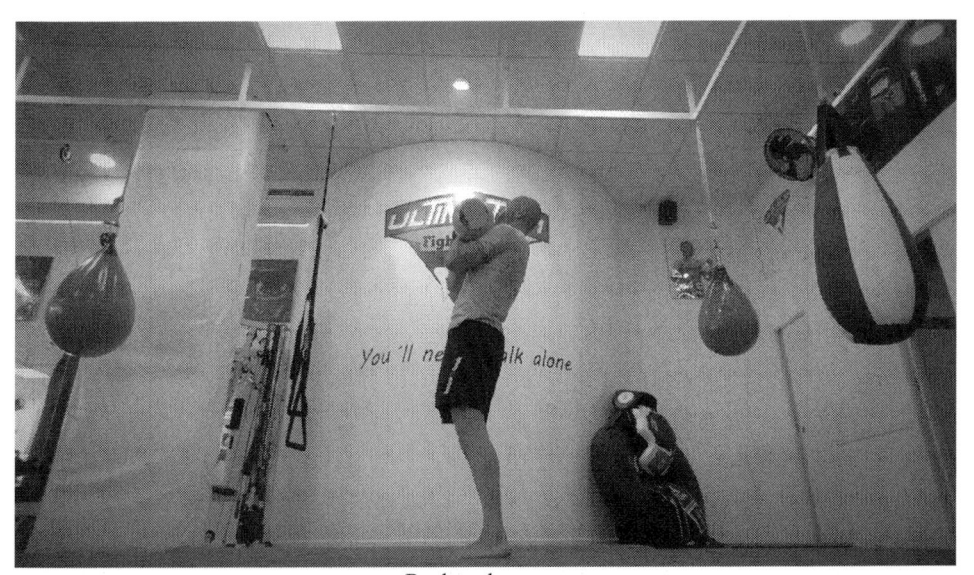

Rack and repeat.

Enjoyed the workout/test? Set a good or bad score, just post here http://bit.ly/kb-wk-link1

The video can be found here http://bit.ly/kb-wk-vid42

THE END OF WORKOUTS AND CHALLENGES

Kettlebell Training Instructions (fundamentals)

Following are 21-days of kettlebell training instructions for anyone that wants to lay the foundations of kettlebell training before attempting any of the workouts. Know that it's important to perfect technique before attempting heavy weight and/or high fast reps (high intensity).

Day 1 Warming up and priming for kettlebell training

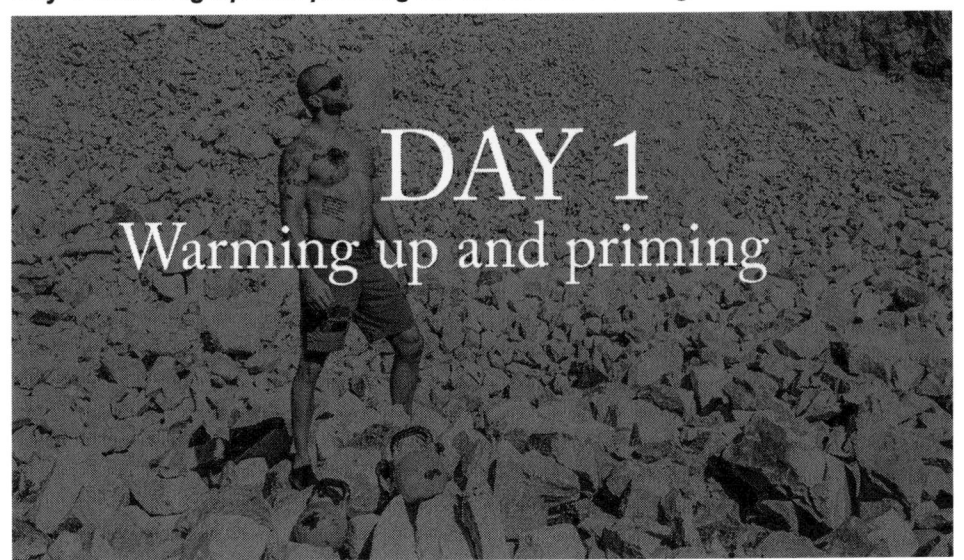

On day 1 you will learn how to warm up for kettlebell training and how super important it is to stay injury free. You will learn that mind-muscle connection is important for an effective and safe workout and that muscle priming is focussing on getting the muscles ready and assists in connecting with them.

I will take you through a **full-body warm up** and **muscle priming routine** for the kettlebell swing.

Dot points:

- Warming up for kettlebell training is super important
- Warm up to stay injury free
- Not one warm-up works for every workout or person
- Full-body warm-ups are best
- Mind-muscle connection is important for an effective and safe workout
- Muscle priming is focussing on getting the muscles ready and assists in connecting with them

Warming up for kettlebells

The full-body warm-up:

1. 10 x single leg hip circles one side
2. 10 x single leg hip circles other side

3. 10 x hip circles one way
4. 10 x hip circles other way
5. 10 x thoracic rotation one side
6. 10 x thoracic rotation other side
7. 10 x arm circled forward
8. 10 x arm circled backward
9. 10 to 20 x jumping jacks use high knees on the second round or complete after the jumping jacks

Single leg hip circles

To perform:

- Stand in a neutral stance
- Decide which hip to circle
- The leg of the non-circling hip should be locked (supporting leg)
- Firmly plant the foot on the ground
- Shift your weight onto the supporting leg
- Contract the gluteals on the supporting side to prevent the hip from dropping
- Lift the knee of the working leg through hip extension into starting position
- Pull the knee as high as possible
- Move the knee laterally out to the side and down creating a quarter of a circle
- Move the knee as for out to the side as possible and feel the stretch in the adductors
- If at this stage you struggle with balance then place the tippy toes on the ground for short support and continue the movement
- If you did not need support then finish the circle through extension and adduction which brings the leg straight under you but not touching the ground
- From there work on the next quarter circle by pulling the knee to the side of the supporting leg (adduction) and raising the knee (hip flexion)
- Feel the adductors working
- Make sure the hips don't drop or shift in any other direction while circling
- Finish the full circle with the last quarter and bring the knee up and back in front of you

Hip circles

To perform:

1. Stand in a neutral stance
2. Keep the spine straight throughout the movements
3. Keep the shoulders at the same level throughout the movement
4. Push the hips forward through hip hyperextension
5. Shift the hips to one side
6. Create slight hip flexion
7. Shift the hips to other side
8. And move the hips back into hip hyperextension
9. Repeat or circle back the other way

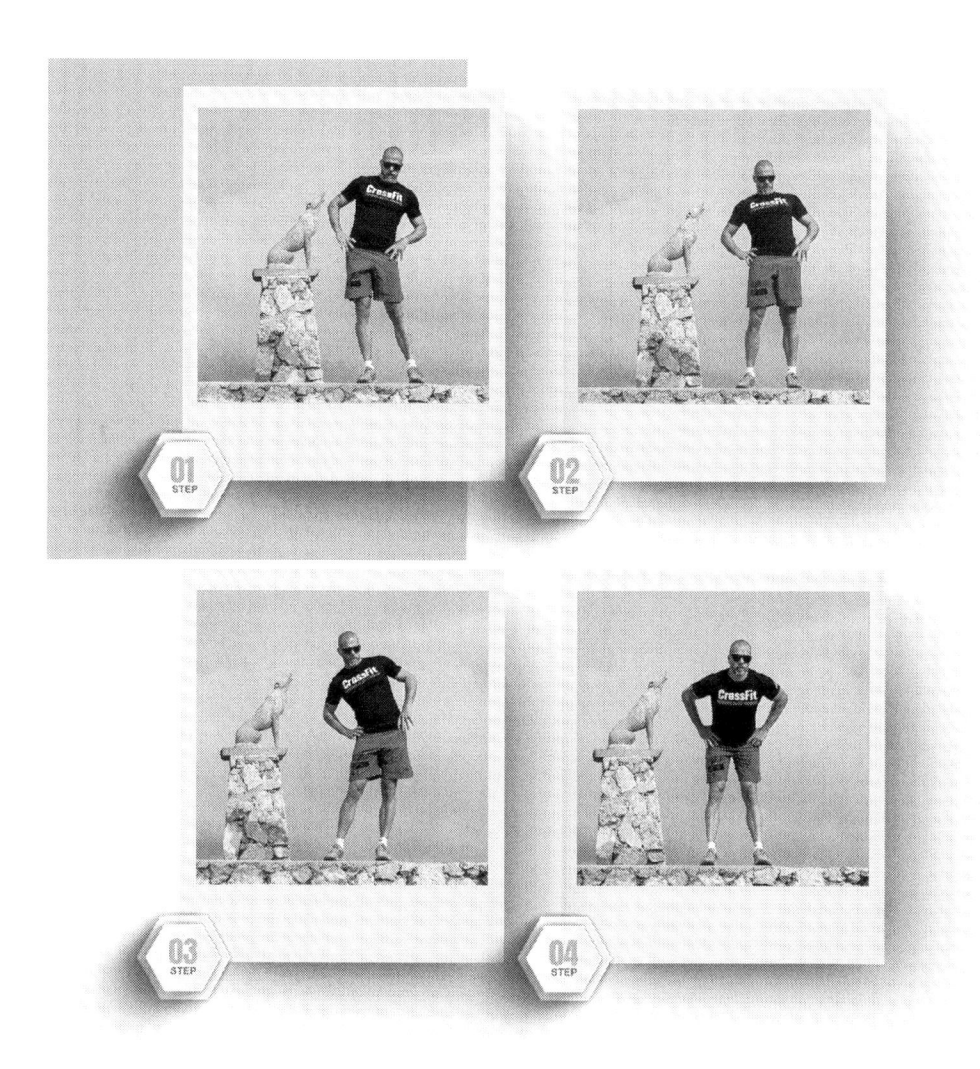

Thoracic rotation

Start with slow controlled movement
Pivot to protect the knees

To perform:

- Stand in a neutral stance
- Lockout the knees with the quads
- Lockout the hips with gluteals
- Think about one of your shoulders and the opposite buttock
  If you start with moving your left shoulder back then you would think about that and the right buttock

- Pull your shoulder back and down toward the buttock
- The movement starts from top vertebrae going down
- Pull the opposite shoulder toward the shoulder that is moving back
- Follow with the head in the direction you're moving
- Reach maximum safe range
- In a controlled movement come back into a neutral starting position
- Perform the same for the opposite side

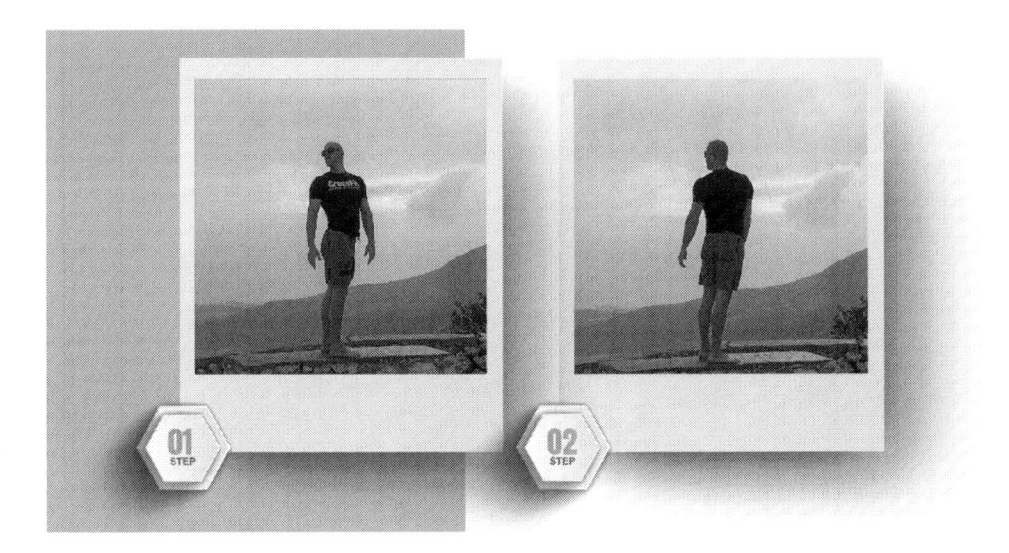

Arm circles

To perform:

- Stand in a neutral stance
- Let the arms hang beside the body
- Arms straight or slightly bend if shoulder flexibility is lacking
- Bring the arms back
- Follow through and create a circular motion forward with both arms

You can also go the opposite direction.

Jumping jacks

Go easy on the overhead position and ease into it as you get warmer.

To perform:

- Stand in a neutral stance
- Let the arms hang beside the body
- Bring the feet apart
- At the same time bring the arms up
- Bring the feet back in
- At the same time bring the arms back beside the body-part
- Repeat

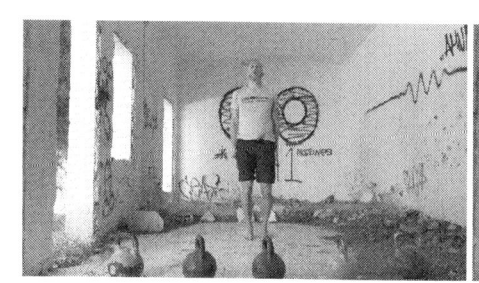

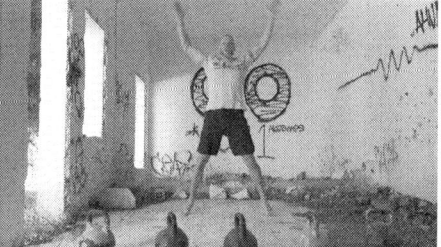

Duration

Your whole warm-up should take 5 to 6 minutes but that also depends on the weather, your state, etc. Increase duration as required.

Task

Your first task is to complete the warm-up as described above, you can do just one round or do more.

Submission

You can film your warm-up for feedback. Submit your video in any way possible. See chapter on *How to submit your assessment*.

Mind-muscle connection and muscle priming

MMC is all about connecting with the right muscles to perform the movement or stabilize for the movement, it is also used to relax the muscles that could be doing part of the work (isolation). Muscle priming is getting the muscles ready that will be doing the work and assists with MMC.

Muscle priming routine for the kettlebell swing:

- Prone bent single leg raises
- Kneeling hip extensions
- Prone back hyperextensions
- Quarter squats
- Calf raises
- Lat pull down
- Scapulae adduction

You're working out to put your muscles under stress. The more muscles you incorporate in your exercise the bigger results you're going to get. Recruit more muscles with MMC.

Prone bent single leg raises

Prone is lying face down.

You're connecting with your gluteus maximus.

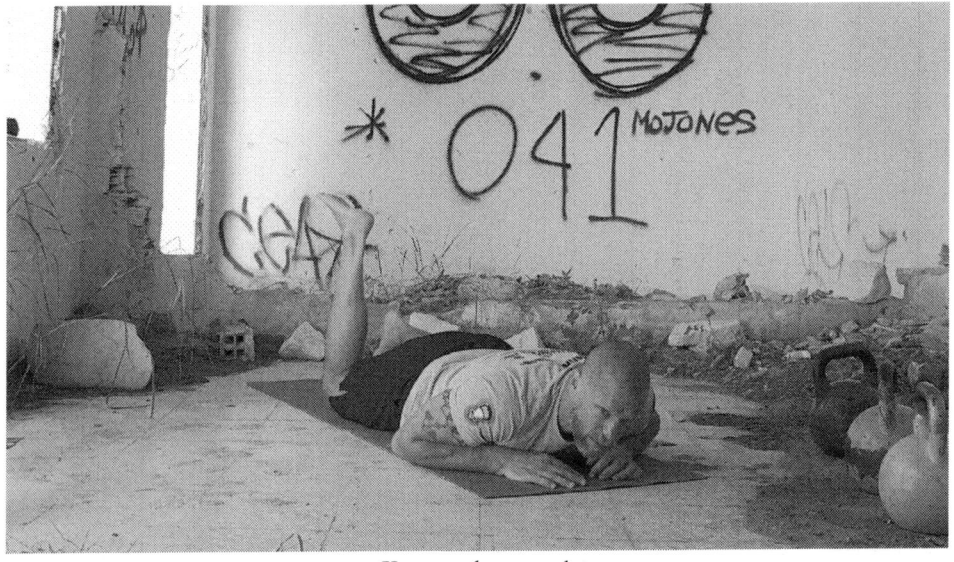

Knee on the ground

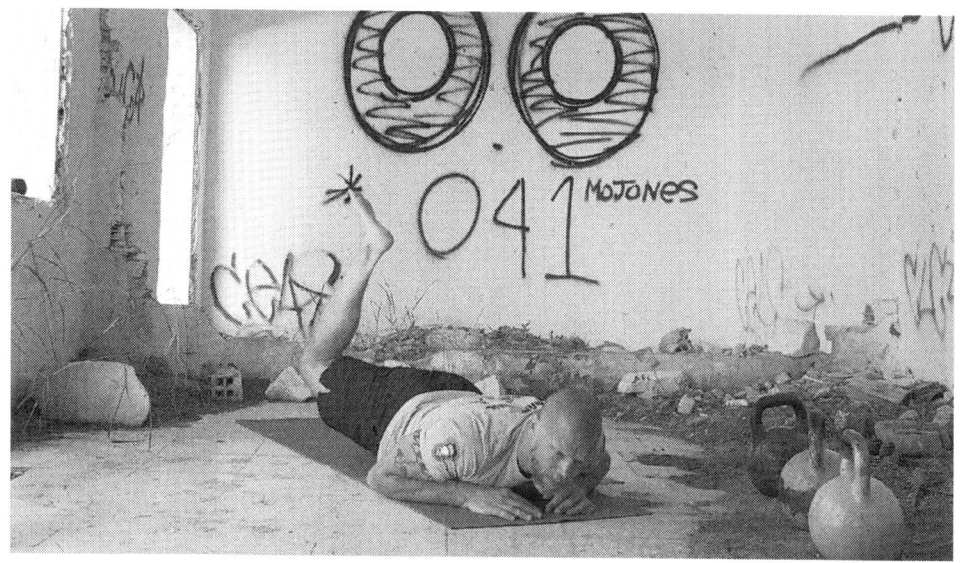

Knee raised and gluteus maximus contracted

Kneeling hip extensions

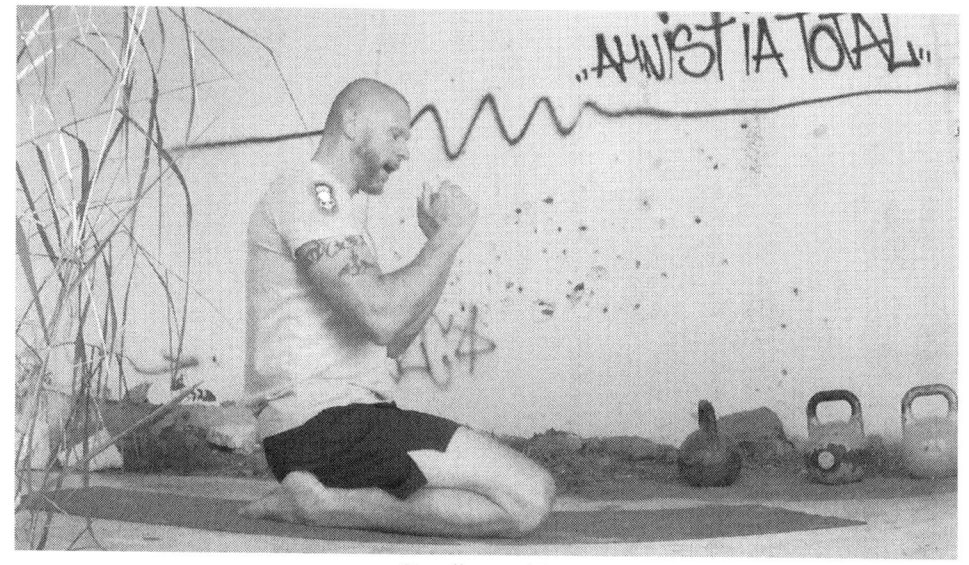

Kneeling position

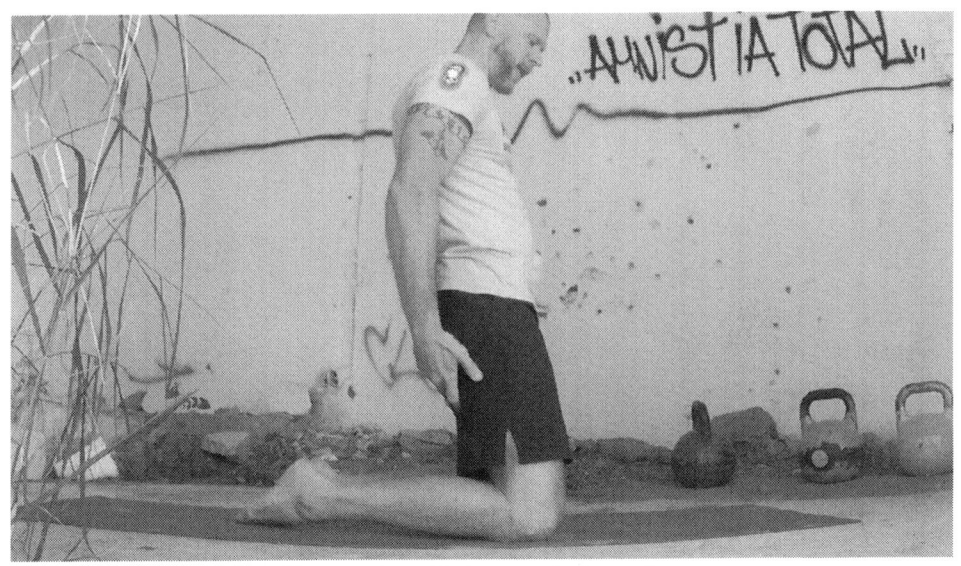

Hip extension with focus on the hamstrings

Prone back hyperextensions

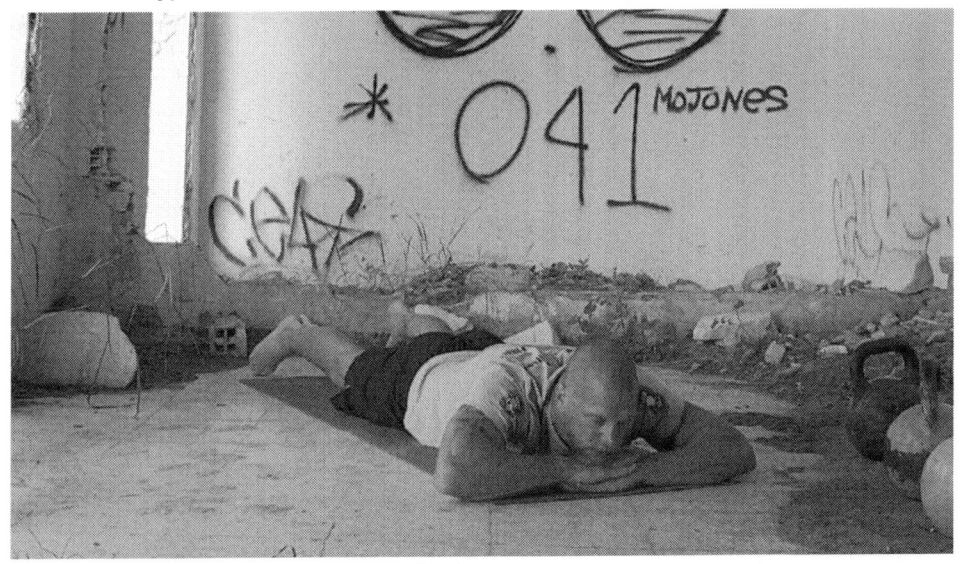

Laying prone

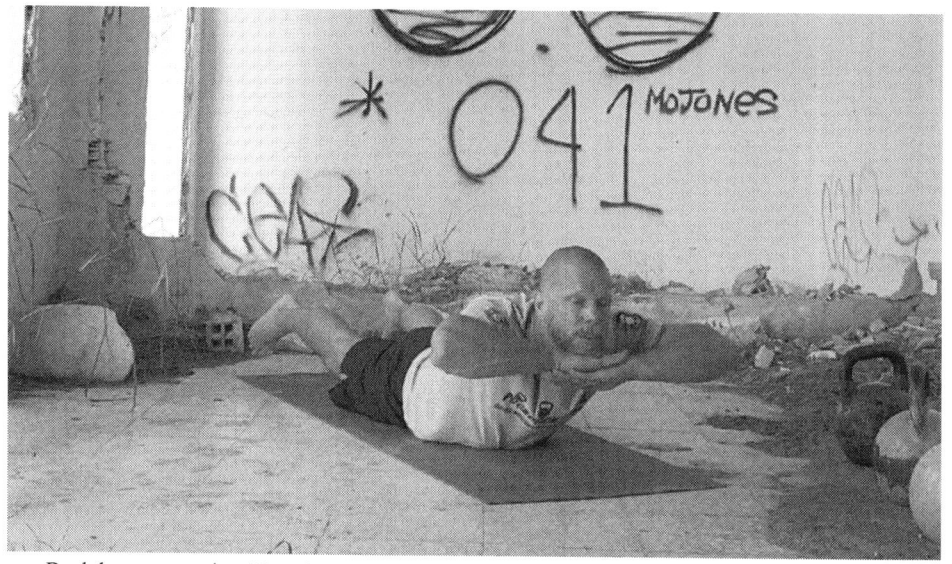

Back hyperextension. You do not need to go as shown, this takes a long time to get flexible. The objective is to connect with the back muscles which stay rigid to protect the spine during the swing.

Quarter squats

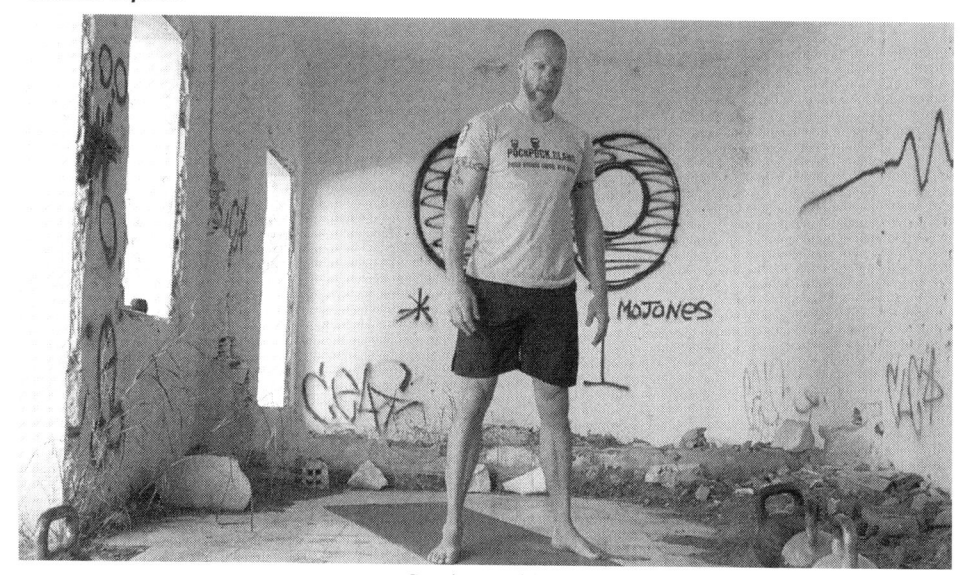

Starting position

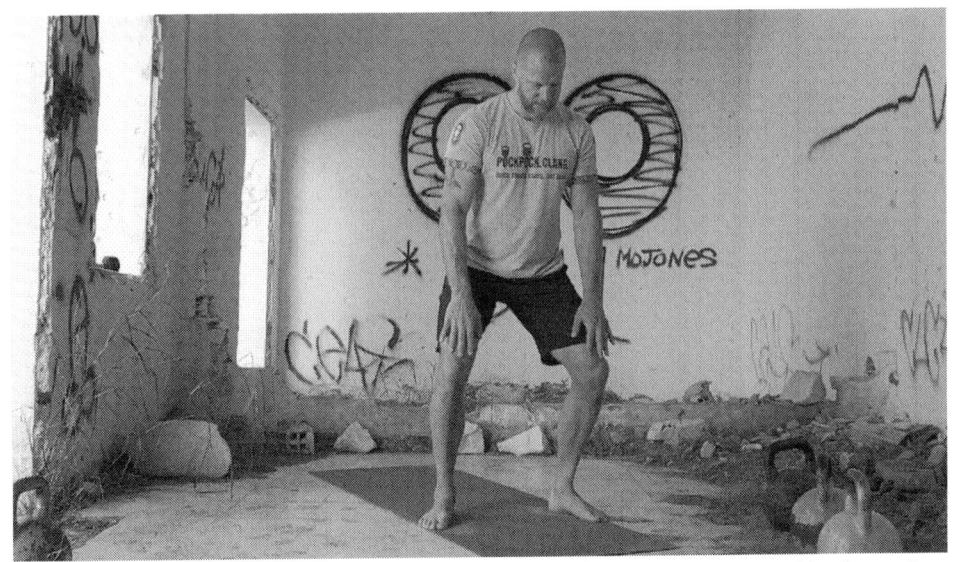

Quarter squat to connect with the area which will extend the knees and move the hips forward.

Calf raises

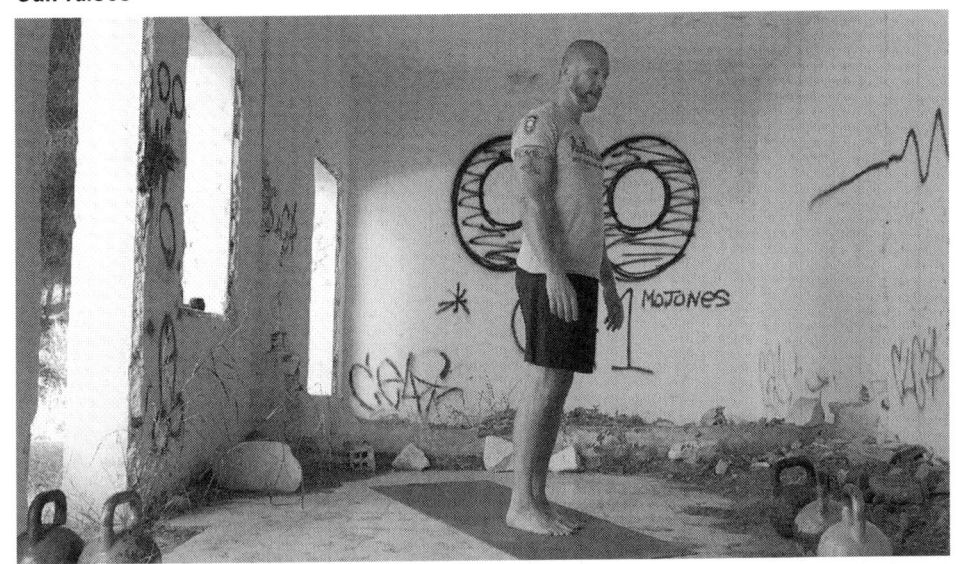

Starting position

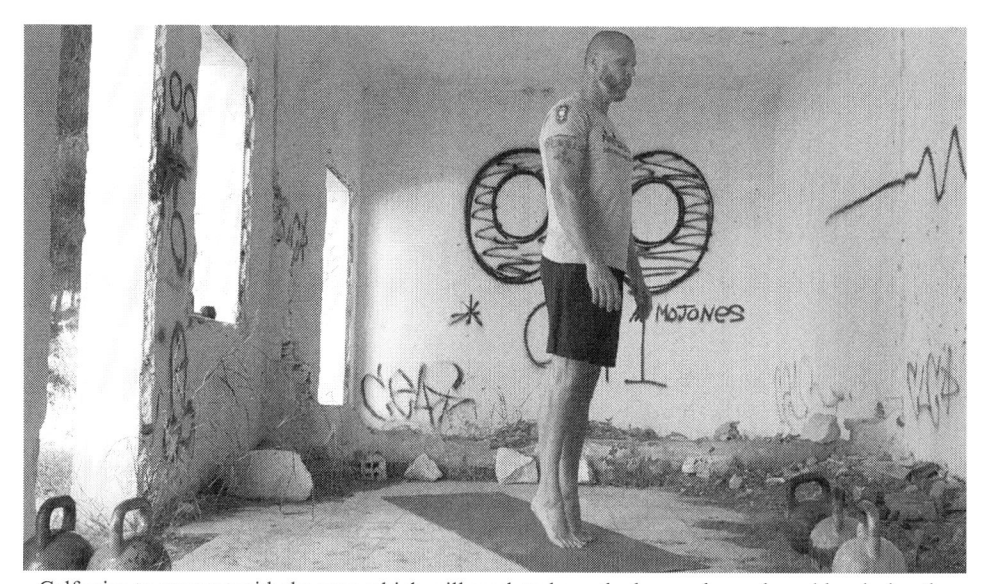

Calf raise to connect with the area which will work to keep the knees above the ankles during the swing.

Lat pull down

Hold on to something and lean to the side, then contract the lat and pull the elbow into the ribs.

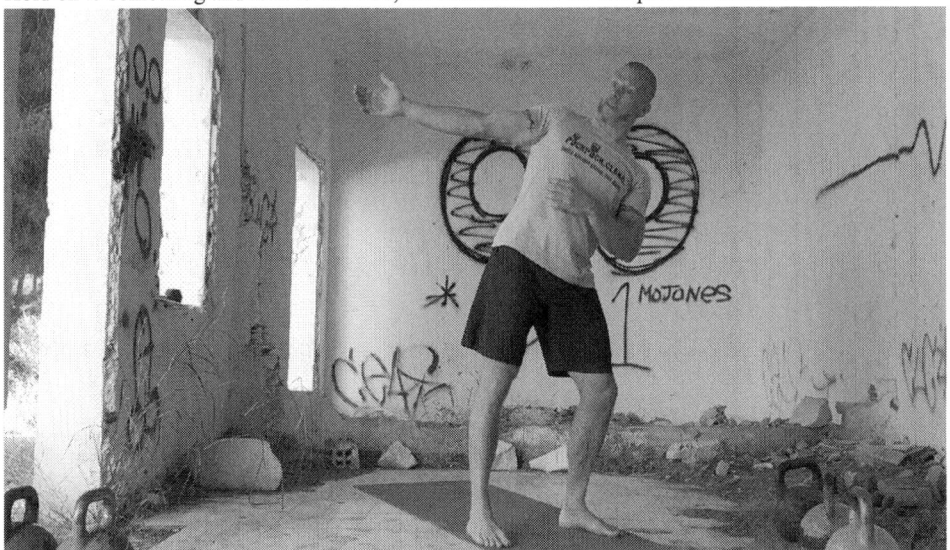

Lean to the side while holding on

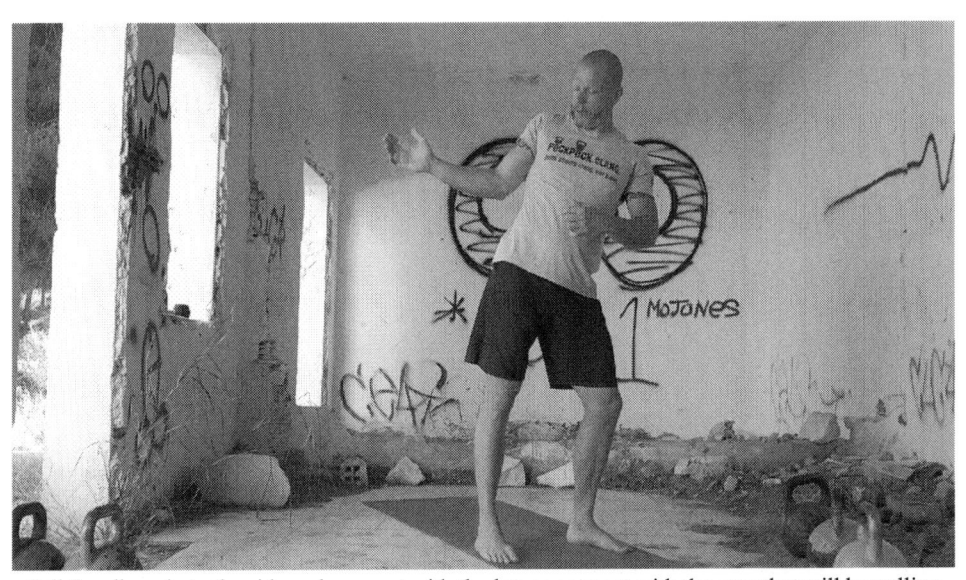

Pull the elbow in to the side and connect with the lats to connect with the area that will be pulling down to protect the shoulders during the swing with slight contraction.

Scapulae adduction

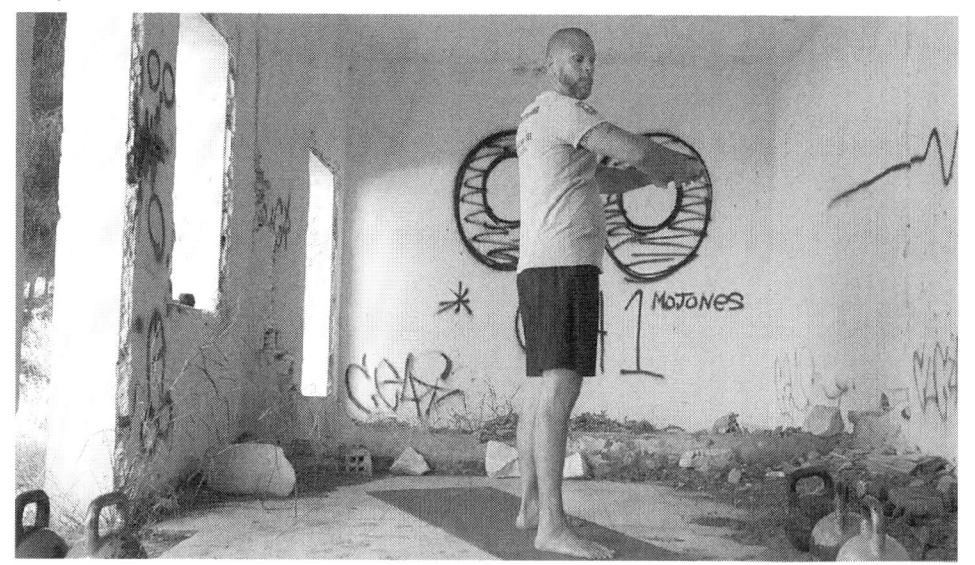

Starting position

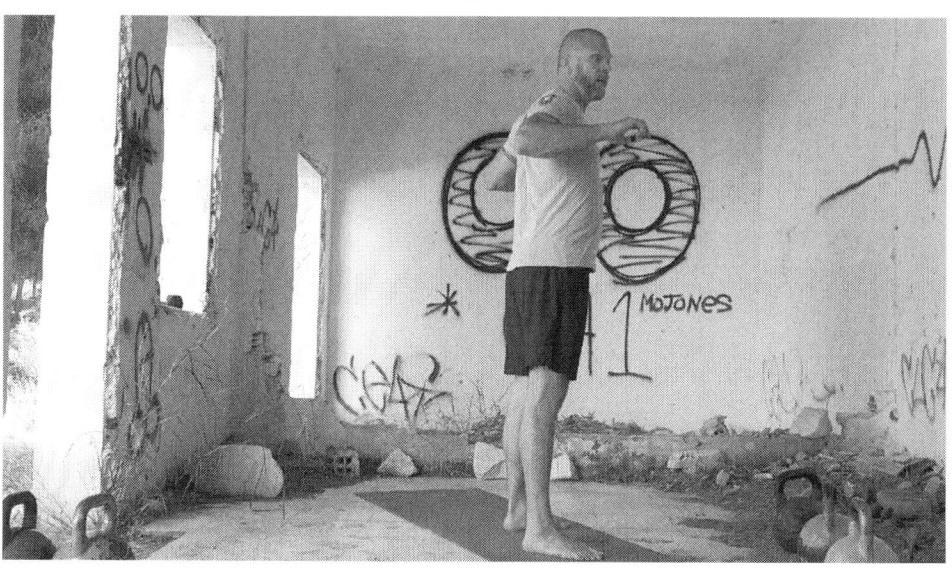

Pull the shoulder blades together and slightly down to connect with the area you want to contract at the top of the swing and slightly during.

Task

Your second task is to complete the muscle priming as per below.

- 5 x prone bent single leg raises each side
- 10 x kneeling hip extension
- 5 x prone back hyperextensions
- 10 seconds static back hyperextension
- 10 x quarter squats
- 10 x calf raises
- 5 x lat pull down each side
- 10 x scapulae adduction

Repeat twice.

Submission

You can film your priming for feedback. Submit your video in any way possible. See chapter on *How to submit your assessment.*

Day 2 Stretching and mobility for kettlebell training

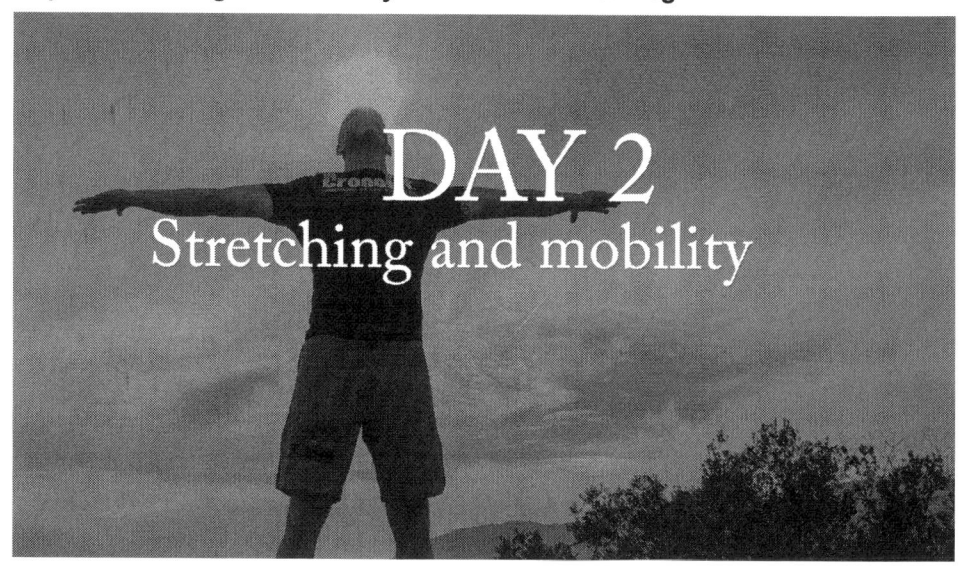

On day 2 you will learn how to stretch and perform some mobility work to increase performance and reduce chance of injury.

Stretching and mobility work is generally performed after working out, however, I recommend you incorporate it as much as you can, before, during, and after.

Dot points:

- Pulse into positions when you're still warming up
- Keep your stretches dynamic at the start of your session
- Increase time in the stretch as you progress through your session
- Internally rotate while kneeling to protect the knee
- Progress step-by-step into the Jefferson curl over a long period of time
- You do not want to feel stress in your lumbar
- The goal of an exercise can change by how you program and perform it
- You never want to feel any torque on the knees

Movements/stretches:

- Reverse lunge
- Reverse lunge arms overhead

- Reverse lunge and twist
- Runners lunge and twist
- Kneeling
- Kneeling and hip extension
- Kneeling and hip flexion with arms overhead
- Kneeling with hip abduction
- Jefferson curl
- Pigeon

Reverse lunge

To perform:

- Stand in a neutral stance
- Decide which leg is going to be supporting and which one is going to lunge back
- Shift your weight onto the supporting side
- Lunge back through sliding or hovering the foot back in position
- The distance back is as far back as possible while keeping the knee above or slightly behind the ankle at the front
- Keep the weight at the front as much as possible
- Use the back leg for balance only
- Aim to gently touch the ground with the back knee
- Spend a short moment in the full lunge position and press the ball of the lunging foot into the ground
- Gently push the hips forward to benefit from the hip flexor stretch
- Your weight is still on the supporting leg
- Press the supporting foot into the ground and contract the quads and gluteals to come back up

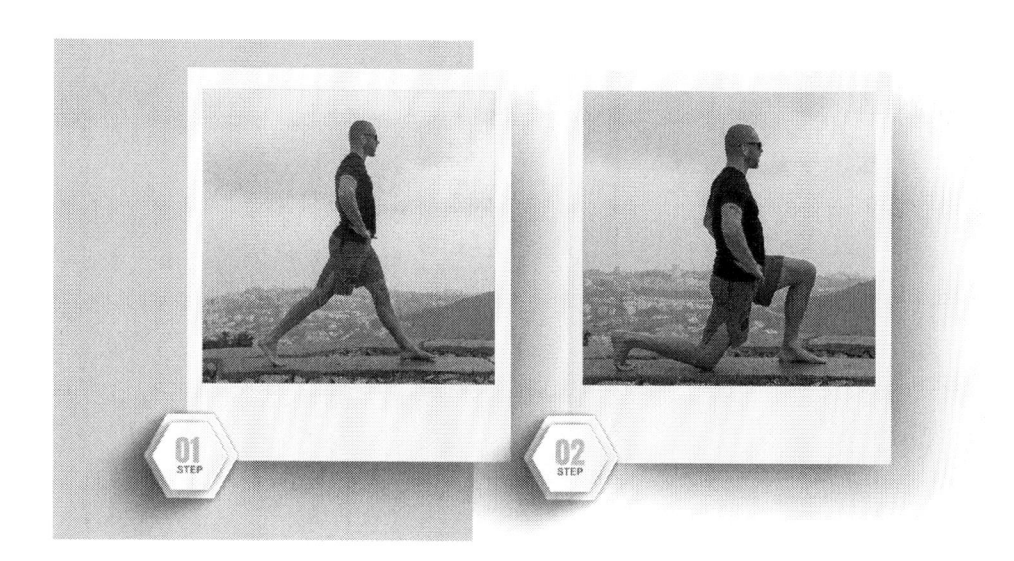

Reverse lunge arms overhead

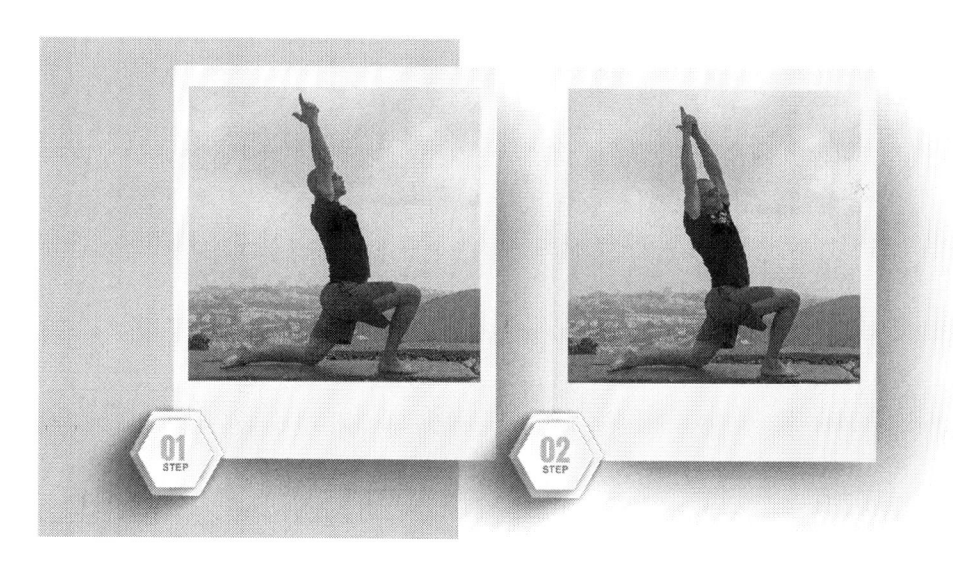

Reverse lunge and twist

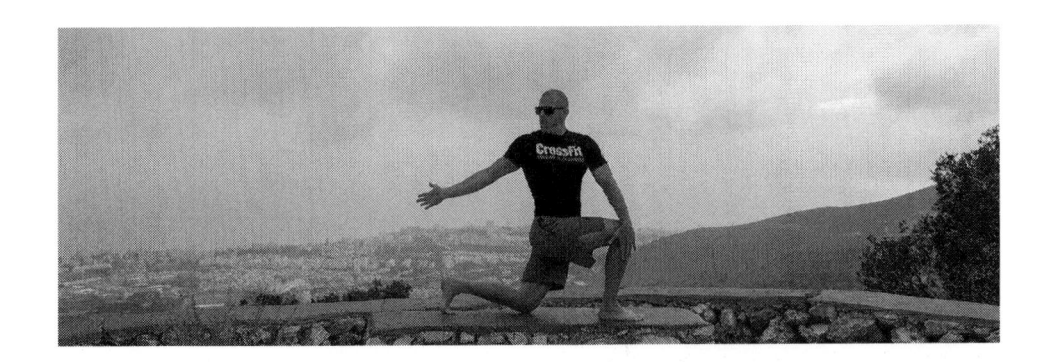

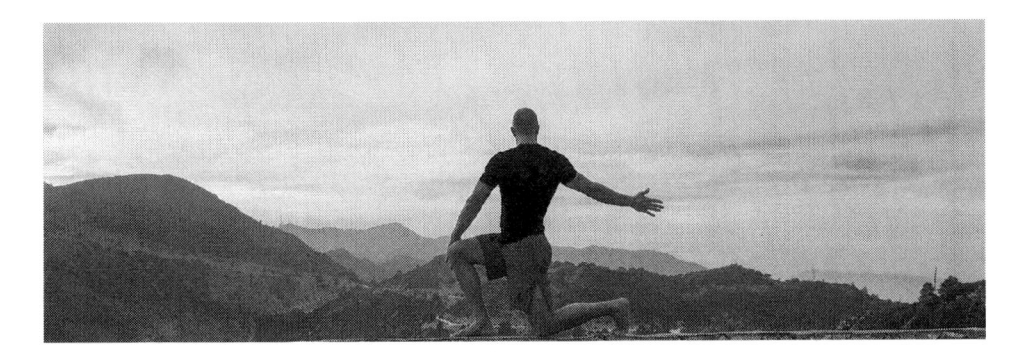

Benefits:

- Strength
- Stability
- Hip flexor stretch
- Ball of the foot stretch

Runners lunge and twist

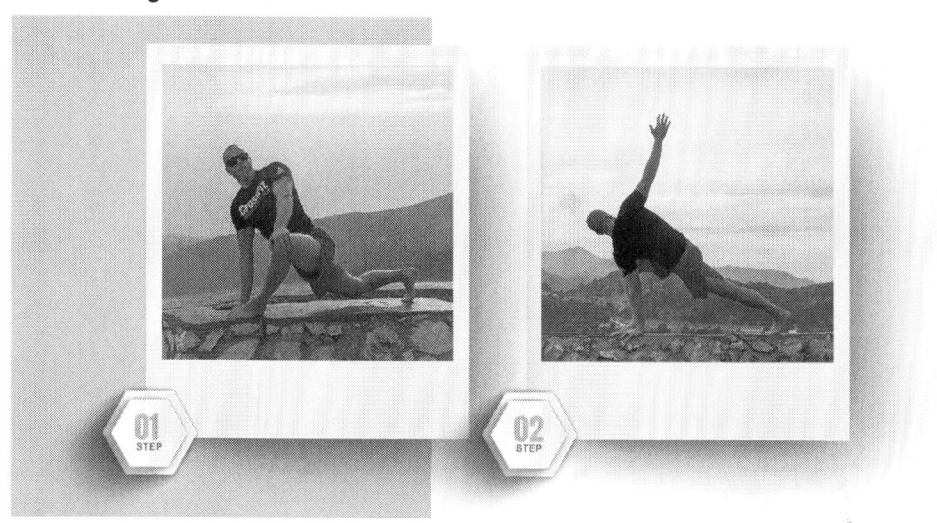

Kneeling

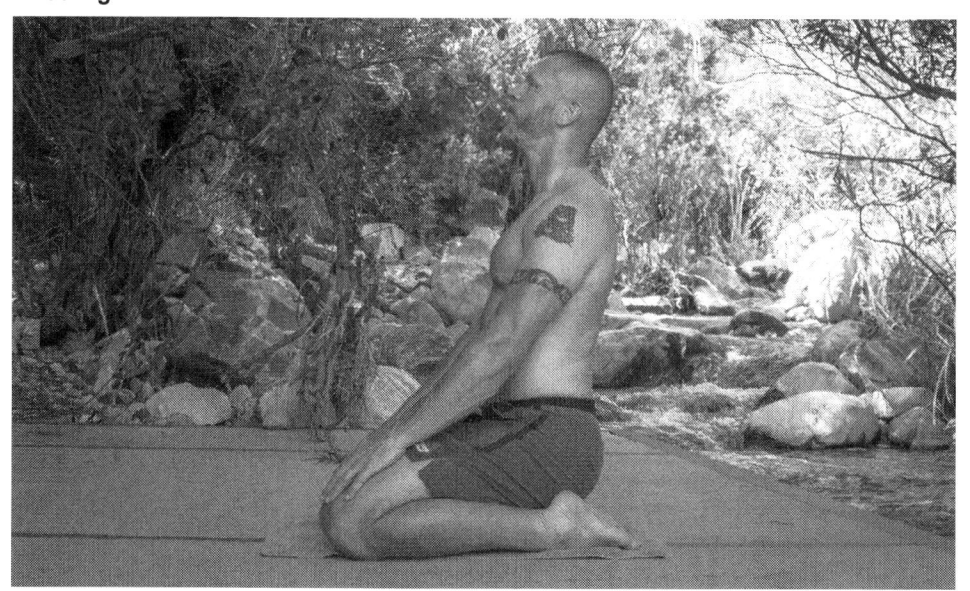

Your goal is to get the dorsum of the feet flat on the ground.

Kneeling and hip extension

You're working up to kneeling and leaning back with hip extension to get a deeper hip flexor stretch.

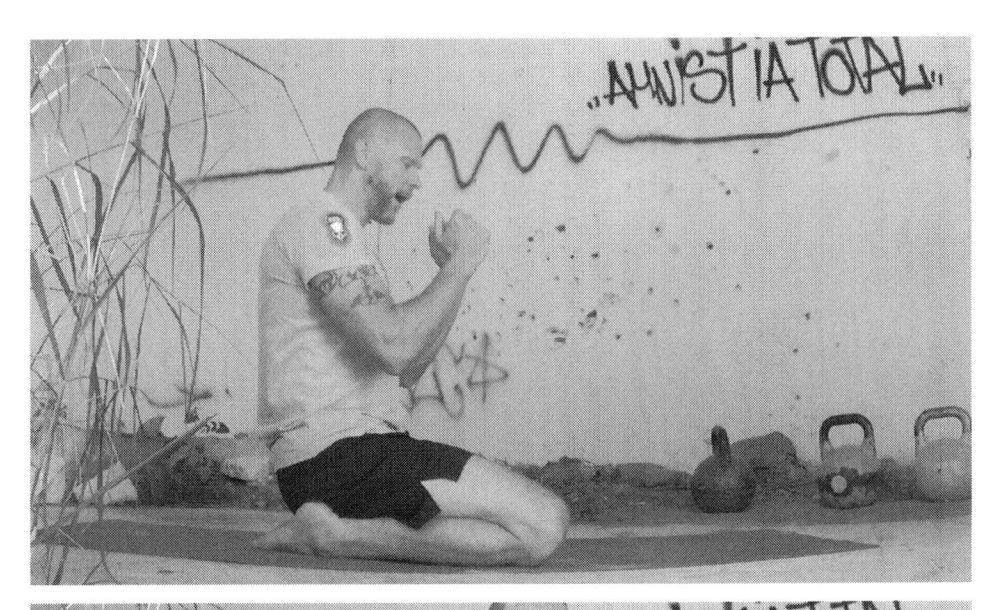

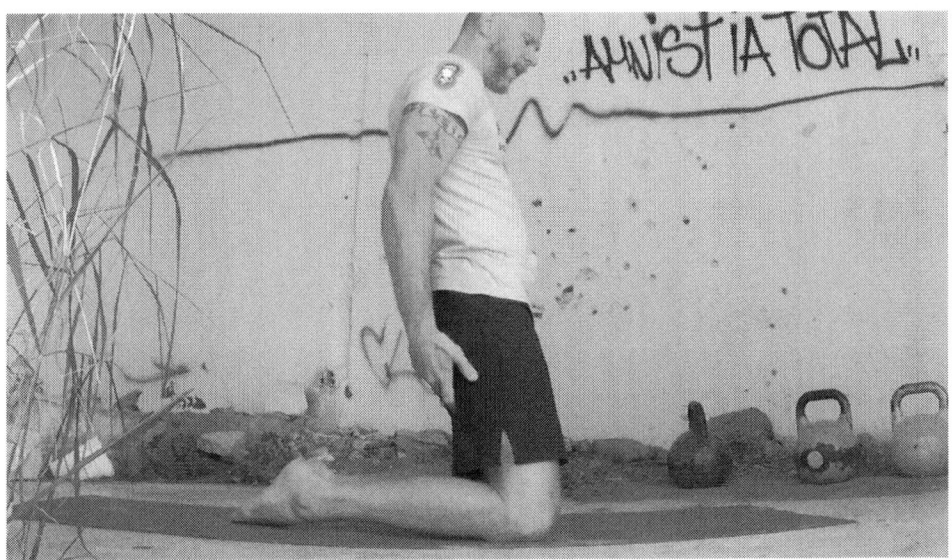

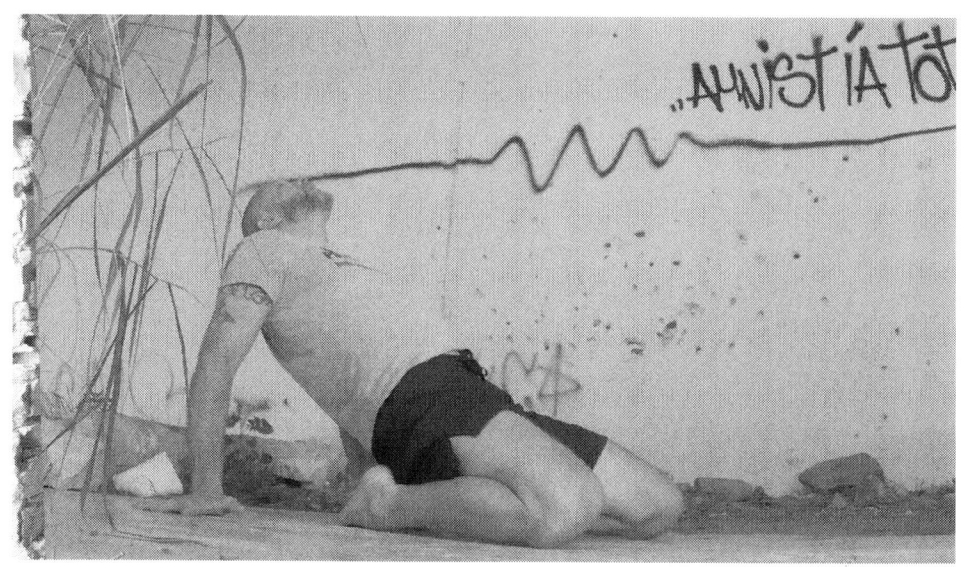

This is where you want to work up to or if you already have the flexibility go straight into this pose.

Kneeling and hip flexion with arms overhead

Same as above staring kneeling position but with the arms overhead, if possible, with the palms together.

Kneeling with hip abduction

Same as above starting kneeling position but with the knees further apart.

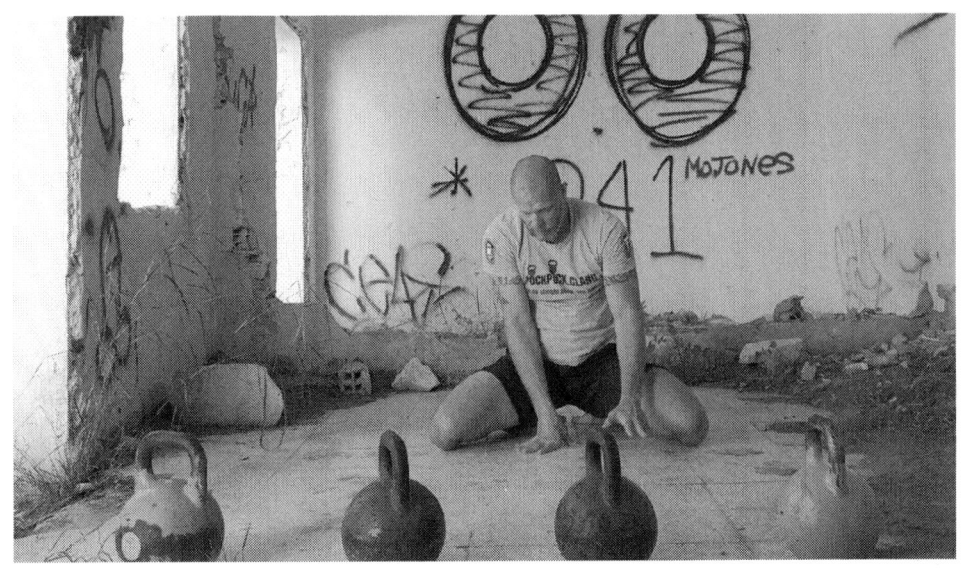

This position is to get into the hip adductors.

Jefferson curl

Step-by-step

- Neutral stance
- Let your arms relax and hang
- Gently press the heels into the ground creating slight tension between the ankles and hips
- Slightly contract the glutes to keep the pelvis aligned vertically
- Start flexing/curling at the top between the thoracic and cervical (neck) spine
- All movement in the spine will be from the top down vertebra by vertebra
- Let your shoulders droop forward
- Your head comes along through flexion at the cervical
- Connect with the muscles at the back and feel each vertebra enter near max flexion
- Continue moving down the thoracic spine
- Leave the lumbar alone and without flexion
- Move to the hips and create hip flexion
- Actively pull the pelvis down toward the ground
- Continue to near max range of hip flexion
- Don't go to the point of pain in the hamstrings
- Keep the legs vertically aligned
- Reach for your toes with the hands
- Don't rush the range
- Time to come back up
- Reverse everything you've done
- Start at the hips
- Pull the pelvis up from the bottom with the hamstrings and adductor magnus
- Pull the pelvis up from the top with the gluteus maximus
- Follow through with each vertebra until in neutral vertical stance

Feel the muscles, engage the muscles, connect with the muscles.

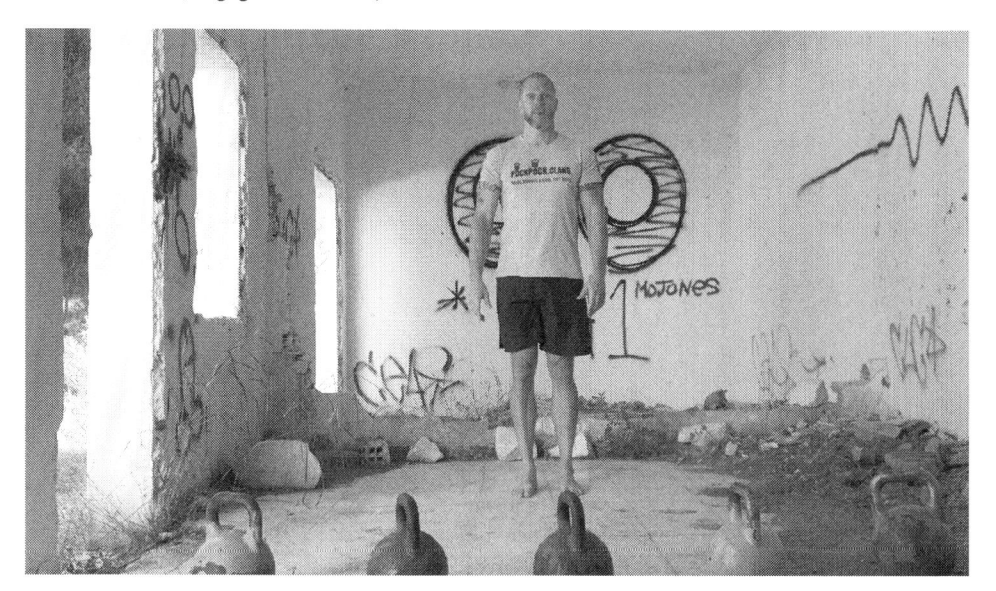

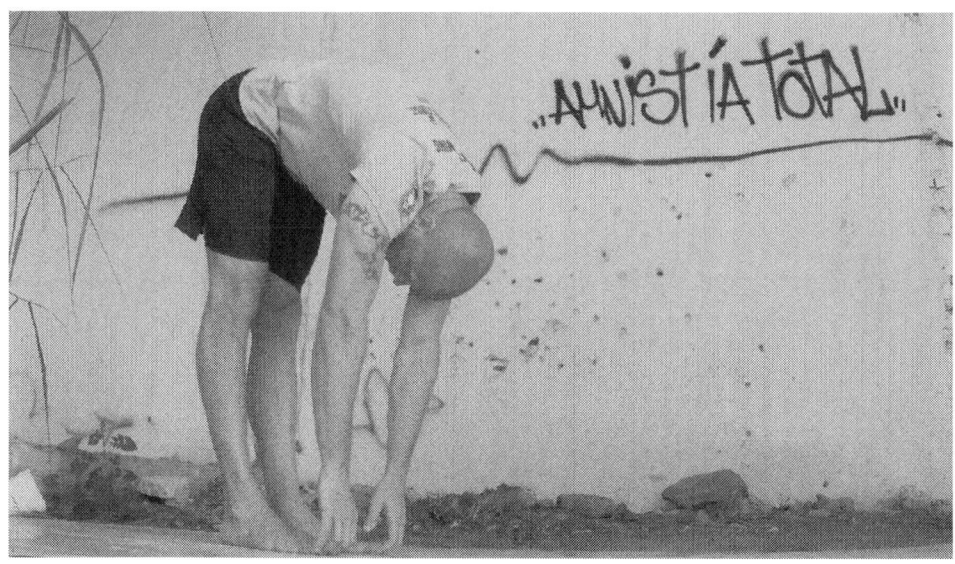

Pigeon

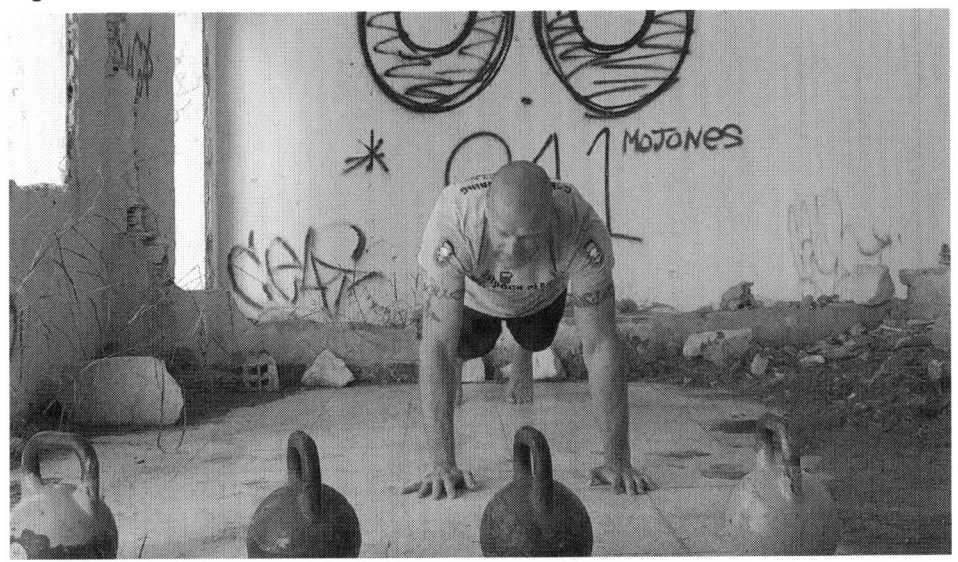

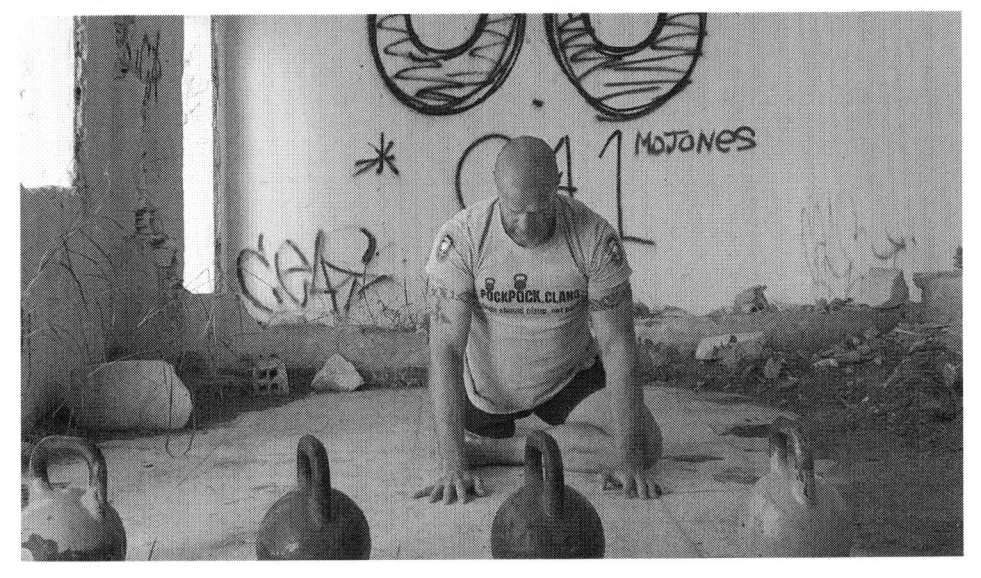

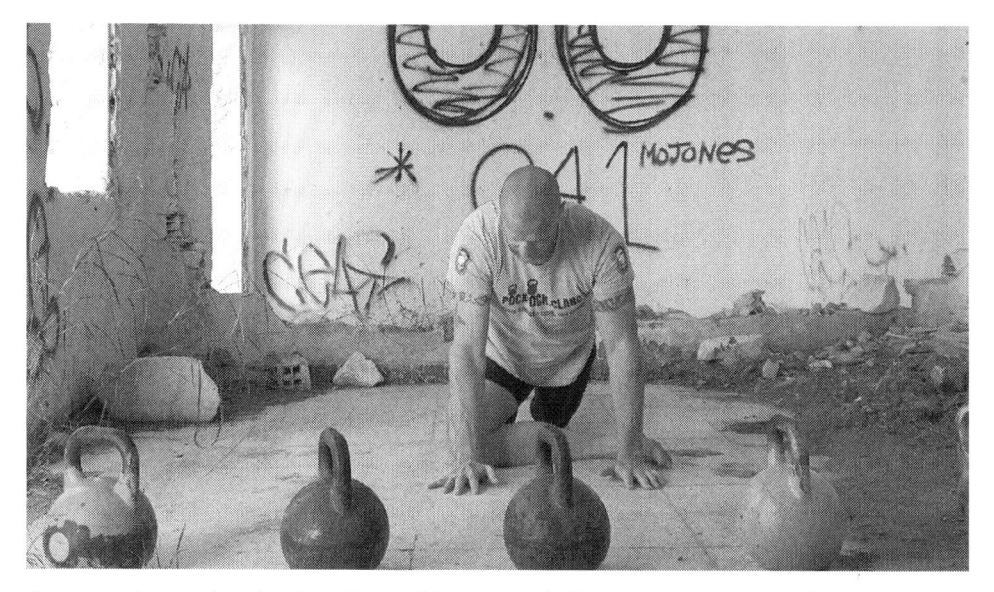

Great stretch to get into the glutes but avoid torque on the knee and create external hip rotation to protect the knees.

Mobility

Mobility is a combination of flexibility, strength, stability, coordination, proprioception, and more, in short, it's defined by how easily you can perform the movement and what ROM can you reach. Slow down your movements to focus on mobility.

Feet

Your feet are super important for balance, performance, stability, spend time on your feet. It's recommended not to train with kettlebells in runners. Ankle circles, calf raises, and Hindu squats are great to train and work on the feet.

Task

Your third task is to complete some stretching and mobility work as per below.

Warm up first

First round:

- 2 x reverse lunge both sides
- 4 x alternating pigeon
- 5 x reverse lunge arms overhead both sides
- 3 x Jefferson curl

- 5 x reverse lunge and twist both sides
- 4 x alternating pigeon
- 3 x runners lunge and twist both sides
- 5 x kneeling and hip extension
- 5 x kneeling and hip flexion with arms overhead
- 3 x Jefferson curl

The first round was more dynamic, moving in and out of positions, and your second round will be slightly longer holds at the end of movements. All movements are to be performed slowly and controlled.

Second round:

- 2 x reverse lunge both sides
- 3 x alternating pigeon
- 2 x reverse lunge arms overhead both sides
- 2 x Jefferson curl
- 2 x reverse lunge and twist both sides
- 3 x alternating pigeon
- 2 x runners lunge and twist both sides
- 4 x kneeling and hip extension
- 3 x kneeling and hip flexion with arms overhead
- 2 x Jefferson curl

Third round:

- Reverse lunge both sides
- Pigeon both sides
- Reverse lunge arms overhead both sides
- Jefferson curl
- Reverse lunge and twist both sides
- Alternating pigeon
- Runners lunge and twist both sides
- Kneeling and hip flexion with arms overhead
- Jefferson curl

10 to 15-second hold for each position.

Submission

You can film your stretching and mobility work for feedback. Submit your video in any way possible. See chapter on How to submit your assessment.

Day 3 Kettlebell anatomy and grip

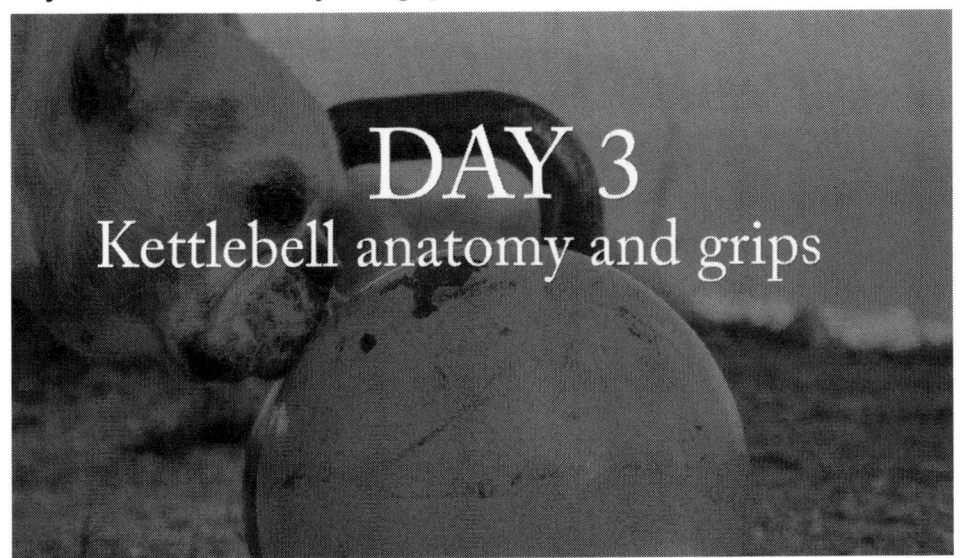

On day 3 you will learn about the anatomy of the kettlebell and grips which is the first important information you should know to progress with your kettlebell training. I'll also cover some exercises for wrist strength.

There are over 25 kettlebell grips, I will cover the common kettlebell grips:

- Hook grip
- Closed hook grip
- Double hand grip
- Closed double hand grip

Kettlebell anatomy:

- Handle
- Horn(s)
- Window
- Bell
- Base

ANATOMY OF THE KETTLEBELL

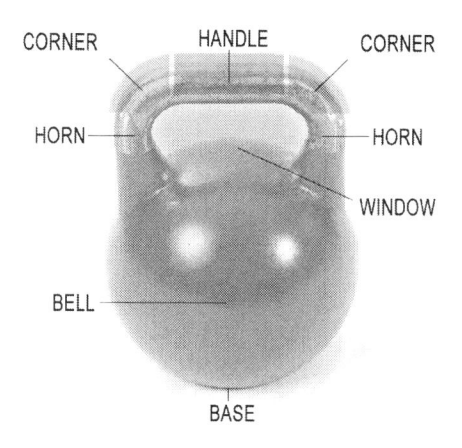

Labels: CORNER, HANDLE, CORNER, HORN, HORN, WINDOW, BELL, BASE

ILLUSTRATED: COMPETITION KETTLEBELL

Grip is usually the first point of failure on high reps snatches or swings with correct technique.

Other points:

- A kettlebell grip should be loose but tight enough to hold on to the kettlebell
- You can work your grip strength by holding the kettlebell in the tips of the fingers
- Wrist strength is often overlooked in training
- You can work on lateral wrist flexion with the kettlebell on the ground and base pointing up
- When you first start training make sure you ease into reps and weight
- Progress slowly and rest enough so you can keep training
- You can work wrist flexion and extension while standing and letting the bell hang next to you
- Stretch your forearms after working out
- Grip is relaxed at the top of the swing

You can download a FREE PDF with over 25 kettlebell grips in it from our website here.

Day 4 Safely lifting the kettlebell with a squat

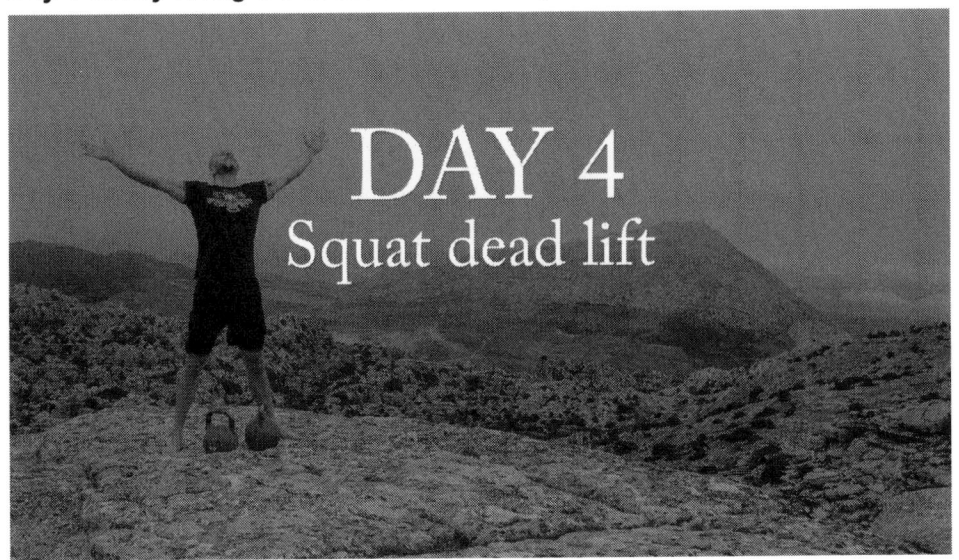

Dot points:

- Deadlift means that the weight starts dead on the ground and is then lifted
- Dead means that the weight is not moving
- Shoulders high and hips low with the squat while pushing the hips toward the ground
- Maintain good aligned between the three joints during the squat
- The knee is a hinge joint that only flexes and extends
- Don't reach out for the weight
- Protect the spine during lifts with a rigid structure
- Perform the hang lift to work on flexibility and range
- If the shoulders come low while the hips stay high then you are not squatting but hip hinging
- Range and technique before weight and reps

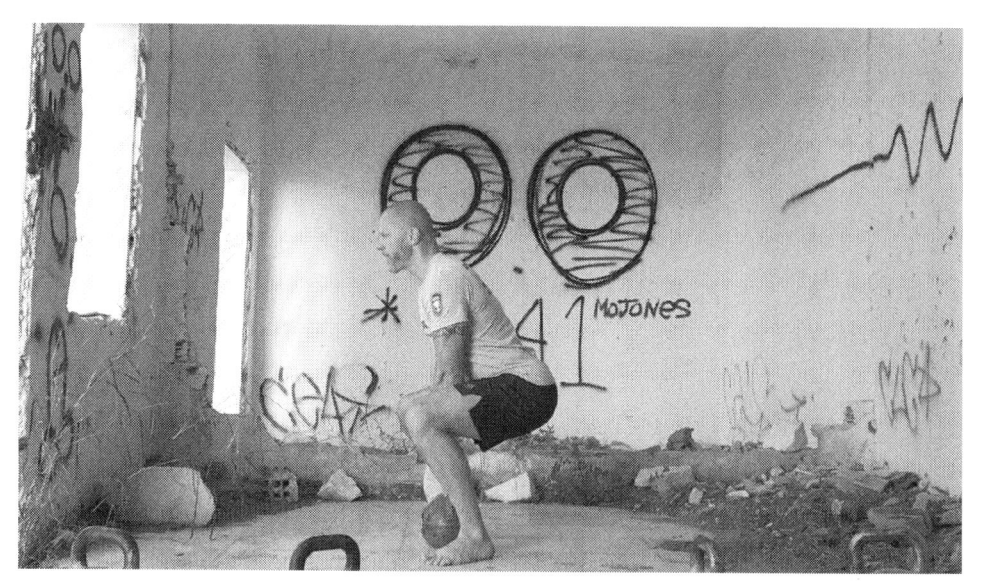

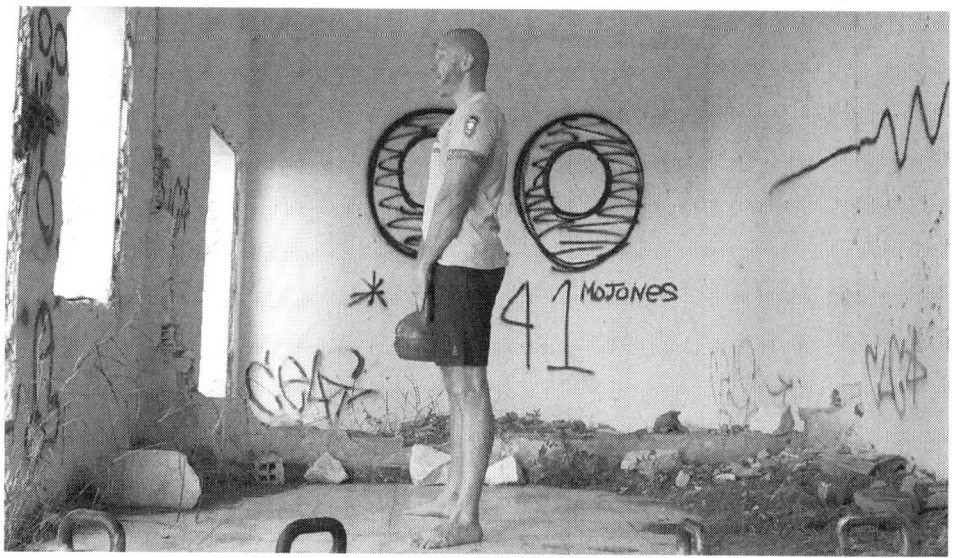

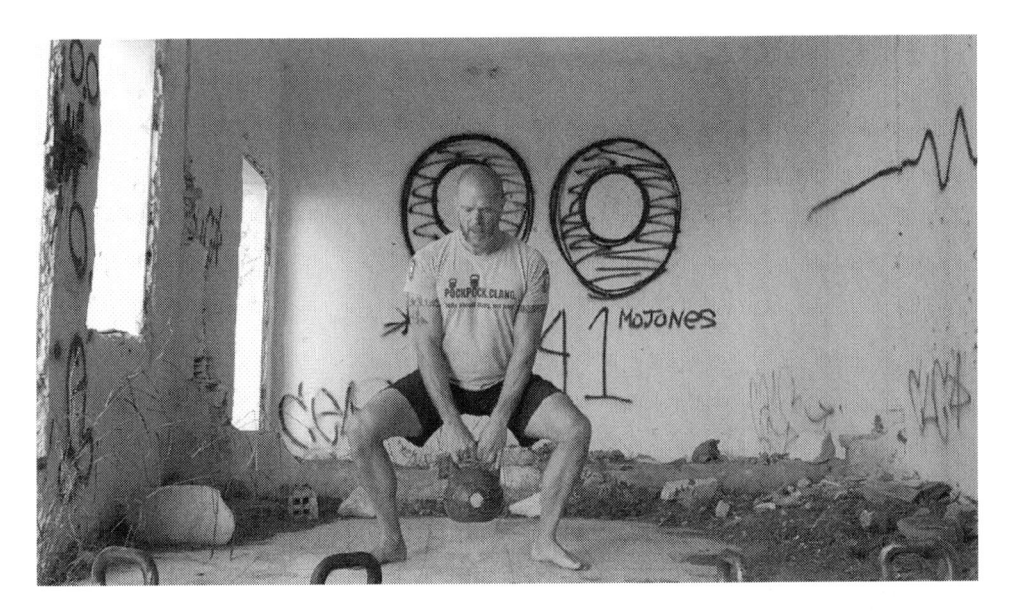

Task

Your fourth task is to complete several sets of the squat dead lift as per below.

Warm up first.

If your form and technique is already close to good then perform 8 reps of the dead lift otherwise regress to 4 reps of the hang lift.

Perform the reps on one side and then rest for 15 to 30 seconds or do 1 minute of mobility work like for example some dynamic pigeon, kneeling hip extensions (focus on working butt to the ground), or reverse lunge and pulse with arms overhead. After the rest you perform a set on the other side. Perform 8 to 12 sets in total.

If you've used your rest time for mobility work then you've already done your stretching for the day, otherwise, end with some stretching.

Submission

You can film your squat dead lift for feedback. Submit your video in any way possible. See chapter on How to submit your assessment.

Day 5 Safely lifting the kettlebell with a hip hinge

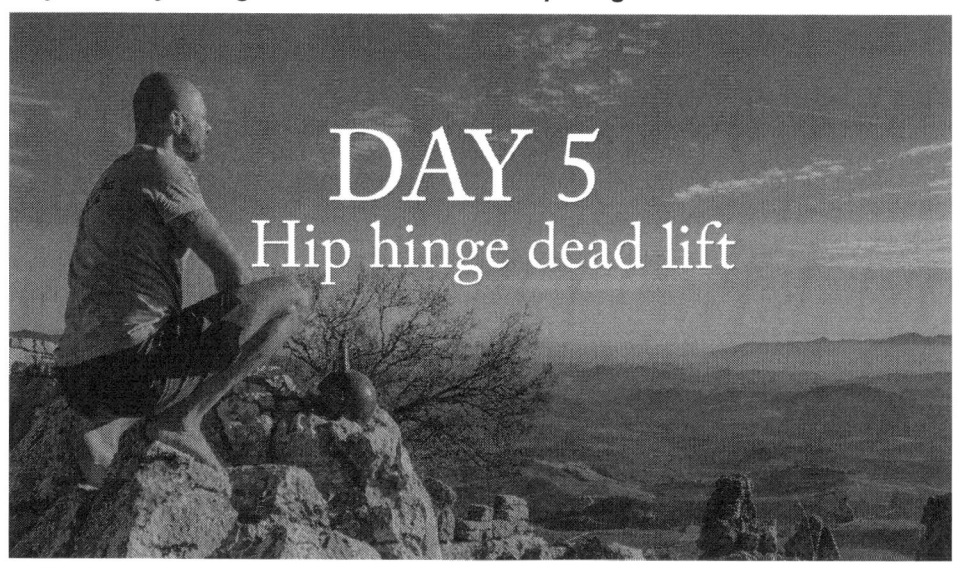

DAY 5
Hip hinge dead lift

Dot points:

- The hip hinge is the most common movement used for deadlifting
- The hip hinge is performed with one or two joints
- The knees stay above the ankles when hinging
- The top of the pelvis is pulled up with the gluteus maximus
- The pull at the bottom of the pelvis is created by the hamstrings (3 muscles) and the adductor magnus
- First master the bodyweight hip hinge before adding weight to the movement
- The weight should be positioned under the shoulder while in the hinge
- Do not bend the back to reach for the weight
- Perform the hip hinge hang lift if you're working on range (3HL)
- Don't hold your breath during the lift
- Brace your core to protect the spine
- Keep your spine straight throughout the lift
- The hip hinge deadlift is better to be performed for strength with slow focussed movement

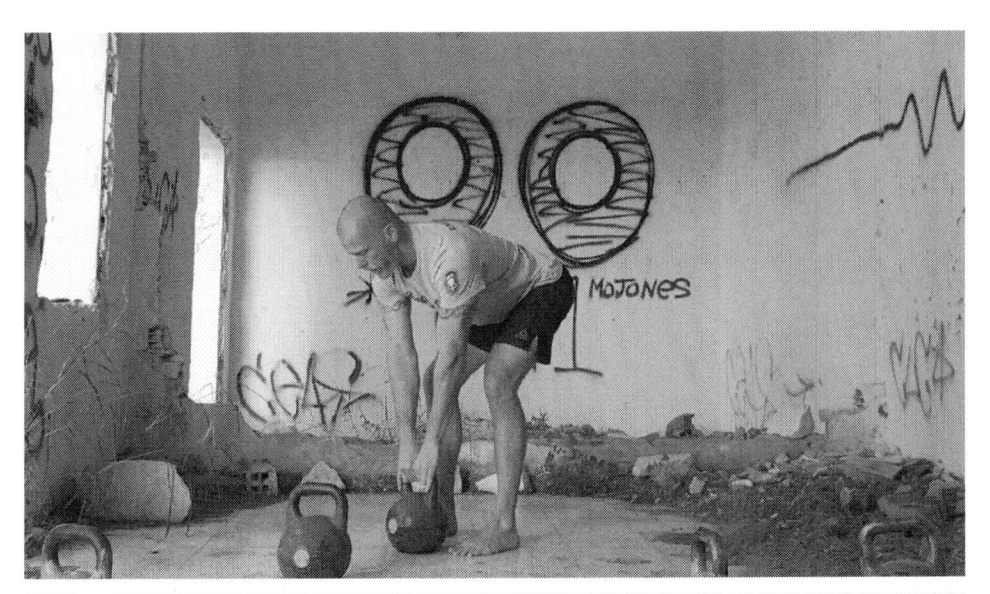

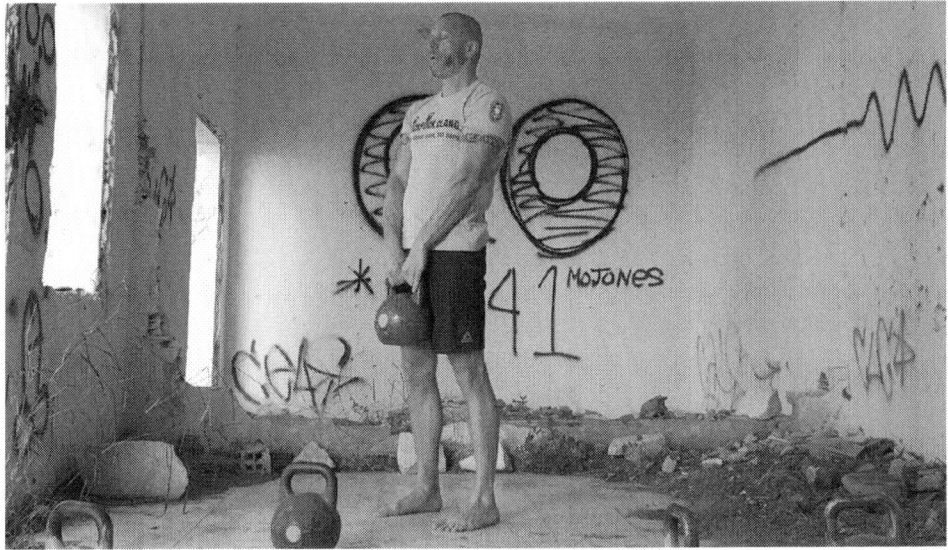

Task

Your fifth task is to complete several sets of the hip hinge dead lift as per below.

Warm up first.

If your form and technique is already close to good then perform 8 reps of the dead lift otherwise regress to 4 reps of the hang lift.

Perform the reps on one side and then rest for 15 to 30 seconds or do 1 minute of mobility work like for example some dynamic pigeon, kneeling hip extensions (focus on working butt to the ground), or reverse lunge and pulse with arms overhead. After the rest you perform a set on the other side. Perform 8 to 12 sets in total.

If you've used your rest time for mobility work then you've already done your stretching for the day, otherwise end with some stretching.

Submission

You can film your hip hinge dead lift for feedback. Submit your video in any way possible. See chapter on How to submit your assessment.

Day 6 Assisted kettlebell clean

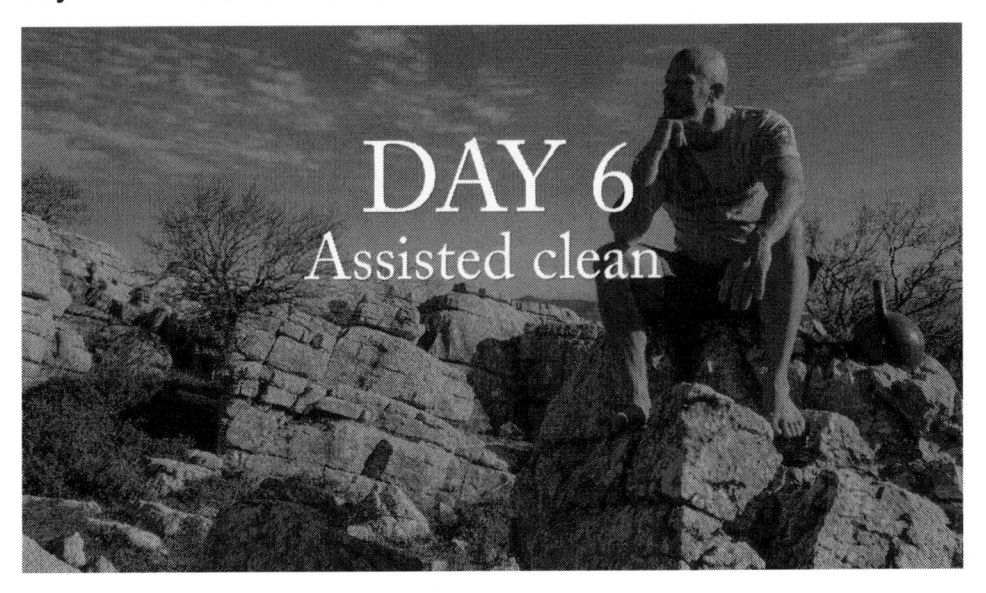

Dot points:

- The assisted clean is performed with a squat
- This drill is super important and will flow through in more advanced progressions
- A clean brings a weight from lower into racking position
- The assisted clean is to be performed slow and controlled to learn the movement and positions
- Eventually you will progress to an explosive movement
- Cleans are explosive apart from the assisted clean which is a drill
- The assisted clean is to teach hand insertion and racking
- Raise the weight with a box if you're working on flexibility
- Open the hand and let the bell come around the hand
- Skip the palm to avoid friction
- No need to look at the weight you know where it is
- Elbow pulled in tight on the rack
- A broken wrist grip is where the line is broken at the wrist
- Racking and bell pressure on the forearm requires some conditioning
- Don't overtrain but gradually increase duration and reps
- Don't put the non working arm/hand on the body during a lift
- Create good form and technique
- Create good habits
- Drill the insert on the ground
- Take note of where the arm should be positioned after the insert

- Use a weight easy enough to handle (light to medium)
- Progress slowly step by step
- Drill drill drill

Assisted clean:
- Squat
- Hook grip
- Lift
- Full extension
- Slight curl
- Assist with the other hand
- Lift the weight up
- Open the hand
- Roll the kettlebell over
- Hand insert
- Rack
- Reverse with assistance
- Pull out
- Hook grip
- Full arm extension into squat
- Lower the weight to dead

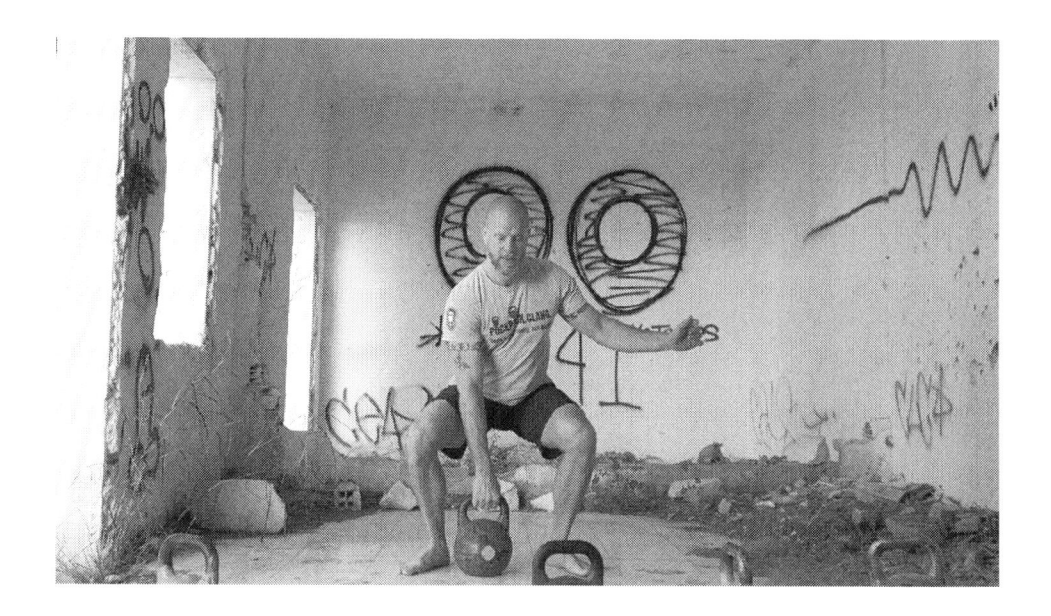

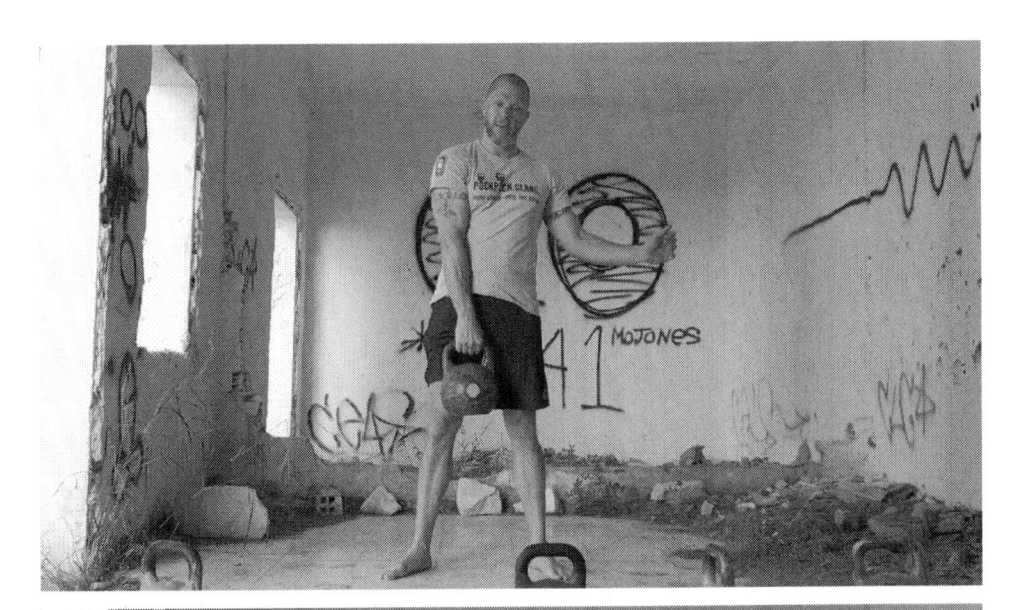

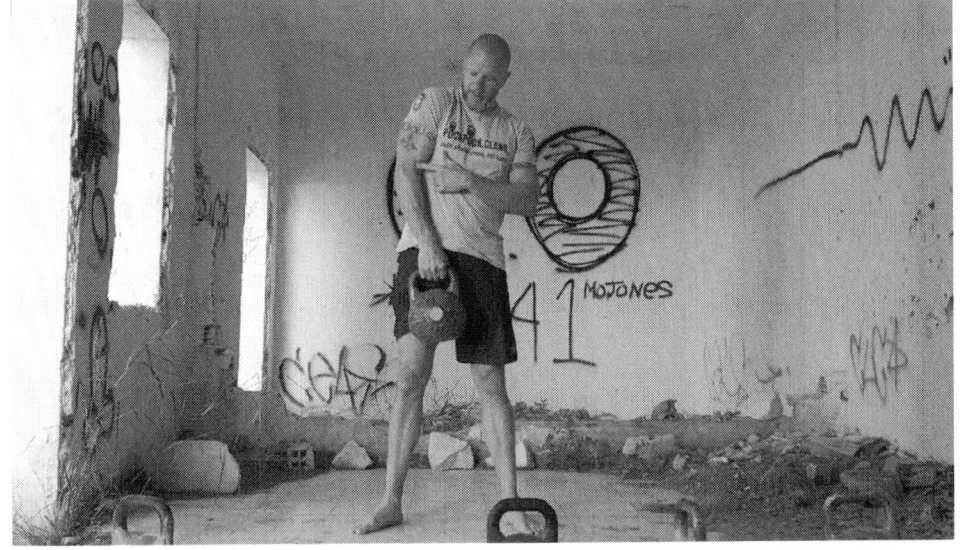

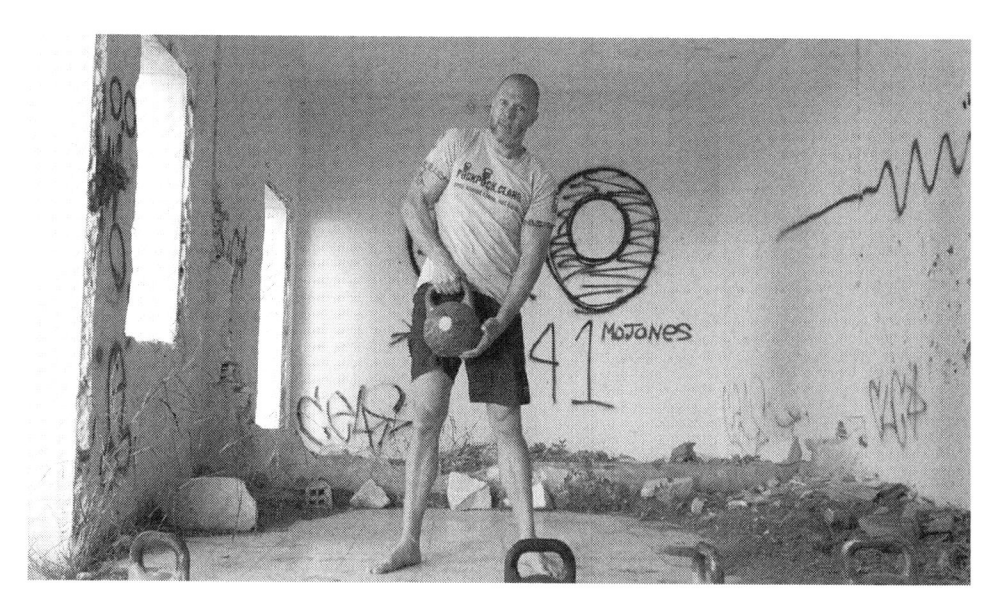

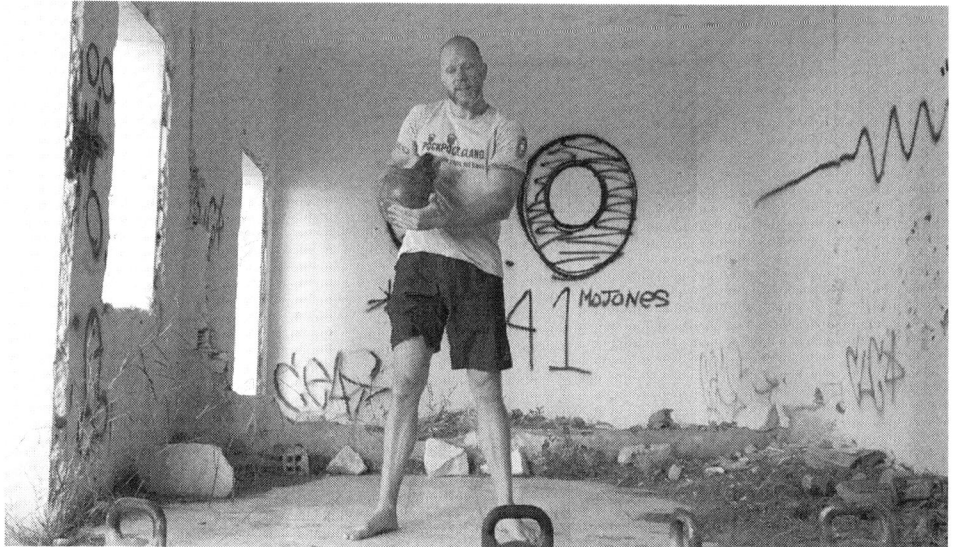

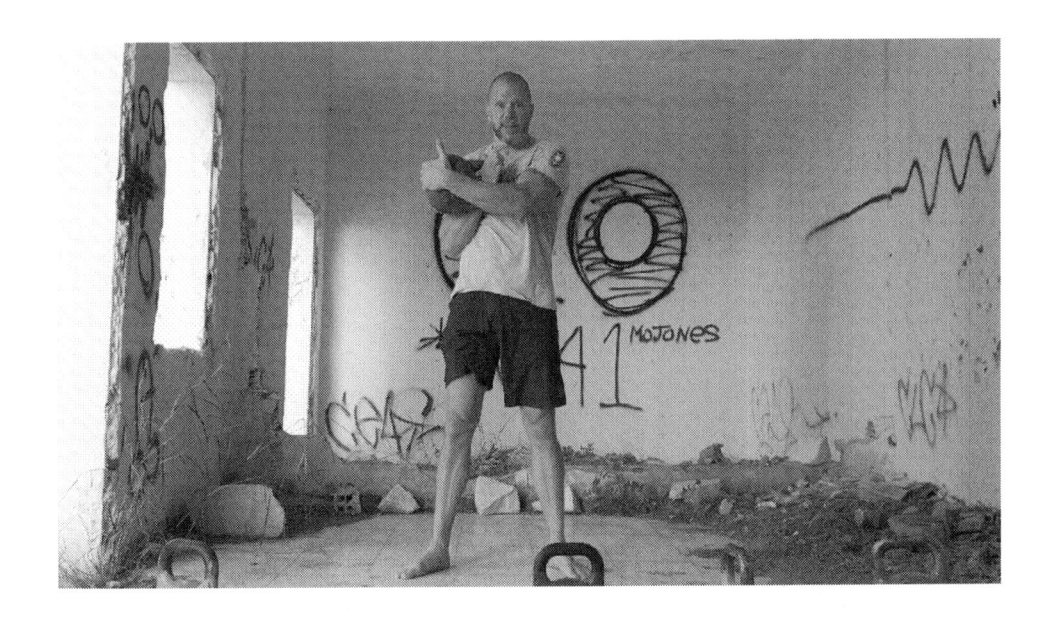

Double hand dead swing clean

The double hand clean is great for beginners but also used with heavy weights or in kettlebell sport where endurance and energy preservation is important. You should wait till hip hinge swing is covered before attempting this one.

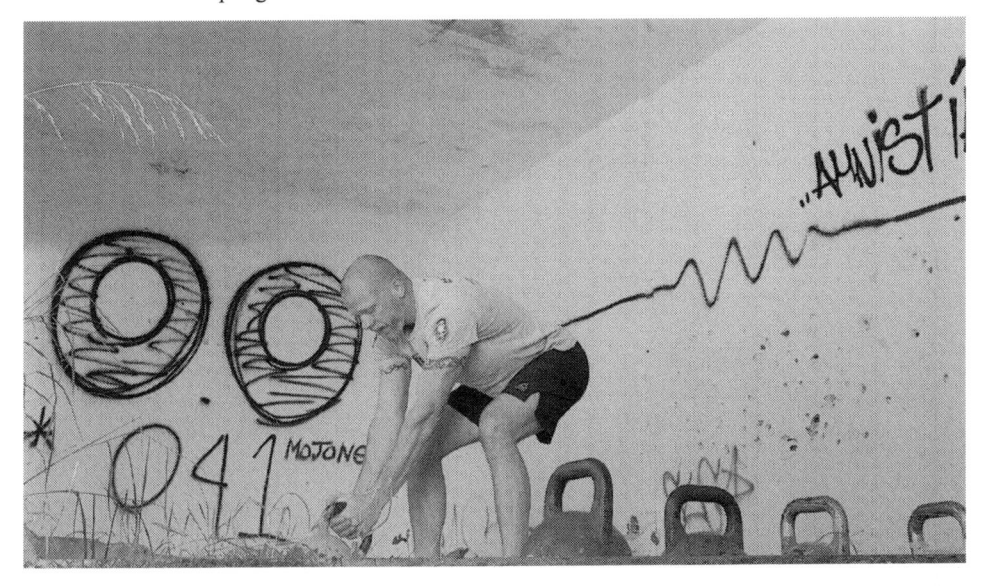

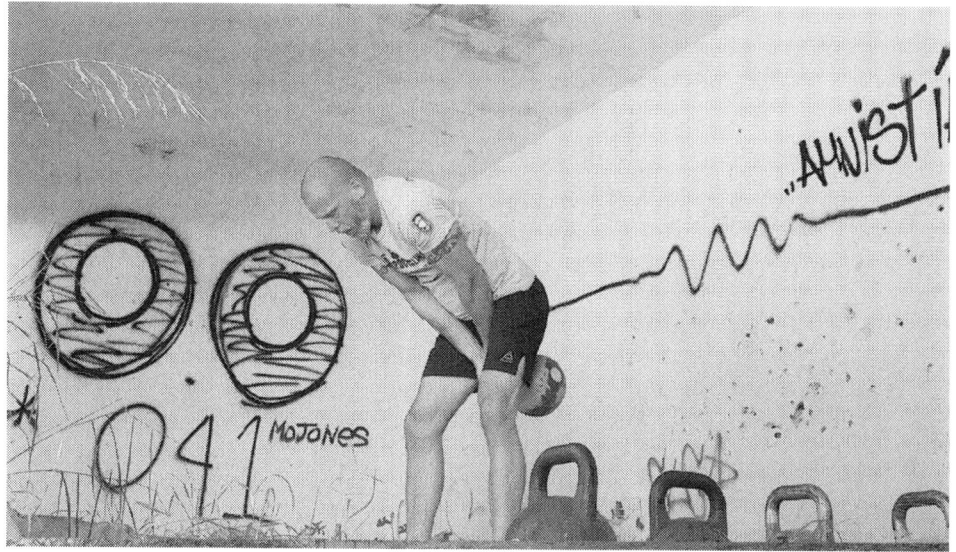

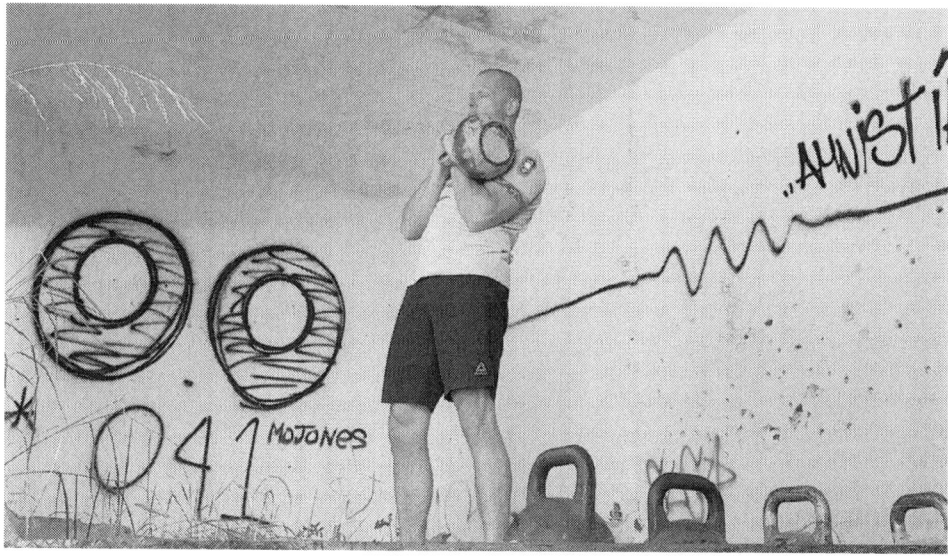

Task

Your sixth task is to complete several sets of the assisted clean as per below.

If in the previous chapters you were doing hang lifts then also perform hang lifts here instead of the dead lift.

Perform four slow reps on one side and repeat on the other. Each rep should take about 10 to 15 seconds. Rest if required, then repeat, work for 4 to 6 minutes. Repeat this drill for as long as you need to master and understand the movement. You can do this 3 times a day with plenty of space in between. You don't really need a warm-up for this drill but you can. You need to use the lightest weight you have available and increase weight over time.

Remember, this exercise is designed for a specific purpose, which is, to learn the most basic and safest lift, but more importantly, to drill the movement which you'll be doing more explosive later on and the hand insertion, feeling how the bell should travel around the hand.

You should film yourself and compare it to the demonstration in the video.

Submission

You can film your assisted clean for feedback. Submit your video in any way possible. See chapter on *How to submit your assessment*.

Day 7 Kettlebell squat swing

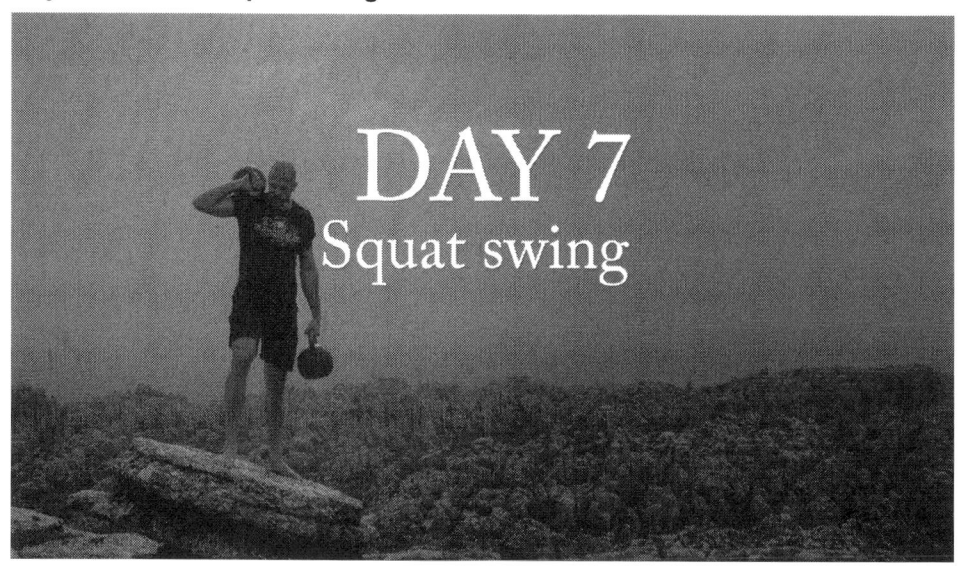

Dot points:

- The kettlebell swing is one of the most popular kettlebell exercises
- There is so much more to kettlebell training than just the swing
- There are many different types of kettlebell swings
- The squat swing is controversial
- A swing is good if its safe and works towards your goals
- It is important to know why you're doing an exercise
- You should also learn the hip hinge swing
- Understand the differences between squat and hip hinge
- The squat swing uses more of the anterior muscles and is less stress on the lower back
- The hip hinge is more isolation of the gluteus maximus and provides more stress on the back (not always a bad thing)
- In the swing your arms are just a pendulum with your shoulder being the pivot
- The only swing that is a shoulder raise is the *American swing*
- Shoulders should be slightly pulled back and down
- Don't pull the kettlebell up with the shoulders
- Drive the weight up with the power from your legs
- To start you bump the weight out and don't worry how high it comes
- If the kettlebell comes too high then the weight is probably too light
- The weight is too heavy if it does not come higher than the hips
- The kettlebell should be a direct extension of your arms at all times
- There should be no bobbing at the end or top of the swing

- If you can see the ground at the bottom of your swing you're probably hip hinging
- You can also start your swing with a dead start (dead swing)
- You need more flexibility for the dead start
- Don't over reach for the kettlebell
- Whether you keep your arms straight or bent depends on the trajectory of the kettlebell
- If the kettlebell trajectory is away from you then the arms should remain straight
- If the kettlebell trajectory is up then you can bent your arms
- Guiding the kettlebell away from you adds more back muscle recruitment
- Bent arm with the trajectory being out and away creates tension/tugs on the elbow flexors

Kettlebell squat swing:

1. Bump the weight out to start
2. Let the weight freely drop down
3. Guide the weight between the legs and towards the ground
4. Bend the three joints for the squat
5. Keep the shoulders high
6. Look ahead
7. Pull the weight back up
8. Come back upright
9. Push the heels into the ground
10. Pull the knees back
11. Extend the hips
12. Let the weight come up and forward
13. Come into full extension
14. The weight reach about chest height
15. Let the weight drop back down
16. Repeat

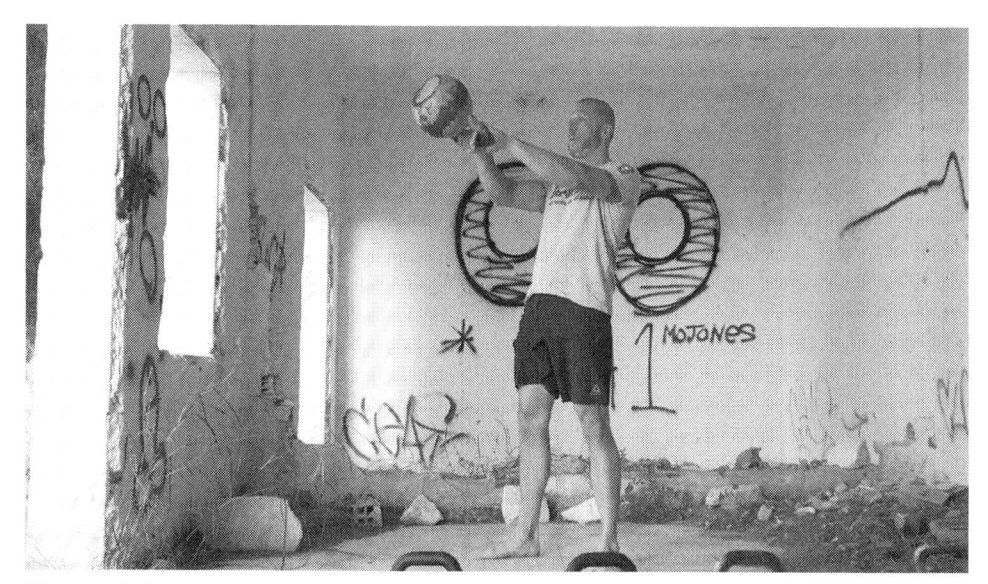

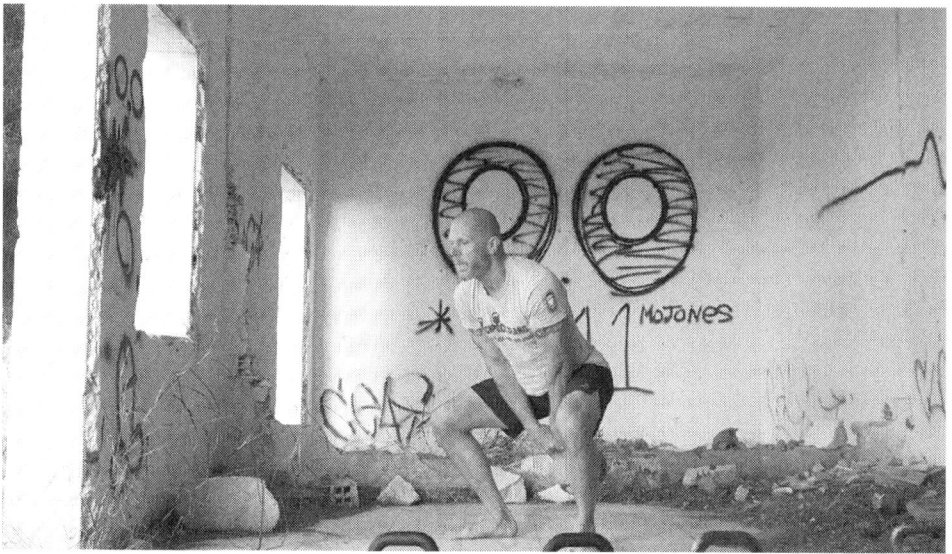

Task

Your seventh task is to complete several sets of the squat swing with double arm as per below.

Start with a dead start if you have the flexibility, if you don't, remember to work on your flexibility.

Pick a weight that allows you to easily get the kettlebell till about chest height but not higher. Pick a weight that requires you to activate the glutes and hammies (hip extensors) but not fatigue them, this is training and not a workout. Your objective is to understand the movement, to analyze the movement, to make notes, and to keep repeating the task over time until you have mastered it.

Perform 8 reps. Put the weight down. Reset. Repeat. Rest when required. Perform 6 rounds. Reduce reps if you're having difficulty, increase reps if things are improving. Aim to work up to sets of 20 reps.

Submission
You can film your kettlebell squat swing for feedback. Submit your video in any way possible. See chapter on *How to submit your assessment*.

Day 8 Kettlebell hip hinge swing

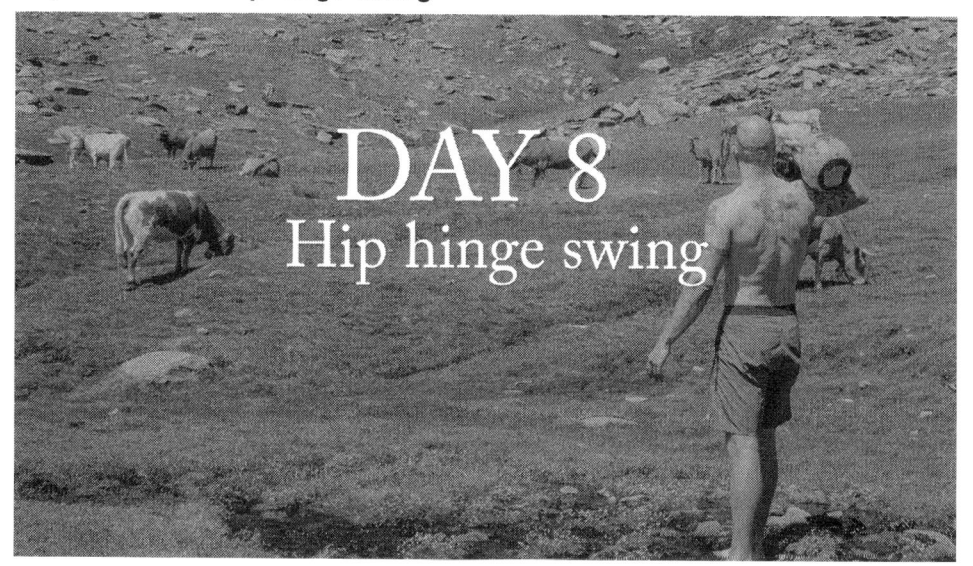

On day 8 you will learn the most common version of the kettlebell swing and I'll talk about how to avoid back aches, what muscles to active and why, and many more tips that are commonly overlooked and will result in back aches when not implemented.

I will also demonstrate how to start the kettlebell swing safety several different ways.

Dot points:

- The hip hinge swing is the most common kettlebell swing
- The movement is wrong when the hip hinge swing is performed with a squat
- Hip hinge and insert
- Pull out and direct the weight forward
- Look ahead at the top of the swing
- Look at the ground in-front at the bottom of the swing
- The hip hinge swing involves two joints for power
- Hips and knees
- The swing can be performed with one joint
- With the hips only it is called the stiff-legged swing
- The swing is going to hurt your back if you do not engage the right muscles intended for the movement

- The right muscles are; gluteus maximus; hamstrings; adductor magnus
- Work on MMC if you experience lower back pain
- Look at technique
- Review programming (reps/weight/rest)
- To protect the lower back you should not follow the kettlebell
- Direct the weight to the back
- Don't let the weight abruptly be stopped by your groin
- Don't let the kettlebell hit your tailbone
- Film and analyze yourself
- Film and ask for form check
- The swing can be started with a dead start (dead swing)
- Do low reps when just starting out
- Stop when you have pain and review muscle priming/MMC
- Focus on technique
- You can breathe twice during the swing
- Breathe out at the top and end
- You can breathe once during the swing
- Breathe in on the way down
- Breathe out on the way up
- Don't hold your breath

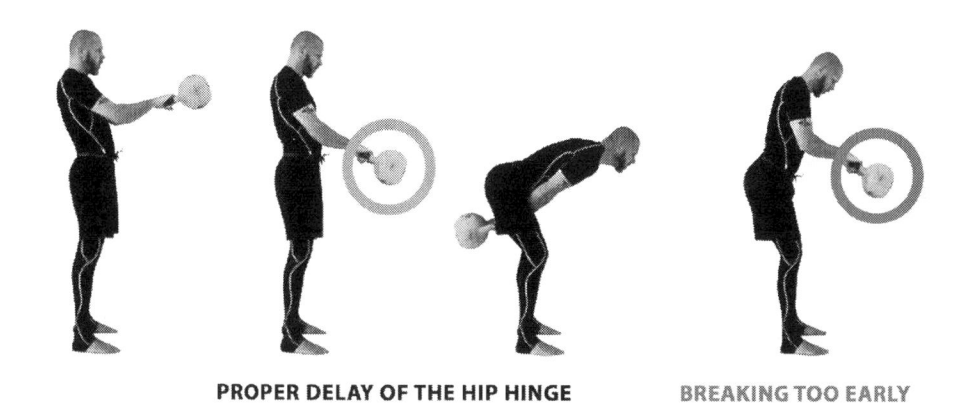

PROPER DELAY OF THE HIP HINGE **BREAKING TOO EARLY**

Kettlebell hip hinge swing:

1. Squat dead lift
2. Bump it out
3. Delay the hinge till the weight is at the right position
4. Insert
5. The weight should come through about knee height
6. Direct the weight to the back
7. Prevent bobbing of the kettlebell
8. Pull the weight back out with the muscles intended
9. Direct the weight forward
10. Come into full extension
11. Wait for the weight to drop back down
12. Delay hip flexion
13. Insert
14. Repeat

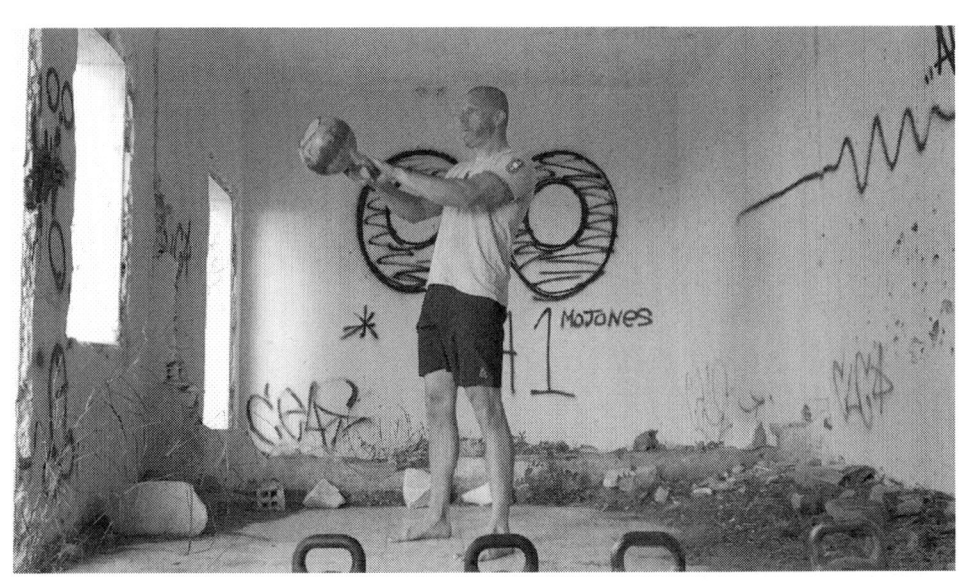

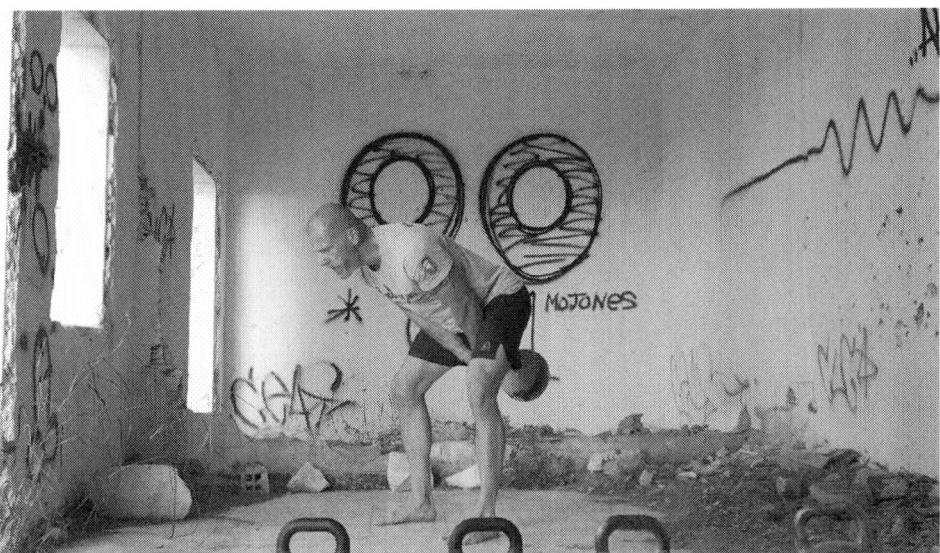

Compare the hip hinge to the squat

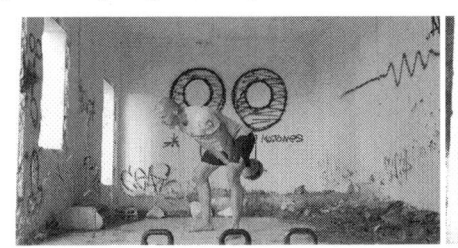

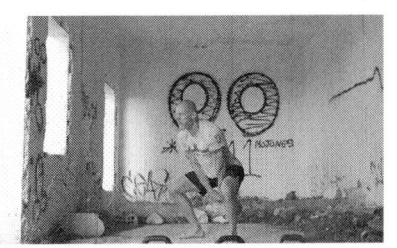

Task

Your eighth task is to complete several sets of the hip hinge swing with double arm as per below.

Start with a dead start if you have the flexibility, if you don't, remember to work on your flexibility.

Pick a weight that allows you to easily get the kettlebell till about chest height but not higher. Pick a weight that requires you to activate the glutes and hammies (hip extensors) but not fatigue them, this is training and not a workout. Your objective is to understand the movement, to analyze the movement, to make notes, and to keep repeating the task over time until you have mastered it.

Perform 6 reps. Put the weight down. Reset. Repeat. Rest when required. Perform 8 rounds. Reduce reps if you're having difficulty, increase reps if things are improving. Aim to work up to sets of 20 reps.

Submission

You can film your hip hinge swing for feedback. Submit your video in any way possible. See chapter on How to submit your assessment.

For more details on the kettlebell swing see chapter on the Kettlebell Swing further in this book.

Day 9 Kettlebell pendulum swing

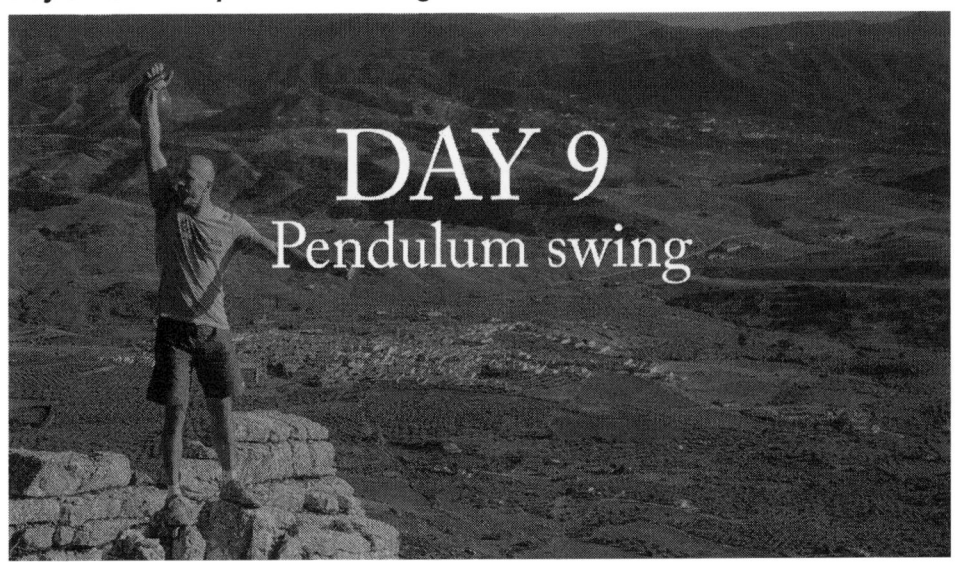

On day 9 you will learn a version of the kettlebell swing that is more advanced but once mastered will open up a whole new world of kettlebell training to you. This version of the swing provides the least resistance to the body and is great for high volume swings. This swing also can improve your clean a lot and gets you ready for snatches in the future.

Dot points:

- There are 3 main movements to perform the swing
- Squat; Hip hinge; Pendulum
- The pendulum swing comes from kettlebell sport
- The pendulum swing is usually performed with one arm
- Make space for the bell
- Stay connected
- Go with the flow
- Don't resist the weight
- This is a push whereas the other two movements are a pull
- Push the arms forward
- Great swing for high volume reps
- Each swing has their own reason for doing them

- The pendulum swing is great for the clean
- There are many different ways to perform the pendulum swing
- The pendulum swing provides the least amount of stress on the body
- Know when to use one over the other

Kettlebell pendulum swing:
- Bump the weight out
- The knees bent
- The arms connect with the body
- The hips are coming back to prevent an abrupt stop
- The knees extend to prevent an abrupt stop
- The shoulders are coming down (hip hinge) to prevent an abrupt stop
- The weight comes back through gravity
- Follow the bell with the hips
- Keep the arms connected
- Push with the hips
- Perform slight hip hyperextension if flexibility allows (stay connected longer)
- The weight does not need to come to any specific height
- Let the weight come back in and through
- Repeat

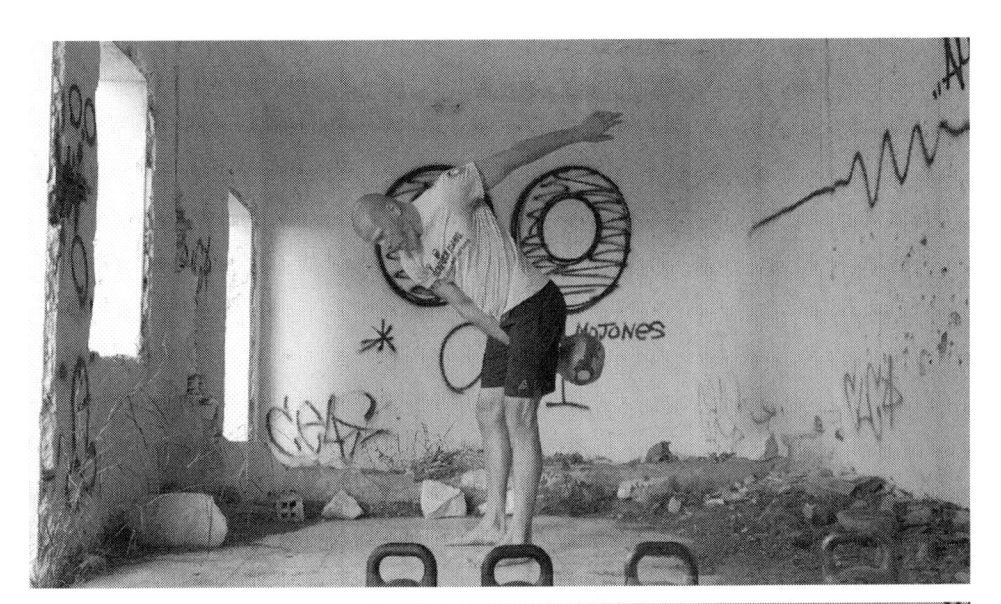

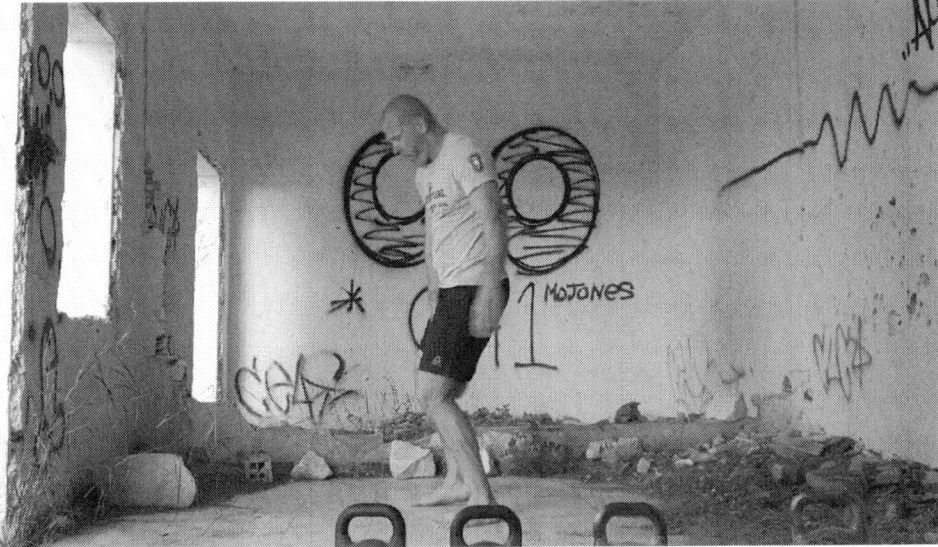

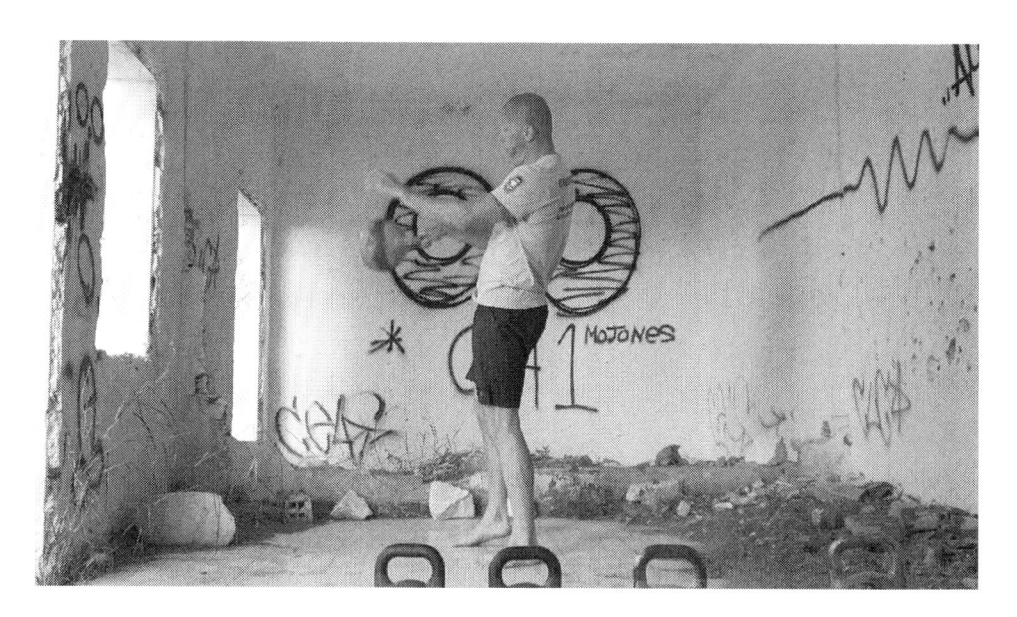

Task

Your ninth task is to complete several sets of the pendulum swing with double arm as per below, but if you find that the swing works better for you with single arm that is fine too, just split the number of reps in half for each side.

Start with a dead start if you have the flexibility, if you don't, remember to work on your flexibility.

Pick a weight that is close to 1/3 heavier than what you've been using for the hip hinge swings. Your objective is to understand the movement, to analyze the movement, to make notes, and to keep repeating the task over time until you have mastered it.

Perform 20 reps. Put the weight down. Reset. Repeat. Rest when required. Perform 6 rounds. Reduce reps if you're having difficulty, increase reps if things are improving. Aim to work up to one set of 60.

Submission

You can film your pendulum swing for feedback. Submit your video in any way possible. See chapter on How to submit your assessment.

Day 10 Double arm swing clean

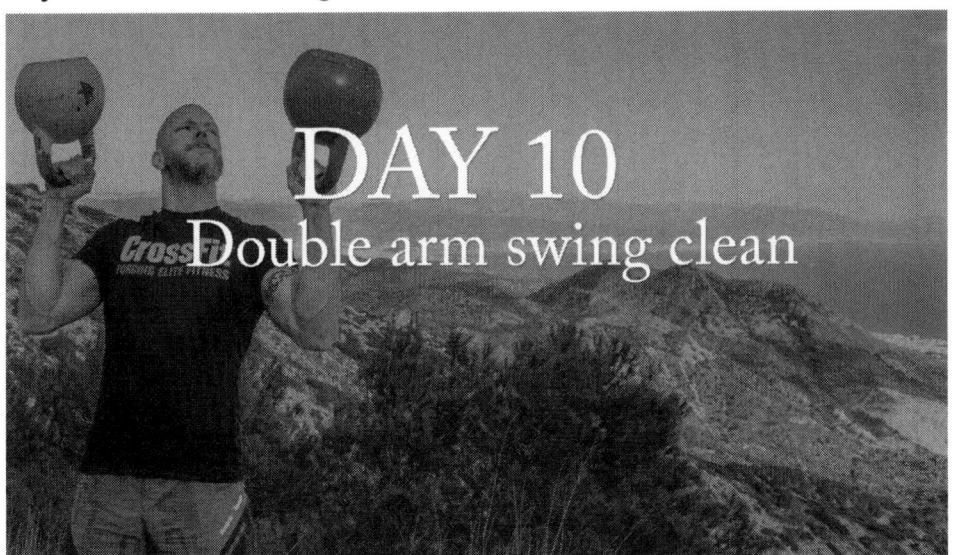

On day 10 you will learn the double arm swing clean which is great to transition into other movements like the squat, press, halo, etc. In other words, once you know this type of clean you can start stringing movements together and create flows.

I will introduce you to some concepts that will help prevent injury when you move on to more complex kettlebell cleans.

The double arm swing clean is great to transition into other movements like the squat, press, halo, etc. In other words, once you know this type of clean you can start stringing movements together and create flows.

Dot points:

- When people refer to a 'clean' they will refer to the most common clean 'they' taught you
- There are many different types of cleans
- Getting specific with naming avoids confusing as to what is asked of the athlete
- Start; Dead swing clean; Swing clean; Hang clean; Dead clean
- Movement; Squat; Hip hinge; Pendulum
- There are over 70 different types/variations of the kettlebell clean
- With a clean you want to keep the weight close to you
- You want the trajectory to be up
- Keeping the elbows in will keep the weight close
- Don't cast the weight out and away from you

- Let the weight drop
- Sometimes a heavier weight for the clean will force you to use correct technique

Double arm swing clean:

- Bump the weight out or start with the weight dead
- Perform the movement to drive the weight up
- Transition the hands from grip on the handle to grip around the bell
- Keep the thumbs pointing up within the window
- Base of the bell should be up but not completely horizontal
- Bring the weight to the chest
- Drop the weight
- Transition into double hand grip
- Move into the backswing
- Repeat

Beginners option is to keep the index finger and thumb closed on both sides which creates a ring around the handle that can be slid across to the horns. Doing so will prevent the need to let go of the kettlebell which can sometimes be daunting for beginners. The grip needs to be loose to be able to slide it across the handle and horns.

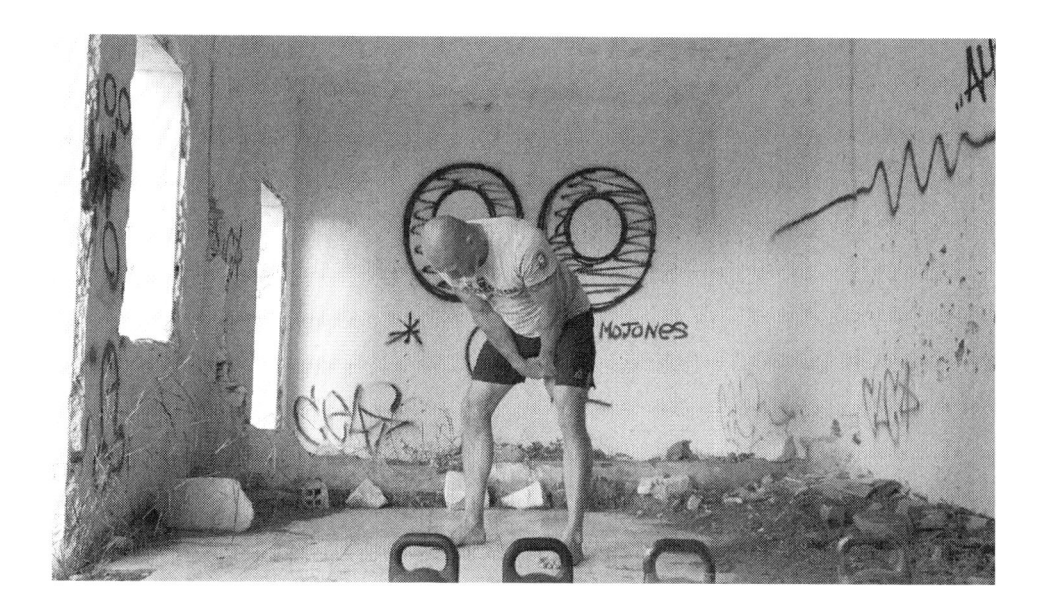

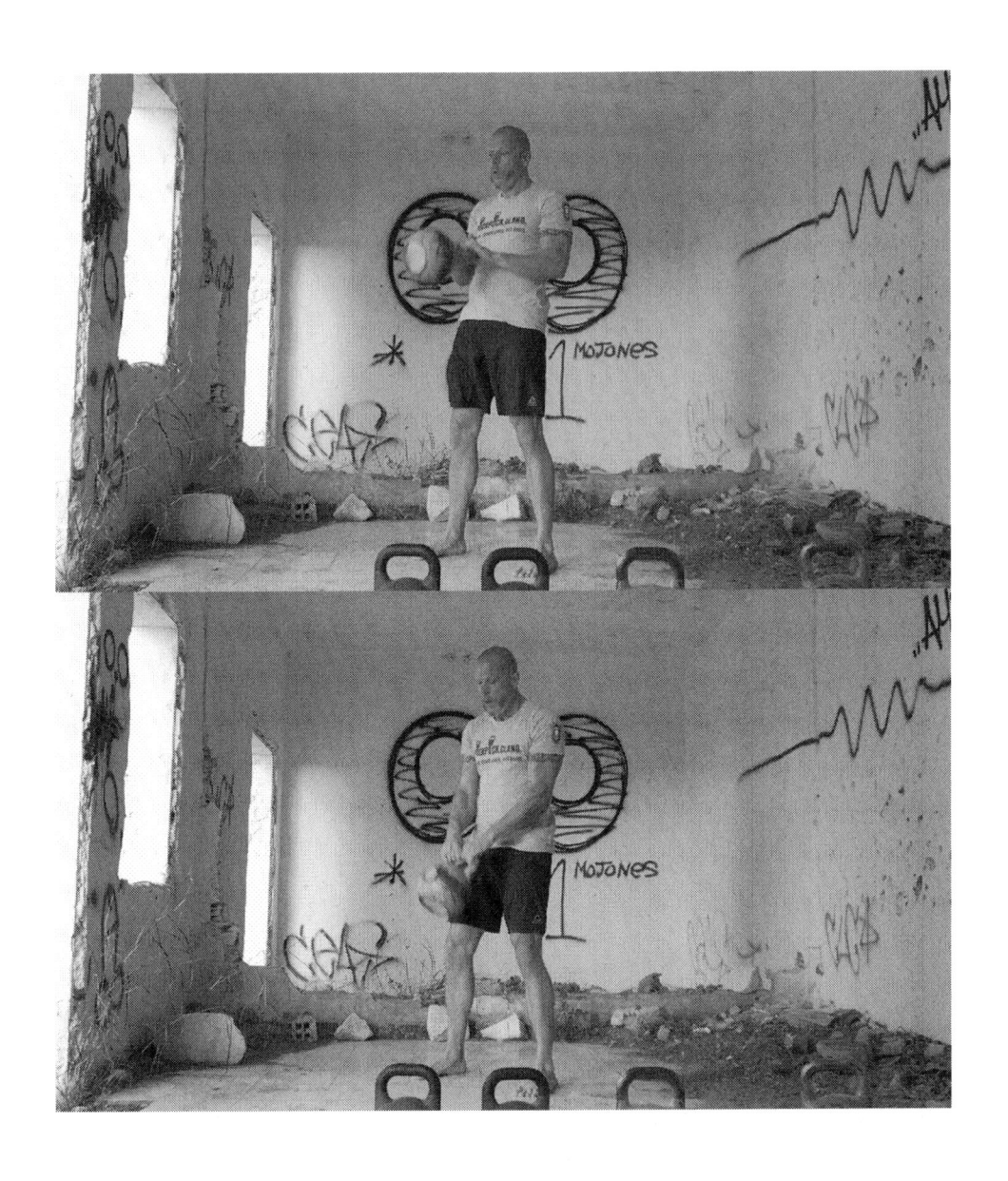

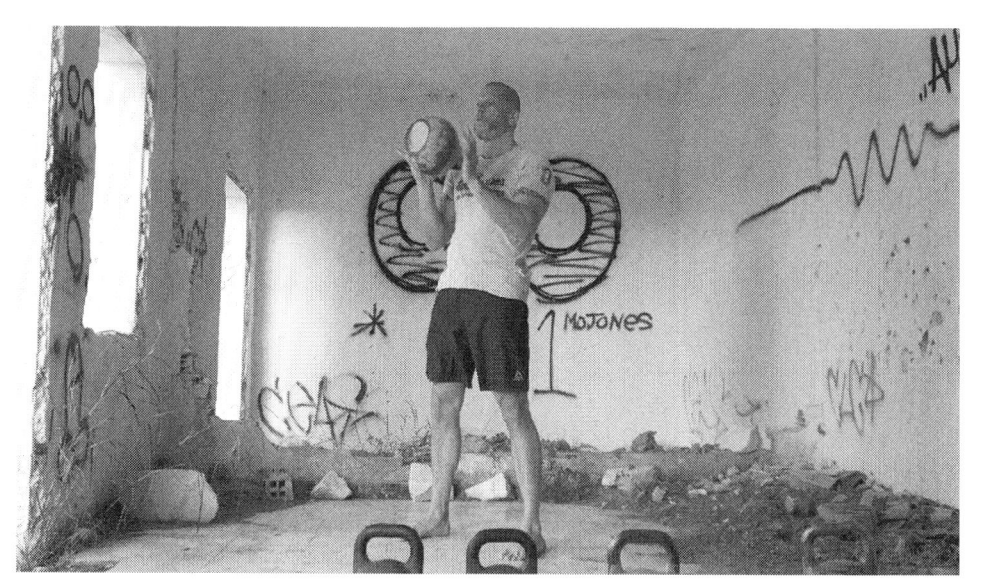

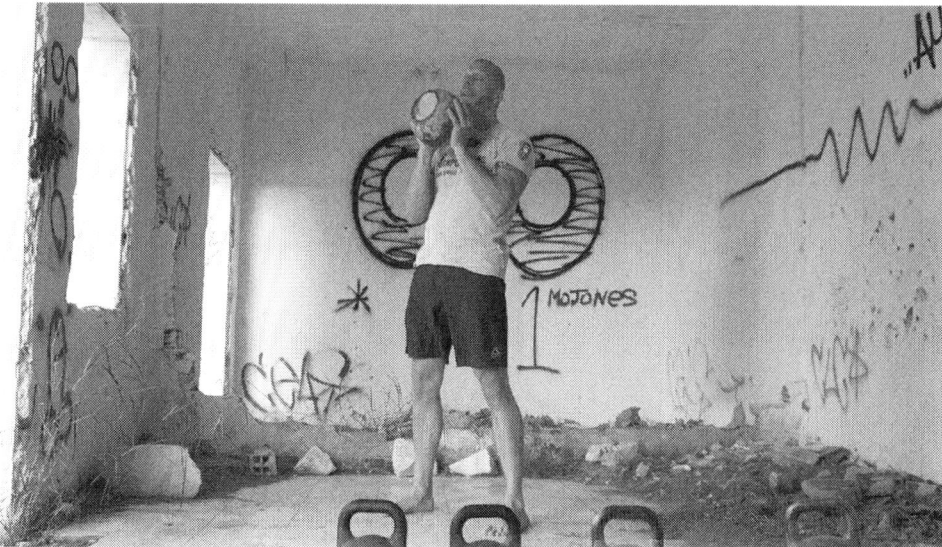

Safety

Catch the weight away from you. When starting out that distance should be great and decreasing as you become more comfortable. If you're not comfortable performing this clean you can just put the weight safely down and lift the bell from the ground in a squat position.

Task

Your tenth task is to complete several sets of the double arm swing clean as per below.

Start with a dead start if you have the flexibility, if you don't, remember to work on your flexibility.

Use the weight that you're currently comfortable swinging with a hip hinge. Your objective is to understand the movement, to analyze the movement, to make notes, and to keep repeating the task over time until you have mastered it.

Perform 6 reps. Put the weight down. Reset. Repeat. Rest when required. Perform 6 rounds. Reduce reps if you're having difficulty, increase reps if things are improving. Aim to work up to one set of 20.

Submission

You can film your double arm swing clean for feedback. Submit your video in any way possible. See chapter on How to submit your assessment.

Day 11 Kettlebell dead clean

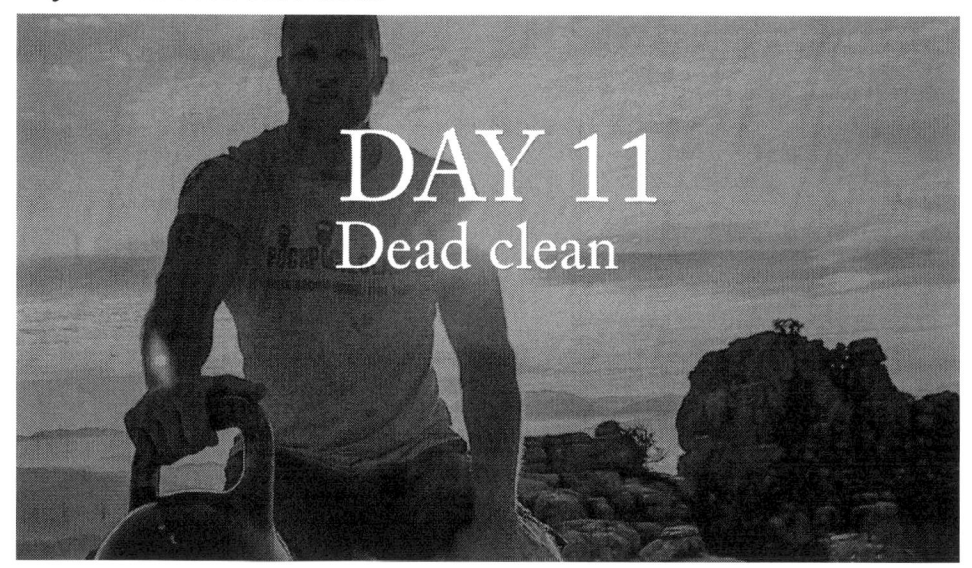

On day 11 you will learn the kettlebell dead clean which is a very explosive movement and great to add to your training. This version of the clean is very similar to the barbell clean in CrossFit. This is where it becomes obvious why you've been drilling the assisted clean.

I will demonstrate this movement step by step and talk about the muscles that need to be engaged and so much more.

Dot points:

- You'll need a heavier kettlebell for this exercise
- The clean brings a kettlebell from a lower position into racking position
- Perform the squat movement to perform this exercise
- This exercise is what you've been drilling the assisted clean for
- The bell comes around the hand and not over the fist
- Make sure you've been drilling the assisted clean
- If you're struggling with the dead clean then drill the assisted clean more
- The weight travel directly up in one straight line looking front and side on
- The weight stays close to you
- Brace the upper trapezius before pulling

- An incorrect clean that's not powered by the legs is called a muscle clean
- Common mistake is bending the arm before coming into full extension
- Clean with your legs and not your arms
- Review your technique if you experience pain or tenderness around the elbow flexors
- Always end up with a good insert and racking position
- Never stay straight while dropping the weight and letting the weight jerk on the shoulders
- If you're working on your flexibility then you can do hang clean to progress to the dead clean
- There should be no rubbing on the palm of the hand
- The skin is bypassed during the insert

Kettlebell dead clean:

1. Bell placed between the feet
2. Squat
3. Look ahead
4. Hook grip
5. Slight tension between you and the weight
6. Think about pulling the weight to the ceiling
7. Press the heels into the ground
8. Pull the knees back
9. Push the hips forward
10. Keep the arm extended for as long as possible
11. Use the power from the legs
12. Don't curl the weight
13. Let the bell travel up further
14. Open up
15. Hand insert
16. Let the bell come around the fist and not over
17. Come into full racking position
18. Loose grip
19. Let the weight drop

20. Pull back and out
21. Hook grip
22. Reduce velocity with the legs
23. Gently place the weight dead on the ground
24. Repeat

Look ahead

No need to look at the kettlebell, maintain good form and alignment, keep your sight ahead, not down.

Extended elbow

Pull with legs, not with the elbow flexors, this means you keep the elbow extended for as long as is required to generate the right amount of power with the legs.

Accelerated pull

The pulling speed needs to increase, accelerate and generate enough power to make the weight float.

Hips low; shoulders high

This is not a hip hinge, it's a squat, drop you hips low and keep your shoulders high.

Float, open + insert

Make the weight float, i.e. get it to the point where it's weightless, then open the hand, let the bell come around, and insert the hand into the window.

Full racking position

End up in full racking position, even if your next rep is another dead clean, complete the full movement and don't get sloppy.

Controlled landing

Don't let the bell just crash on the floor, control the descent and gently put the kettlebell back dead on the ground.

Drop + pull-out

Let the kettlebell drop back down, pull the hand back out, transition back into hook grip.

Drop + pull back

While the bell drops, pull the elbow back, keeping it where it is means that the bell will move away from the body, you want a direct path back down.

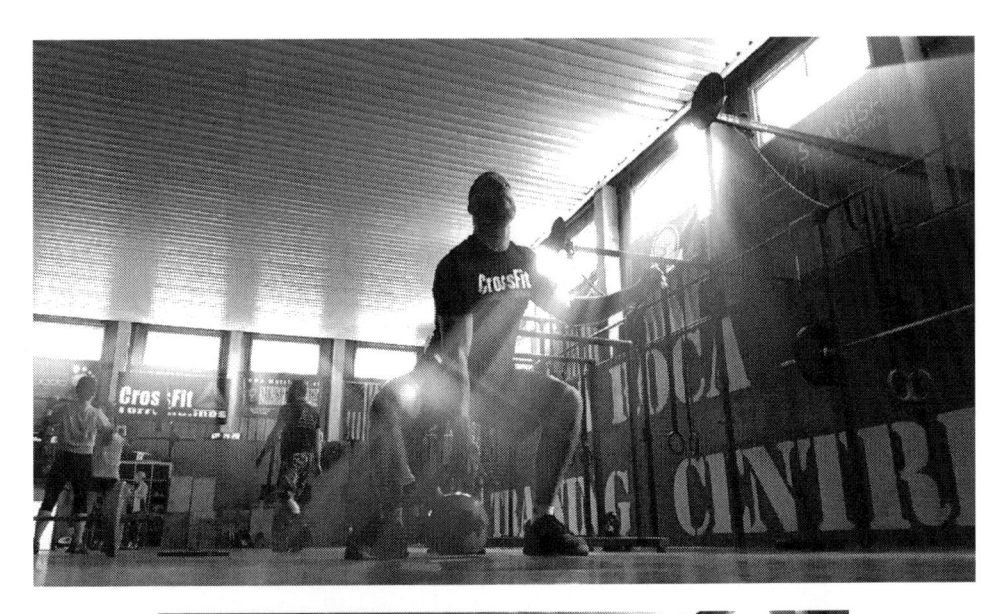

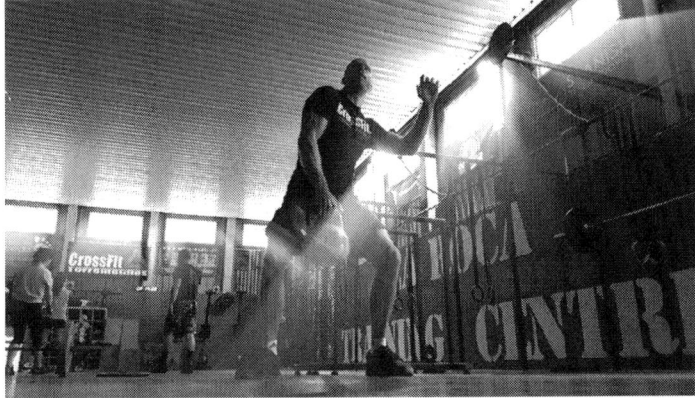

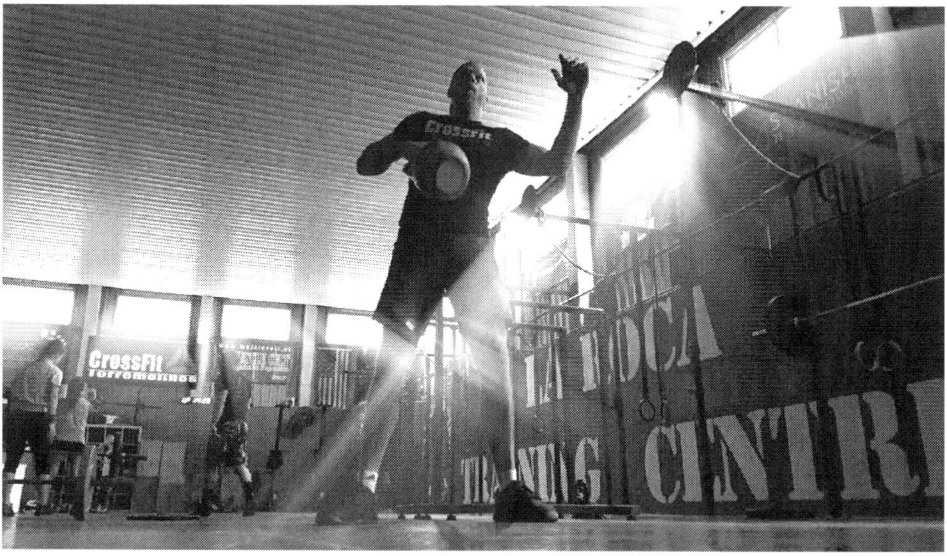
CrossFit
CrossFit
Torremolinos

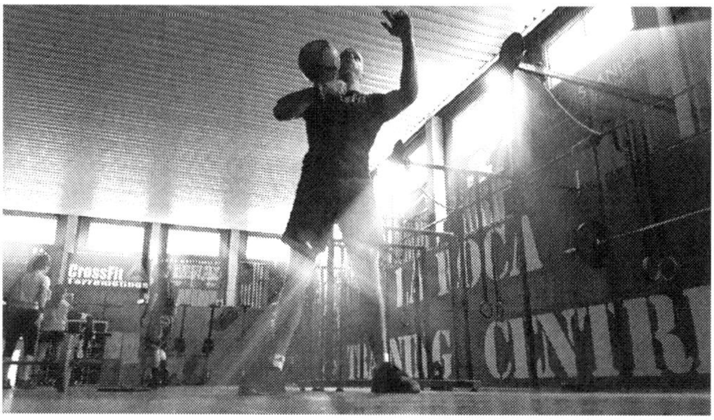
CrossFit

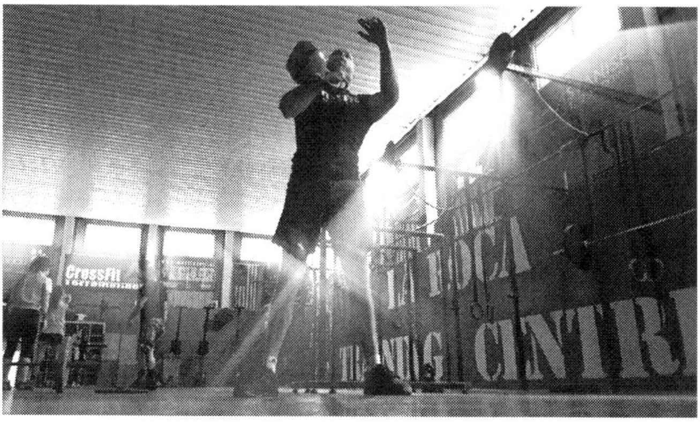
CrossFit

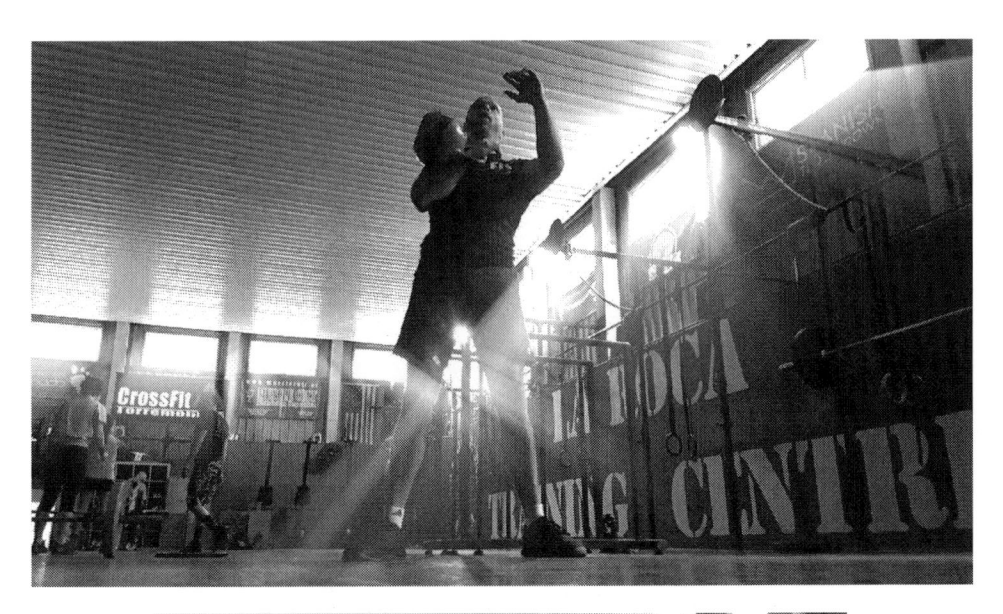

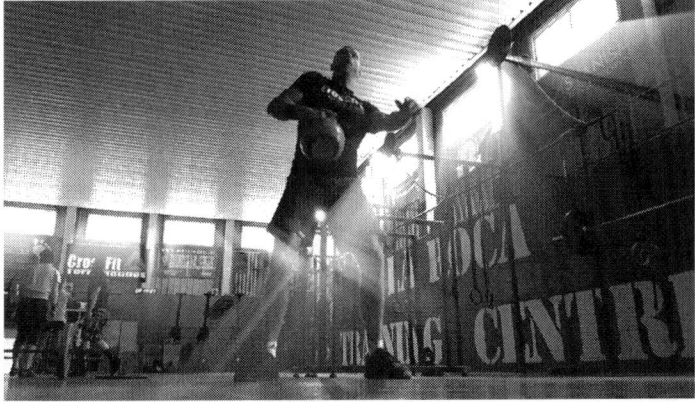

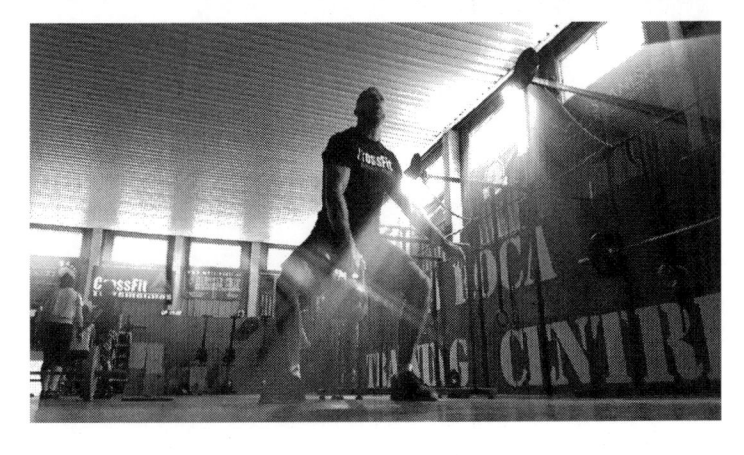

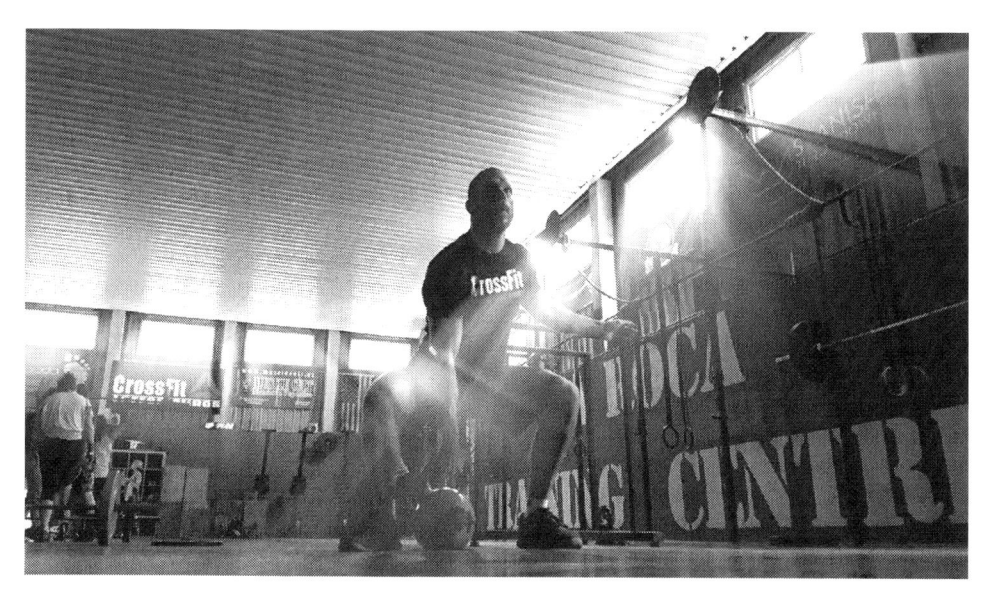

Common mistakes

Swinging

The kettlebell should go up and down in one straight path, the kettlebell should not move away from the body, when it's away from the body and then needs to land between the feet, it will turn into a swing.

Curling

This is a clean, not a curl, a clean is always powered by the lower-body, hence, no bicep curling, no matter how light the weight is. Bicep curling will not only promote bad technique, but also bring along a host of other issues, like tendon injury etc.

Light weight

Using a weight too light promotes bad technique, the weight needs to provide adequate resistance to be able to give the legs the resistance they need to become explosive and have good technique.

Tight grip

Employ a loose hook grip, transition into racking grip, back into hook grip, never hold the kettlebell handle tight.

Task

Your eleventh task is to complete as per below.

Train your dead clean and work your way up over time:

1. 12kg/26.4lbs
2. 16kg/35.2lbs
3. 20kg/44lbs

Duration and sets:

- 2 reps each side
  1 set and 10 seconds rest
  Repeat 4 times

- 4 reps each side
  1 set and 15 seconds rest
  Repeat 4 times

- 6 reps each side
  1 set and 20 seconds rest
  Repeat 4 times

Program each progression until you feel comfortable. For example, the first week you might do 3 days of 12kg and 2 reps. The next week you increase the reps to 4 and so on. At the end you move up in weight for the next 3 weeks until you've completed 20kgs.

Submission

You can film your dead clean for feedback. Submit your video in any way possible. See chapter on How to submit your assessment.

Day 12 Kettlebell swing clean

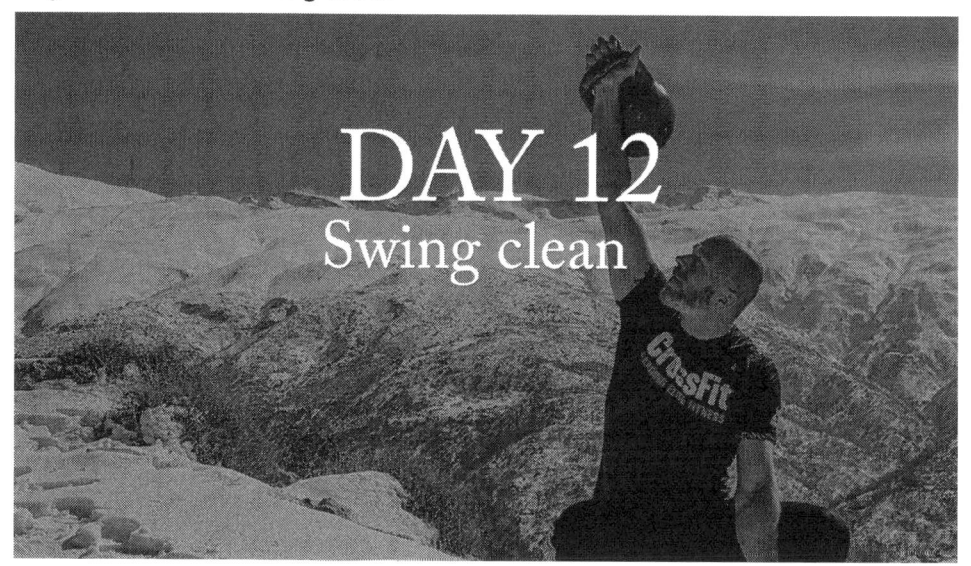

On day 12 you will learn the most common version of the kettlebell clean, the swing clean. The swing clean clean is the most common clean used for clean and press, clean and jerk, etc. I will demonstrate that you can swing clean with a squat, hip hinge, and pendulum so that you can create the clean that works and feels good for you.

Dot points:

- The same concept as with the dead clean applies and you want to drive that weight up
- Use the legs to clean and at the top open up to perform a hand insert
- You can clean with; Hip hinge; Squat; Pendulum
- Keep the weight close to you
- A good drill is the towel drill to practice elbow to body proximity
- If the towel falls then your elbow was not in the right place

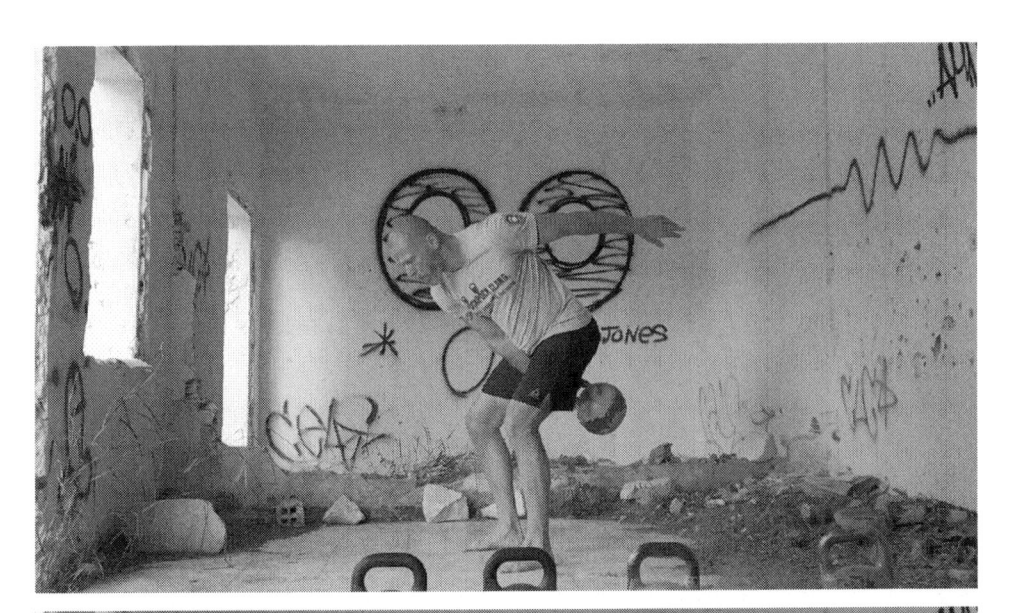

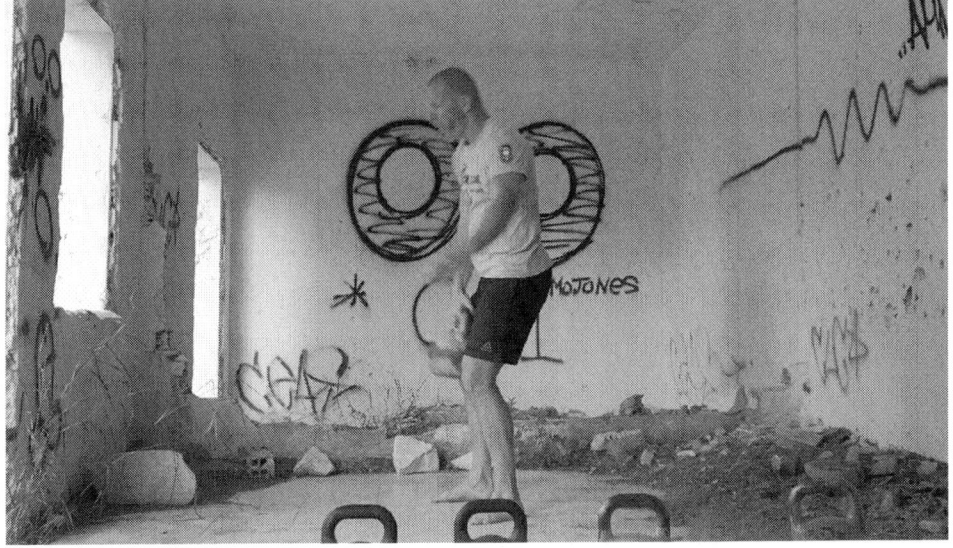

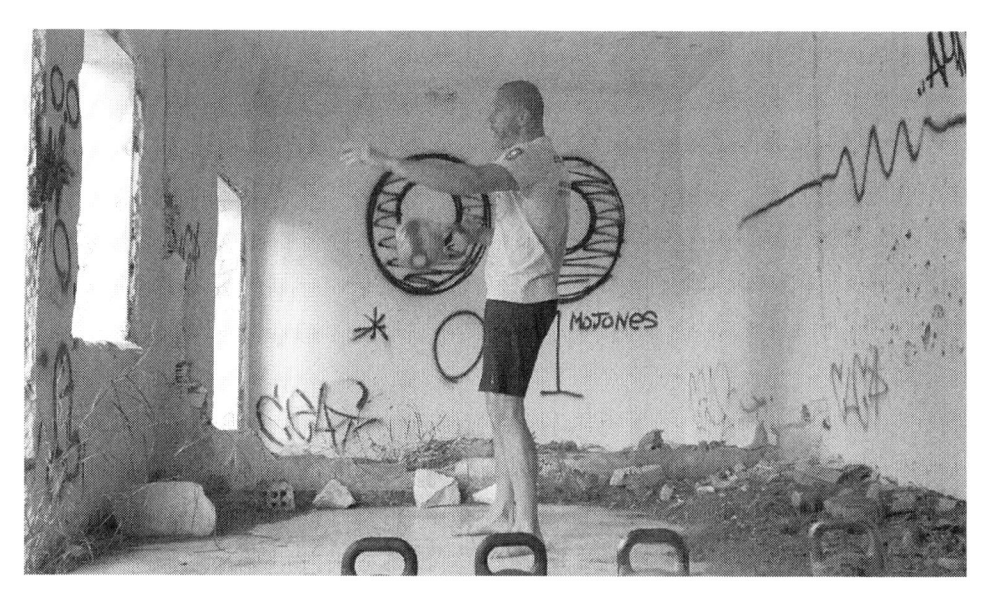

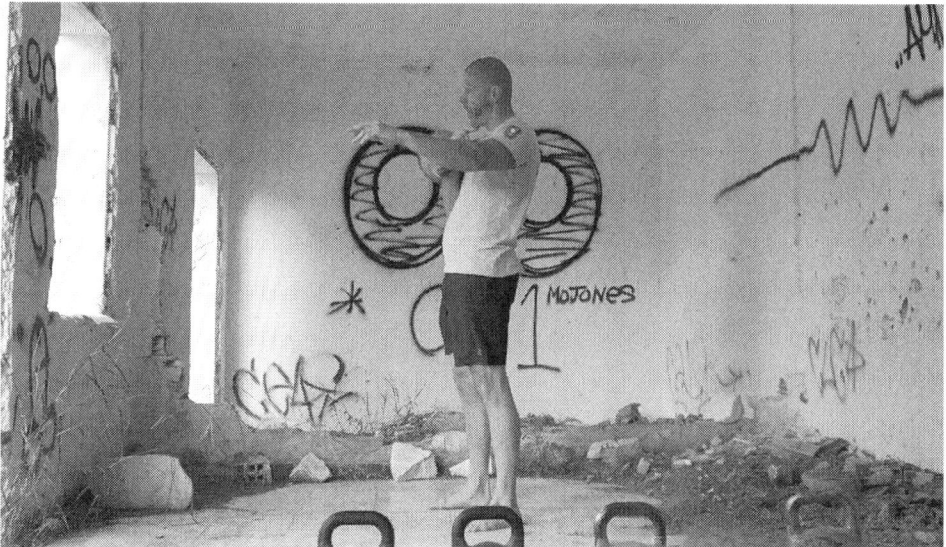

Task

Your twelfth task is to complete as per below.

Train your swing clean and work your way up over time:

1. 8kg/17.6lbs
2. 12kg/26.4lbs

3. 16kg/35.2lbs

Duration and sets:

- 4 reps each side
  1 set and 10 seconds rest
  Repeat 4 times

- 6 reps each side
  1 set and 20 seconds rest
  Repeat 4 times

- 8 reps each side
  1 set and 30 seconds rest
  Repeat 4 times

Program each progression until you feel comfortable. For example, the first week you might do 3 days of 8kg and 4 reps. The next week you increase the reps to 6 and so on. At the end you move up in weight for the next 3 weeks until you've completed 16kgs. Perform double kettlebells if you want to take it a step further. 4 reps each side would just become 4 reps one time.

Submission

You can film your swing clean for feedback. Submit your video in any way possible. See chapter on How to submit your assessment.

Day 13 Kettlebell racking

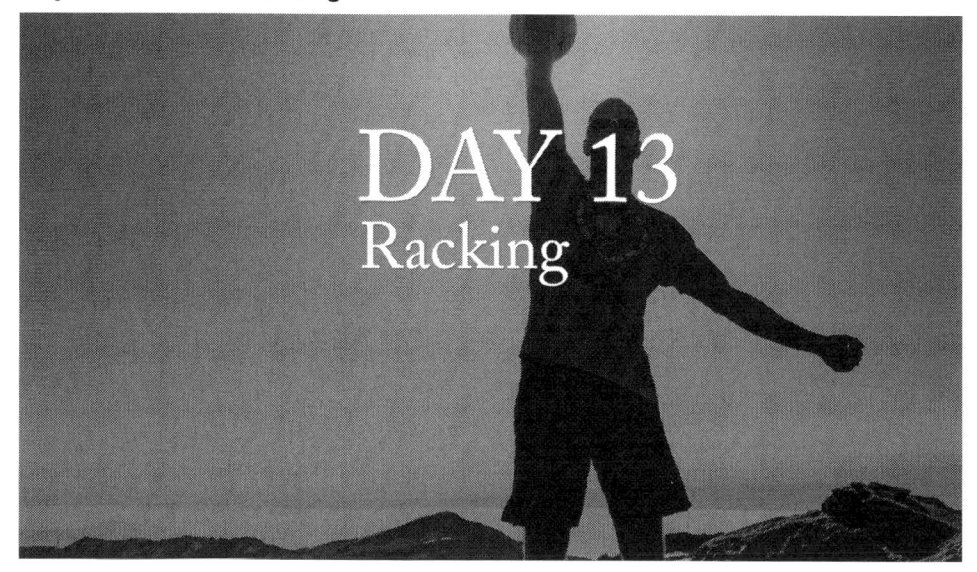

On day 13 you will learn how to rack a kettlebell properly and with the least amount of effort. Racking is what happens after the clean or after bring the kettlebell down from overhead. Racking may seem unimportant and simple, but it's not, it's super important to get your racking right and I will explain why and show you how to get your rack right. I will also cover racking for females.

Dot points:

- Kettlebell racking happens after you clean a kettlebell
- The rack can be a resting or transitional position
- A bad racking position can burn out the shoulders or affect the forearm
- With a transitional rack your elbow should be tucked/pulled into your obliques/ribs
- Use your latissimus dorsi to pull the elbow/arm in
- Rest the bell on the biceps and forearm
- A little bit of space at the bottom of the elbow is ok for a transitional rack
- For jerking or push pressing you want to rest the elbow on the ilium to transfer power
- For resting you want to rest the elbow on the ilium
- During sport/endurance/high volume reps you want to use a good rack to be able to rest with the bell up

- A disconnected arm means shoulder flexion which means additional and unnecessary work
- Let the weight rest on your skeletal system and not your muscular system
- Although it might look like it's bad for the lumbar there is actually no movement in the lumbar
- All range is created through hip hyper extension and extension plus flexion in the thoracic
- A good rack requires flexibility in the hips and thoracic
- Squeeze the gluteus maximus to pull the top of the pelvis back
- Let the top of the femur come slightly forward
- Getting better range in the hip flexors takes time
- Hip hyper extension and crunch
- A rounded back is not a problem because we're not pressing
- You want to rack with just enough contraction to obtain a good posture
- The weight naturally wants to fall away from the body which requires work to pull in
- Make space to let the weight rest on/above the legs
- The cradle rack is an option for females with larger breasts
- The rack is a position you need to learn properly

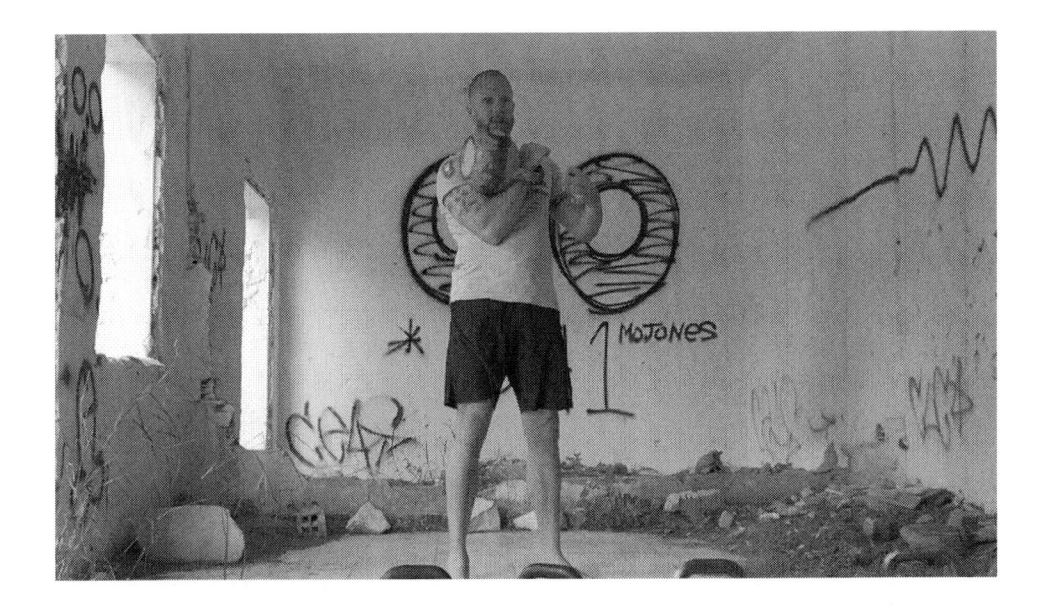

Task

Your thirteenth task is to complete as per below.

Drill your racking and work your way up over time:

1. 8kg/17.6lbs
2. 12kg/26.4lbs
3. 16kg/35.2lbs

Duration and sets:

- 15s each side
  1 set and 30 seconds rest
  Repeat 4 times

- 30s each side
  1 set and 45 seconds rest
  Repeat 4 times

- 45s each side
  1 set and 60 seconds rest
  Repeat 4 times

- 60s each side
  1 side and 30 seconds rest
  Repeat 4 times

Program each progression until you feel comfortable. For example, the first week you might do 3 days of 8kg and 15s work. The next week you increase the time under the rack to 30s and so on. At the end you move up in weight for the next 4 weeks until you've completed double 16kgs. Perform double kettlebells if you want to take it a step further. 15s each side would just become 15s one time.

Submission

You can film your racking for feedback. Submit your video in any way possible. See chapter on How to submit your assessment.

Day 14 Kettlebell pressing

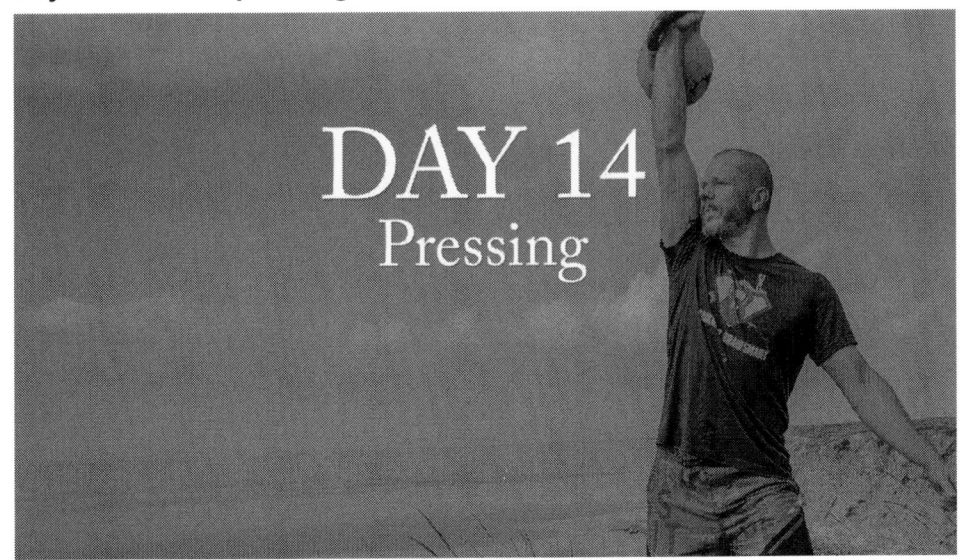

On day 14 you will learn how to press a kettlebell overhead. Before pressing you need to clean and rack, hence the reason I've covered the clean and rack first. I will demonstrate and string all three things together, cleaning, racking, and pressing. With all 3 of these under your belt you can already being to create little full body workouts for yourself like, clean, rack, squat, and press.

Dot points:

- Before you can press you will need to clean and rack
- I'm covering the overhead press but there is also the chest press which is not covered
- Before you press create tension and lock everything out so not to lose power during the press
- Tension and locking out creates a stable base to press from but also recruits more muscles
- Protect your lower back through gluteus maximus contraction (and hamstrings)
- As the bell comes overhead you're moving underneath it
- You want to end up directly under the kettlebell
- It's ok to work on overhead range with a light weight
- The triceps lock out the elbow
- Keep the shoulder safe through lat engagement and pulling the scapulae slightly down

- Once overhead let the weight rest on the skeletal system but keep pressing up
- Obtain a good overhead lockout on each rep
- Work on full range for mobility and flexibility
- Full range means longer under tension which is good for strength
- Keep the elbow under the weight during the press

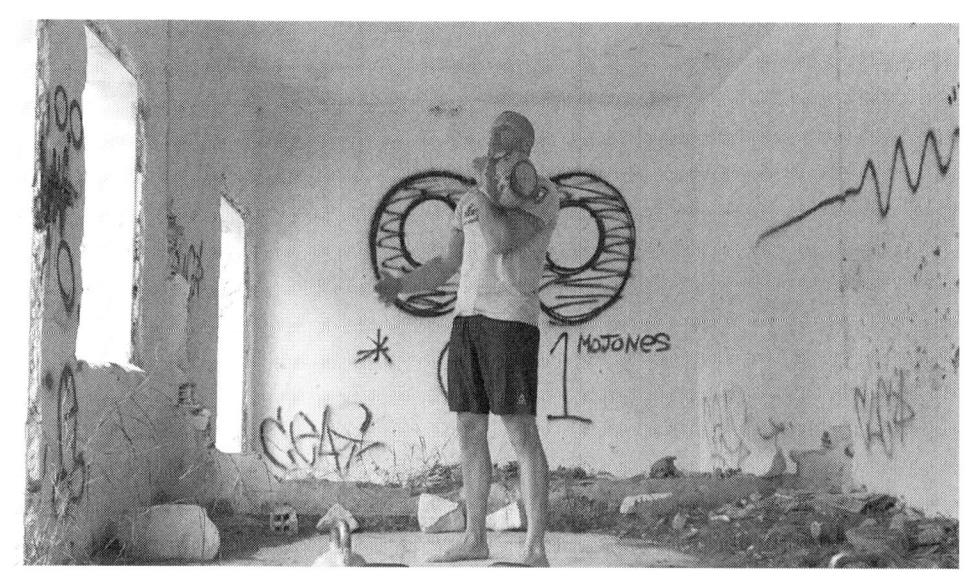

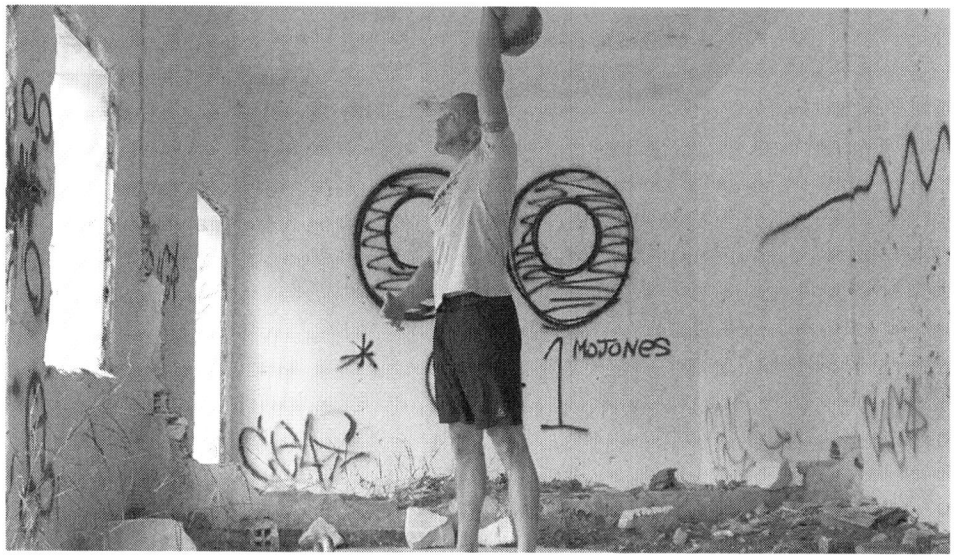

Task

Your fourteenth task is to complete as per below.

Train your press and work your way up over time:

1. 8kg/17.6lbs
2. 12kg/26.4lbs
3. 16kg/35.2lbs

Duration and sets:

- 4 reps each side
  1 set and 10 seconds rest
  Repeat 4 times

- 6 reps each side
  1 set and 15 seconds rest
  Repeat 4 times

- 8 reps each side
  1 set and 20 seconds rest
  Repeat 4 times

Submission

You can film your pressing for feedback. Submit your video in any way possible. See chapter on How to submit your assessment.

Day 15 Kettlebell rowing

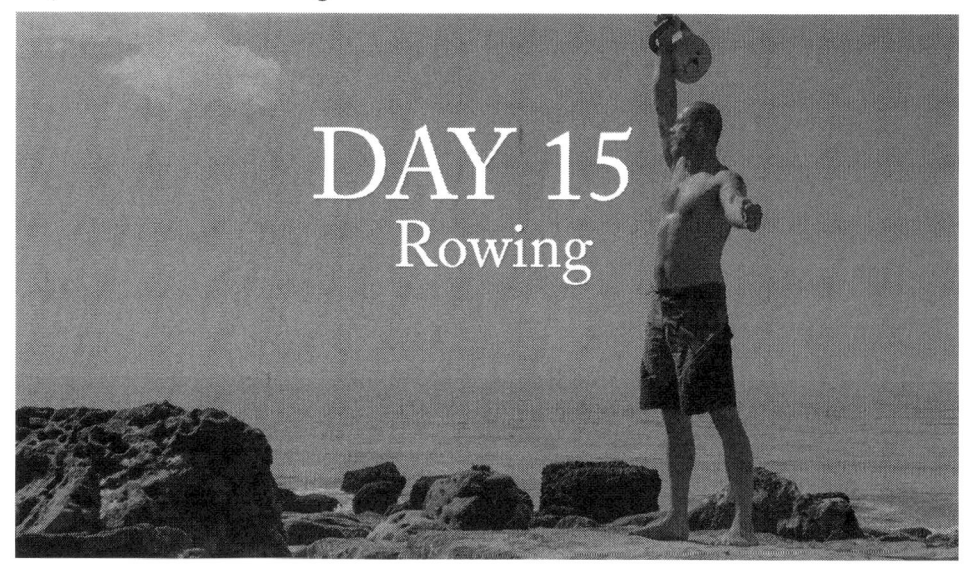

On day 15 you will learn how to perform the bent-over row which is a must do exercise to work the muscles in the back. Rowing is great to work the rear delts but also works lots of other muscles in the back including the all important erector spinae muscle groups.

Dot points:

- The row as demonstrated targets the rear delts but other muscles of the back are involved
- You can row while supporting the torso or without
- Rowing without support challenges the core muscles more
- Rowing with support allows you to isolate and focus on the row more
- Relax the elbow flexors while rowing
- Pull the elbow back into the hip and past
- If the weight starts dead on the ground it's a dead row
- If your hand is coming toward the shoulder you're curling instead of rowing
- Control the movement and get out of it what you're working out for
- Master the movement first and then go high reps and heavier weight
- Nothing but the arms that are working should be moving

- The row demonstrated is the safest in regards to angle between the elbow and ribs
- The bigger the angle between the elbow and ribs the more emphasis will be placed on the middle of the back
- The closer your elbow is to the body the safer it is for beginners
- There are many more ways to perform the kettlebell row

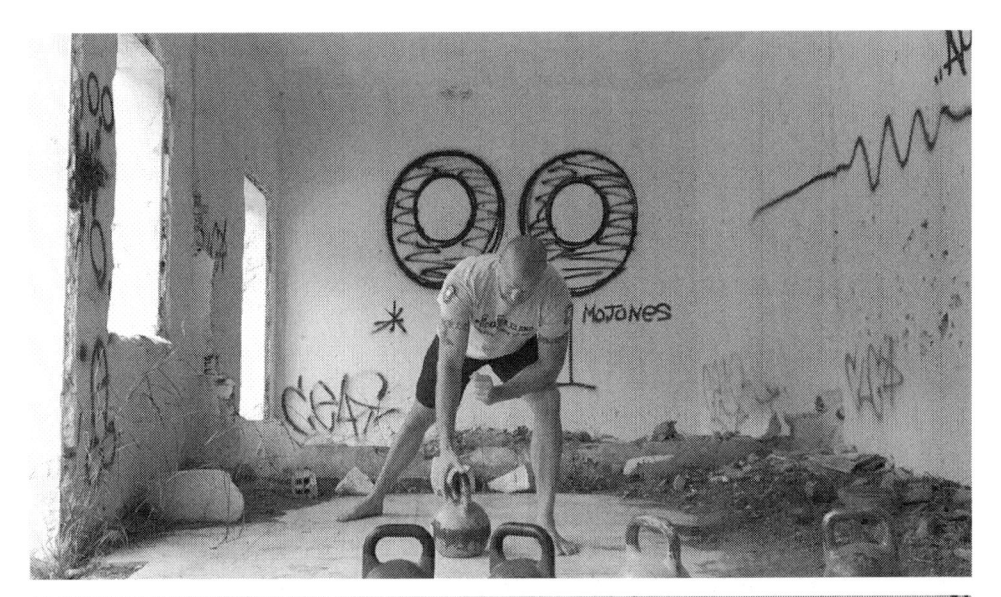

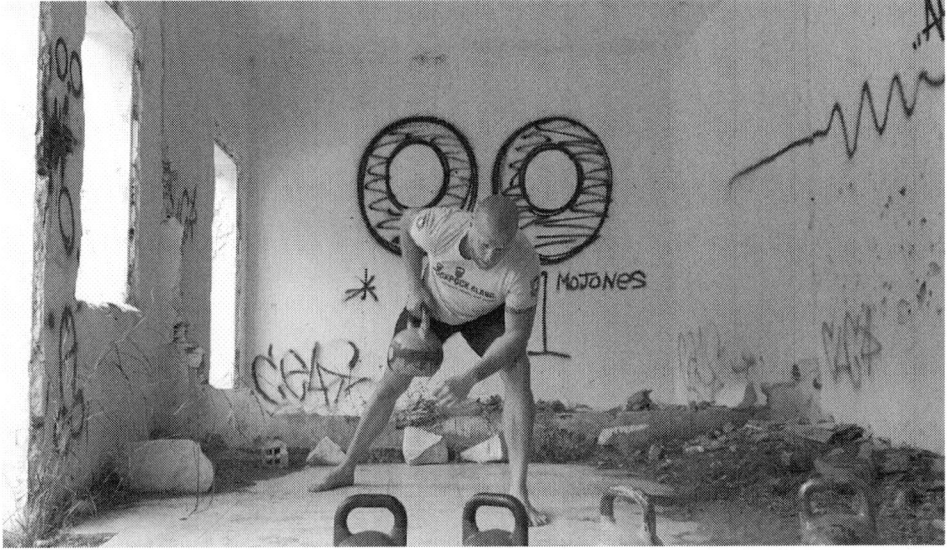

Task

Your fifteenth task is to complete as per below.

Train your row and work your way up over time:

1. 8kg/17.6lbs
2. 12kg/26.4lbs
3. 16kg/35.2lbs

Duration and sets:

- 4 reps each side
  1 set and 10 seconds rest
  Repeat 4 times

- 6 reps each side
  1 set and 15 seconds rest
  Repeat 4 times

- 8 reps each side
  1 set and 20 seconds rest
  Repeat 4 times

If you can find a couple of seconds to rate the book on Amazon I would really appreciate it. go.cavemantraining.com/kbwc-link19

Day 16 Kettlebell American swing

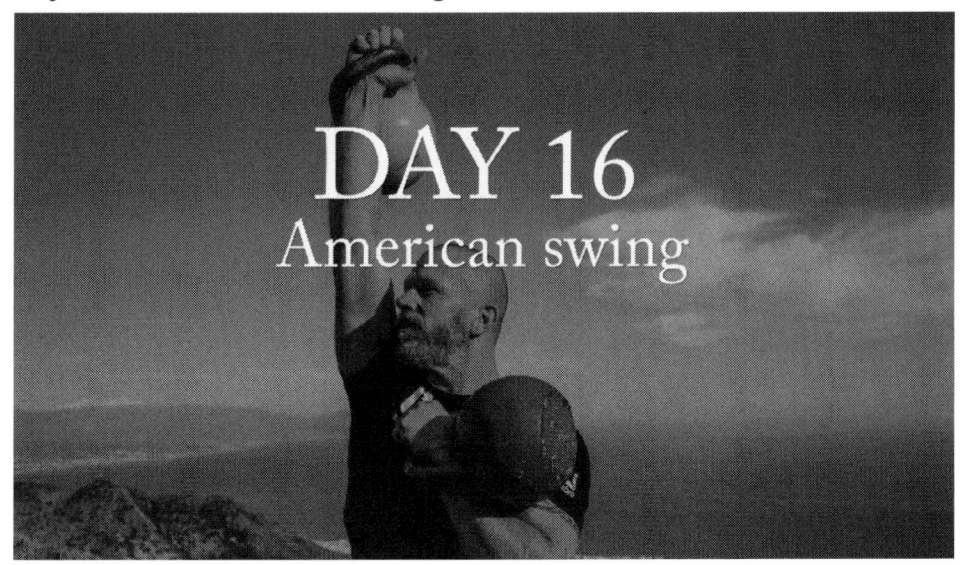

On day 16 you will learn how to perform the American swing which is the most popular version of the swing in CrossFit. The objective and height of this swing is completely different to the previous versions of the swing that I covered.

Dot points:

- The American swing is a swing that does involve a shoulder raise
- This version of the swing is created by CrossFit
- Before you do this exercise you need to check if you can safely/easily bring your arms above your head with a close grip
- The American swing is great if you want to work your shoulders and legs at the same time
- The swing can be performed with a squat, hip hinge, or pendulum

The American swing:

- Perform a swing
- Follow through with a shoulder raise
- Lock the arms out overhead
- Let the bell drop back with slightly bent arms to keep the drop closer
- Guide into the backswing and repeat

You can also replace the raise with a press out and treat this as a double arm snatch.

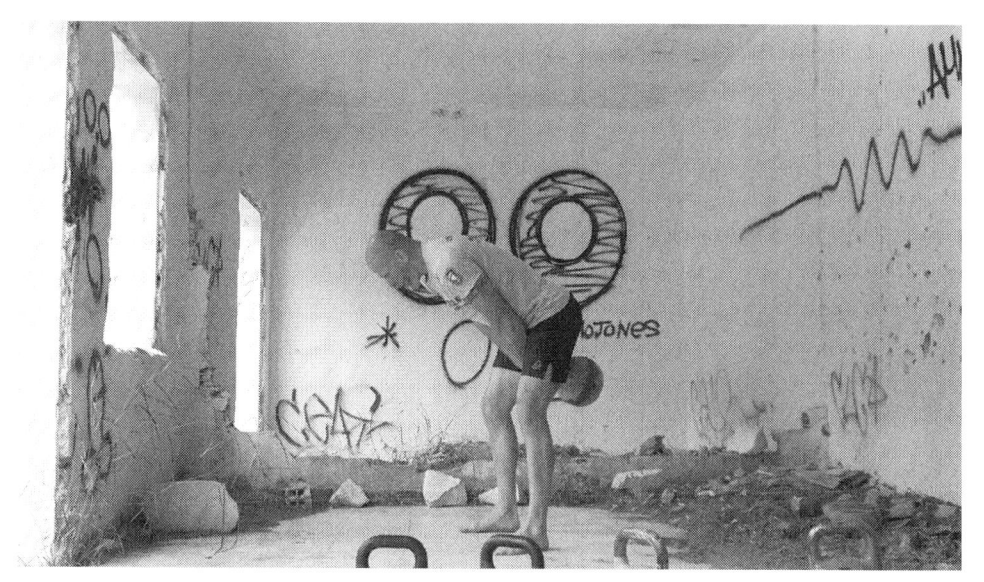

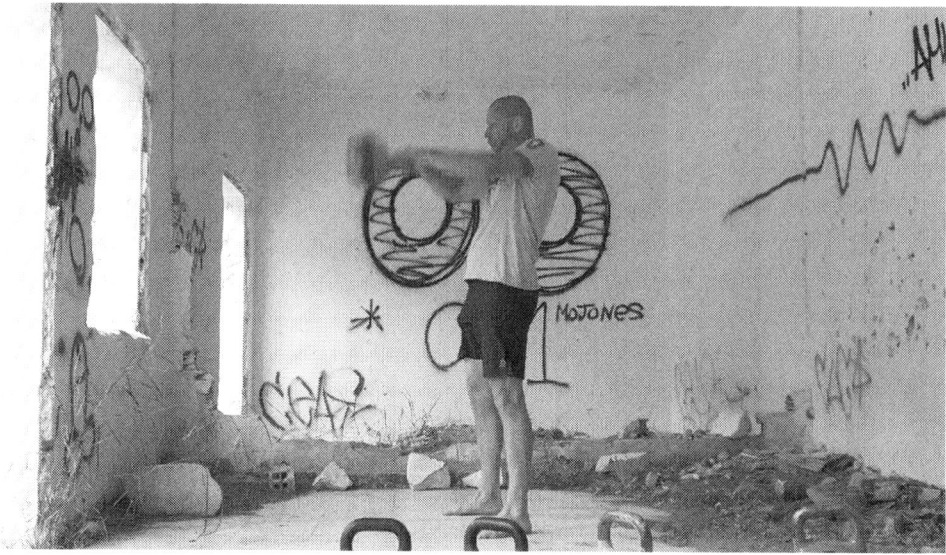

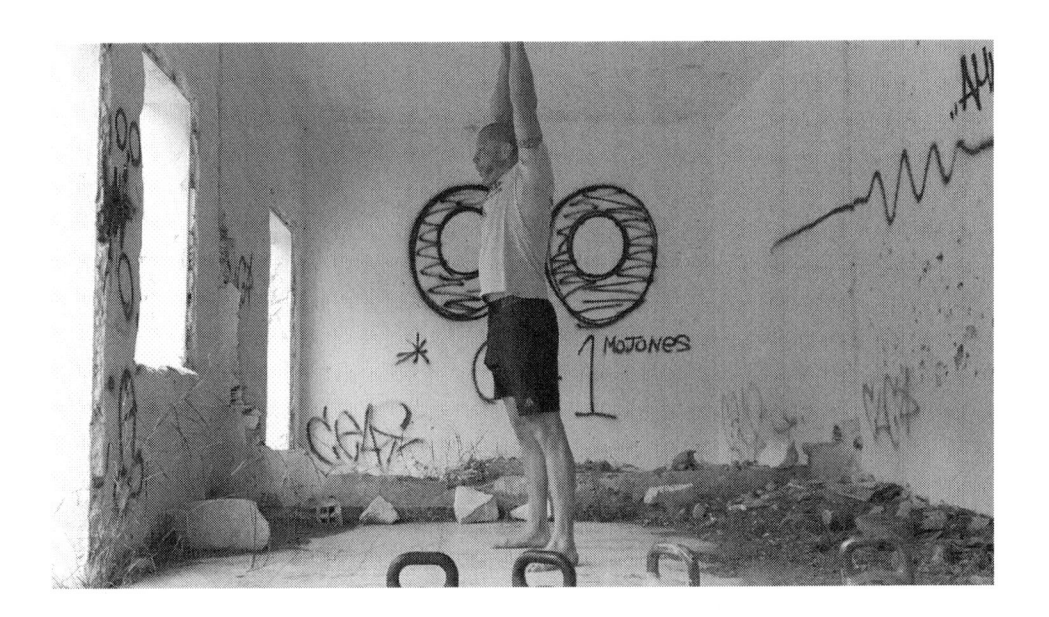

Day 17 Double kettlebell dead swing clean

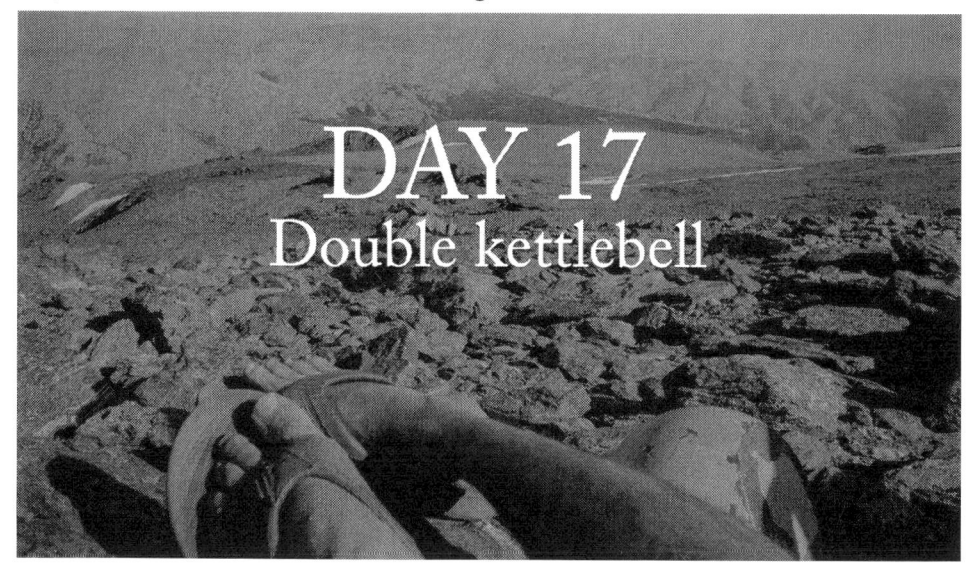

On day 17 you will learn how to clean double kettlebells to lay a basic foundation to start working with double kettlebells when you've mastered all previous steps. However, double kettlebell sounds complex and advanced, but in some cases I've found that people actually get the technique quicker when working with two bells, hence, I like to include it in this course to see if it works for you.

Dot points:

- Double kettlebell work is great to add additional weight to your workout
- Some double bell exercises are but not limited to; front squat; shoulder press; swing; etc.
- How the arm is rotated (where the thumb points) has an effect on the clean
- The effect it has is not covered but you should know that there is so much more to learn about the clean for efficiency
- Safety racking grip is the grip you should implement with double kettlebells
- There is a free PDF you can download which has over 25+ kettlebell grips including the flat hand and others for double bell
- When working with two kettlebells your legs need to be further apart
- Don't get your fingers caught in between the handles when working with double kettlebells

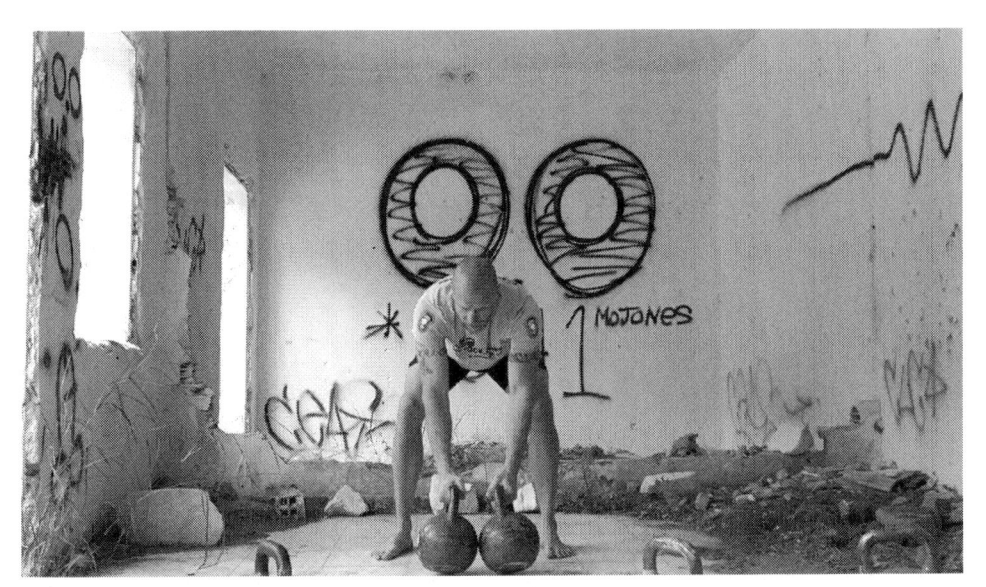

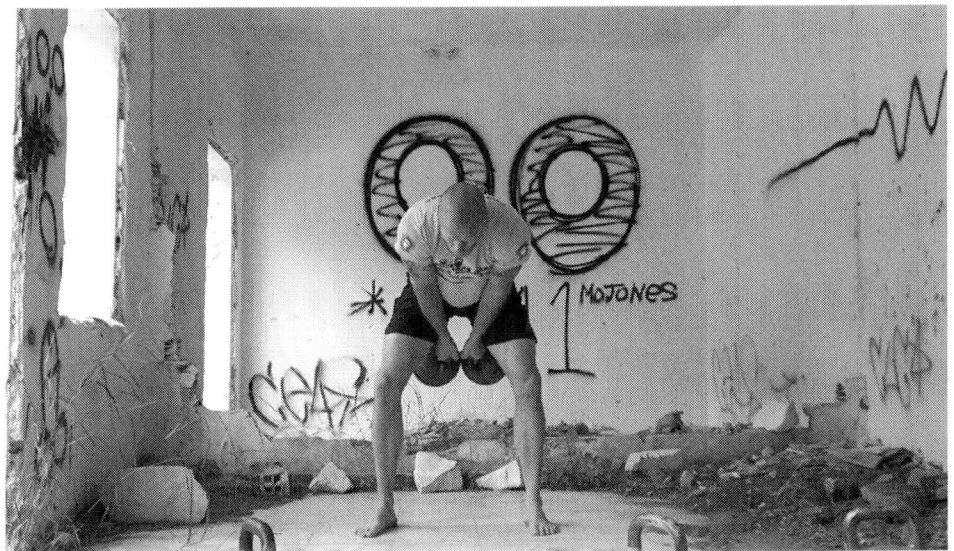

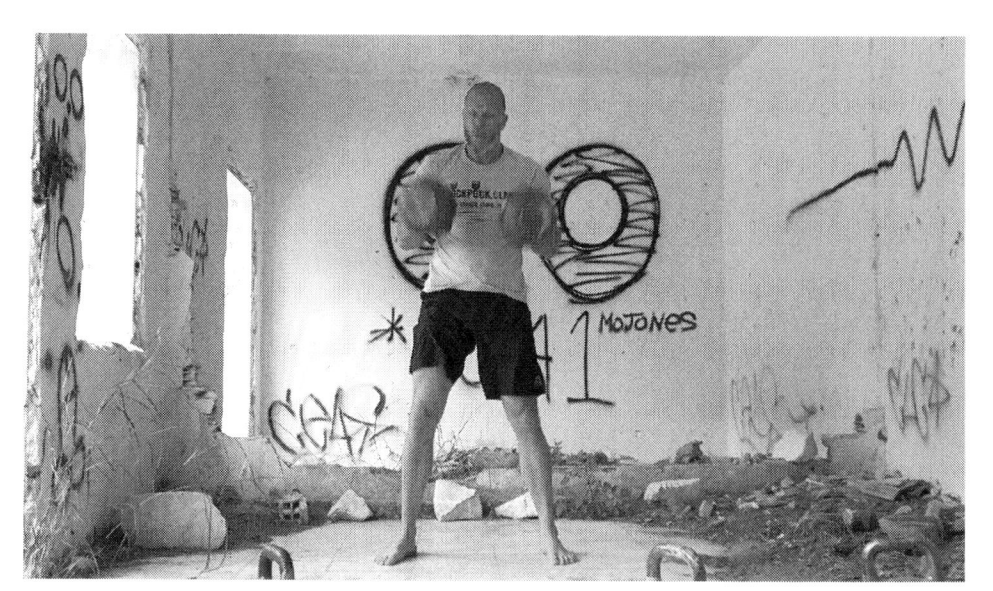

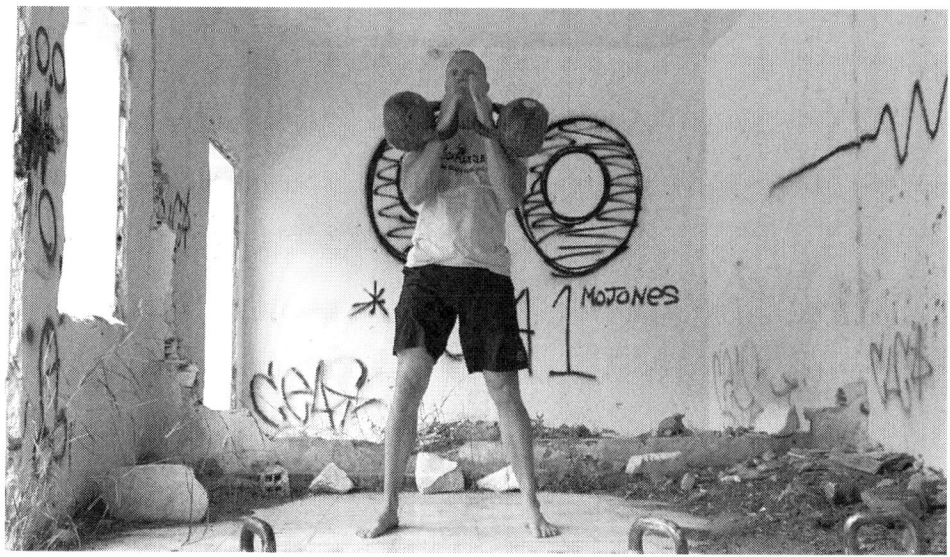

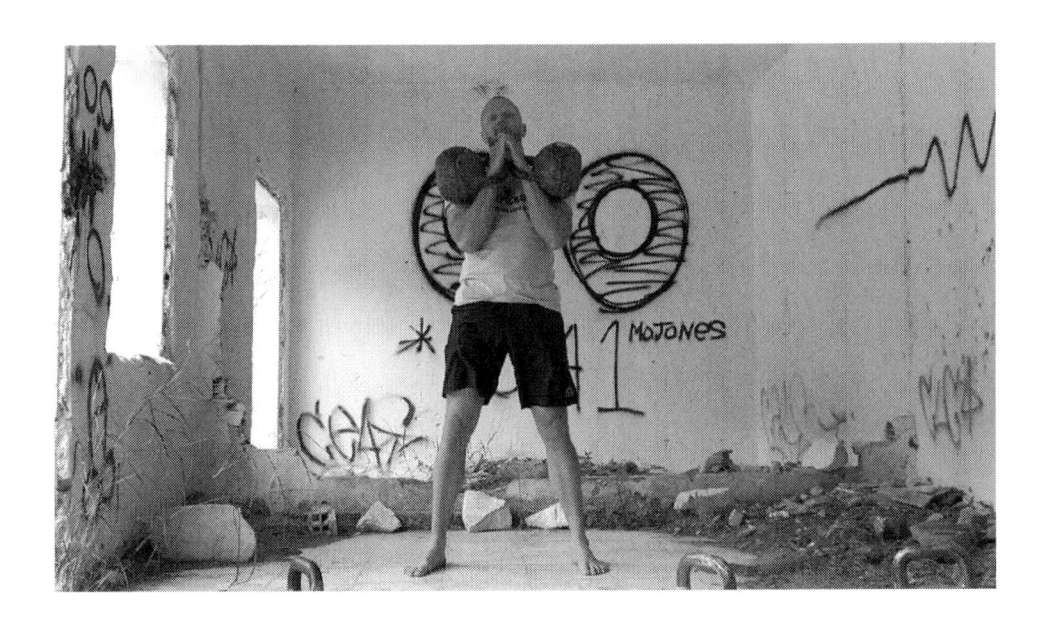

Day 18 Recap and additional kettlebell tips

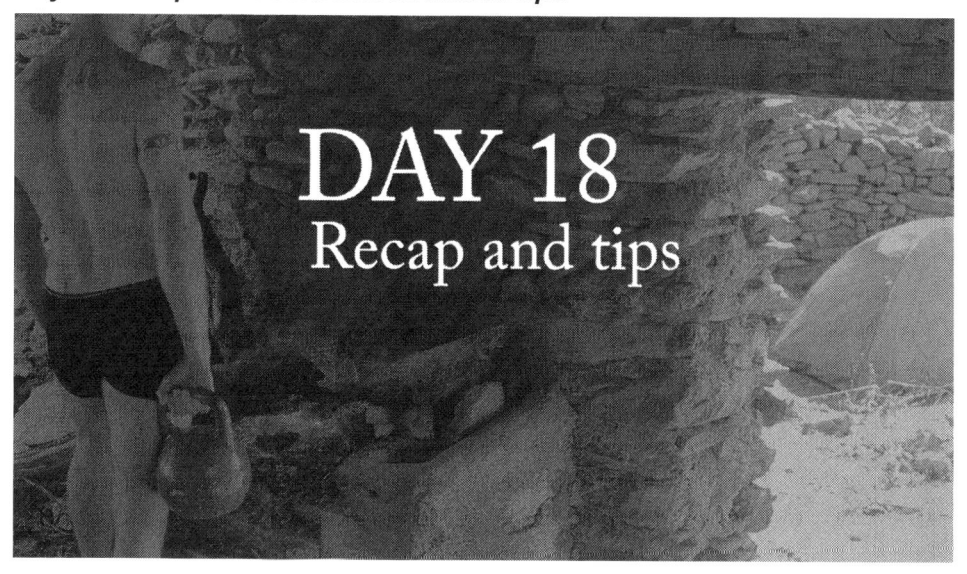

On day 18 I will recap some of the previous days and add additional tips for most of them.

Dot points:

- Warming up and muscle priming are super important
- Mobility work and stretches should become part of your regular training
- Kettlebell grips and assisted clean should be drilled often
- With the dead clean you want to get the power generation right to avoid banging
- If you do come too high you want to come toward and catch the bell
- Don't wait for the bell to bang when it went too high
- This early catch should only be used when working on getting the power
- Don't cast your bell out with the clean to avoid a jolt on the shoulder or lower back
- Move yourself away from the bell to create counter balance
- You need good thoracic and hip mobility to be able to perform this correctly
- Don't follow the kettlebell
- Let the weight drop naturally and guide it back
- Tensing the other arm creates even tension throughout the upper body

- Don't press away from you but up and back to overhead
- If you've progressed with strength and technique you can start looking at pressing away (more advanced)

Day 19 Kettlebell programming and goals

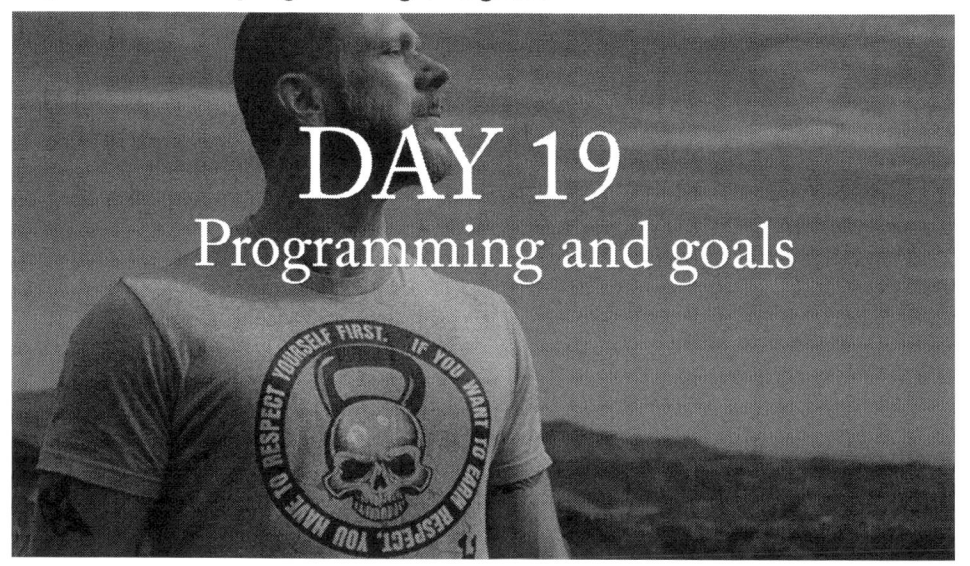

On day 19 I cover some information about basic programming and goals.

Dot points:

- Setting goals in training is important even if those goals are generic training
- Proper programming will help you reach your goals correctly and safely
- Programming involves choosing the right exercises
- Programming for safety involves choosing the right weights and reps
- Identify your goals and write them down
- Figure out how to program to reach those goals
- Training without goals is training for generic fitness
- There is nothing wrong with training for generic fitness
- Find someone to help you reach your goals or do your own research on the topic
- To train for cardiovascular endurance you take lighter weight and work with higher reps
- To train for strength or hypertrophy you go heavier with lower reps and more rest
- To train for flexibility and increased range of motion you program exercises that can challenge your range

- The kettlebell is a weight and can help to reach just about any goal with the right technique and programming behind you
- Due to the design of the kettlebell it is more versatile and optimal for functional movements
- Proper programming is not easy
- To program properly you should learn about muscles and their function
- Think joints not muscles to understand what does what
- Increase weight gradually
- Increase complexity gradually
- Increase rest as you go up with weight
- Control the concentric and eccentric phase and own the movement
- If you're progressing to speed reps then leave the hip hinge deadlift for slow reps for now
- Master the exercise before entering the world of high intensity

TAKE NOTE

The recommendations made in regards to programming are for **beginners**, i.e. assuming you still need to work on strength, coordination, form and technique but still wanting a cardio workout.

Low reps per exercise and muscle groups but performing longer unbroken durations to work on cardio. Once advanced, you can perform longer sets per exercise.

The idea is to increase speed but not to overload muscles and work with bad form and technique, we want to avoid that at all cost. However, once you have mastered an exercise and can identify when form and technique go bad, then it's time to go for longer.

Longer sets are great to work on technique but not under the umbrella of getting is as many reps as possible within the defined amount of time, or getting in a set amount of reps as fast possible. All these types of training are good, but not when you're needing to focus on technique and have other areas to improve upon first.

Day 20 Kettlebell workout

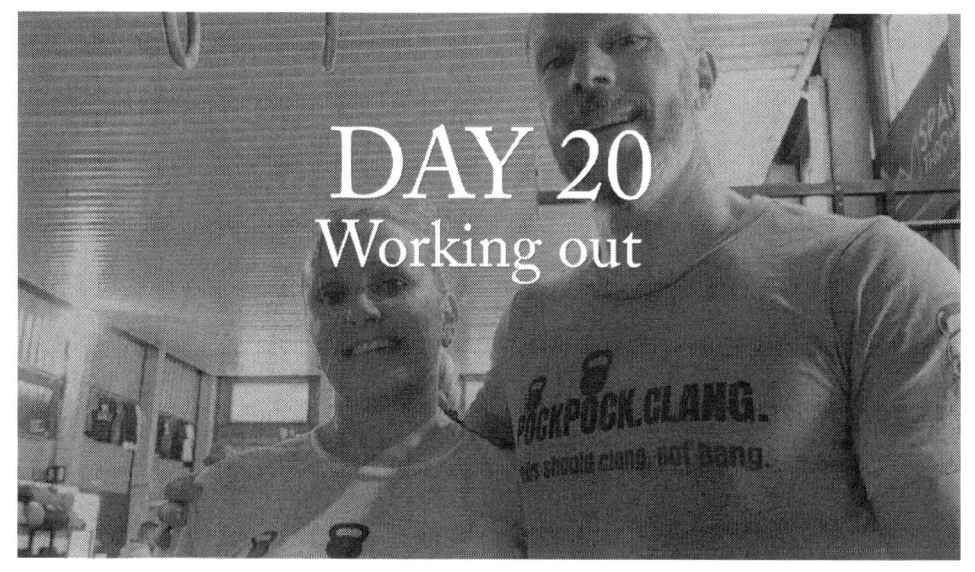

On day 20 you will learn how to string all exercises together and create a few different workouts you can complete.

Workout 1

- Squat dead lift
- Hip hinge dead lift
- Dead swing double arm clean
- Squat
- Press
- Squat thruster (if you feel you're ready)
- Transition to upside down horn grip
- Halo 2 x each side
- Return dead to the ground with a reverse dead swing

Repeat 4 times
Rest 1 minute or include mobility exercises
Work for 20 to 30 minutes.

Notes

The one bell double arm press requires more flexibility than a one arm press. This version of the press is great to work on overhead mobility but you need to progress gently, remember that you can just press half way, next week a bit further, and so on. The double arm press is great to make a heavy weight light enough to press.

If you don't feel comfortable with the transition for the halo grip then add the extra time and relax, put the weight down and pick it up as shown, don't use another complex in the air transition.

Over time you can increase the reps and instead of 1 repetition you can do 2, for example, first 2 weeks you do 1 rep of each exercise, week 3 and 4 you do 2 reps of each exercise, week 5 and 6 you do 3 reps of each exercise and so on till about 6 to 8 reps exercise. You can also increase duration of the workout.

Workout 2

This workout is slightly more advanced than the first one and is programmed more for cardio and endurance.

- One arm swing
- One arm clean
- One arm strict press

Switch at will.

Work for 5 or 10 minutes
Rest in rack

Notes

Rest or reduce weight if you can no longer perform a strict press. Chose your weight carefully at the start.

Create your own workout

Put your own workout together with the exercises you've learned. Feel free to post a copy of your workout with the goals, weight, reps, rest, etc.

I have put together many other beginners workouts for you which you can view on YouTube.

8-minute kettlebell workout www.youtube.com/watch?v=Z75BlIc3zlM

Kettlebell Workout WKV 3 Beginner youtu.be/fOnQgLWwqhY

The Basics—Kettlebell Beginner Workout 3 Exercises youtu.be/jkXtJEF7GuQ

Beginner Workout For Total Body WKV1 youtu.be/rZ_pSdcQIIU

Simple Kettlebell Workout 10 min. Kettlebell youtu.be/ygmFTFdfke8

8 Minute Kettlebell Workout youtu.be/e0q4kHO4okU

Kettlebell Strength Workout - THE BIG FOUR youtu.be/mUyu6haFo8c

This last one is a bit more advanced but still contains all the exercises you've learned in this book but it's performed with two kettlebells. You can perform this with one kettlebell and just double the rounds.

Day 21 Common kettlebell injuries and annoyances

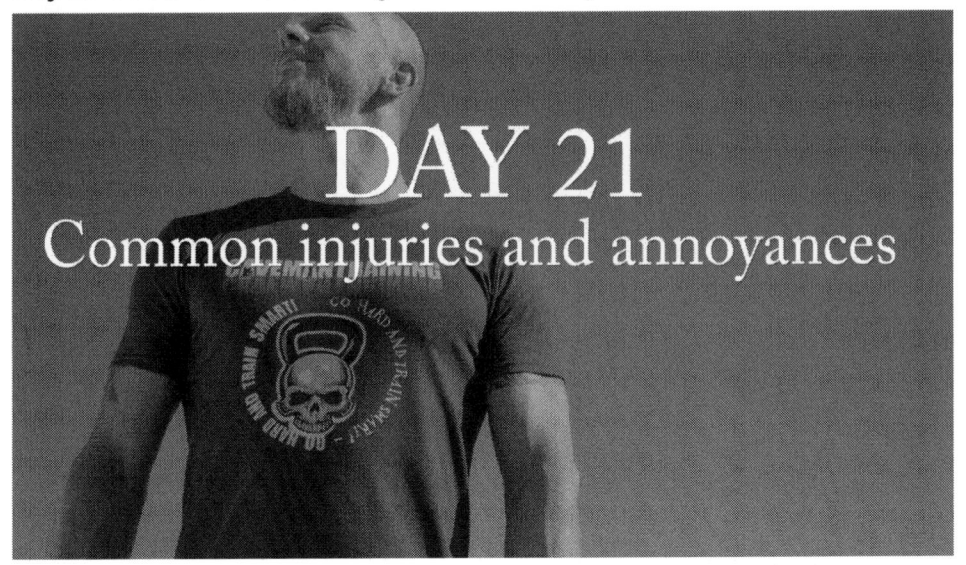

On day 21 you will learn how to avoid common injuries and annoyances with kettlebell training.

Dot points:

- The broken wrist grip is where you don't obtain a good hand insert
- Pressing with a broken wrist grip affects the wrists and can cause injury or pain
- Focus on the assisted clean drill
- Don't work with a broken wrist grip even if the weight is light
- Take your time to get the hand insert right if you intend to train with kettlebells for a long time
- Lower back problems are common with the kettlebell because of the dynamic movements
- The kettlebell is not at fault and neither are the exercises
- The kettlebell requires respect and dedication
- Don't throw the kettlebell out and follow it
- Don't lift with the back but use the muscles intended
- Go back to MMC and muscle priming if back aches occur
- Look at programming when aches occur

- Don't hold the kettlebell too tight or let it flip over the fist
- Kettlebell training does not need to hurt if you invest the time
- Maintain the calluses on your hands
- Work on technique and do not wear gloves
- If you have blisters you need to look at your technique or programming
- Friction occurs in the hand when you don't open up during the clean or the kettlebell bobs during swinging
- The handle does not need to rub when moving directly from hook grip into the 45 degree angle
- Bypass your skin during the clean and insert
- The kettlebell should remain a direct extension of your arm during the swing
- In the beginning you can't avoid mild bruising on your forearm as there has never been a weight resting on it before
- Additional pressure on the forearm can be created by too much wrist flexion
- Grabbing the handle in the middle will result in the middle of the bell providing unnecessary pressure on the forearm

Got back pain?

Don't blame the kettlebell. The kettlebell is just another weight like a dumbbell or barbell.

If you're experiencing lower back pain after a kettlebell workout it could be due to many things, some of the common ones are:

Incorrect technique

Too many reps

Too heavy

Not enough rest

Insufficient recovery

Bad programming

Overtraining

I will explain several simple techniques how to avoid back pain from kettlebell swings and other exercises like cleans, deadlifts, and snatches.

>Don't follow the kettlebell
>
>Contract the gluteus maximus to raise the pelvis
>
>Progress safely
>
>Rest between sets
>
>Let the body recover fully after intense workouts

I will go into more details on the two major causes for tight or lower back pain.

1) Following the kettlebell

Following the kettlebell prematurely is cause number one for lower back problems during kettlebell training! There are several kettlebell exercises in which we let the weight come away from us at the front in a ballistic movement, those are (but not limited to):

- Kettlebell swing
- kettlebell snatch
- Kettlebell clean

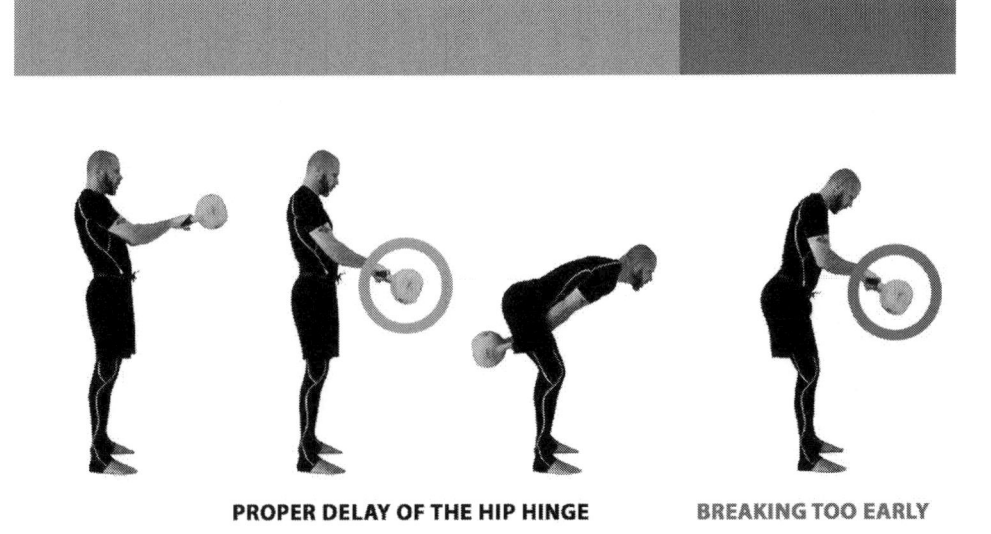

PROPER DELAY OF THE HIP HINGE   **BREAKING TOO EARLY**

2) The Kettlebell Drop

When the kettlebell comes from overhead or racked, it's called 'The Drop'. Following photo is the drop from full snatch. The weight is kept as close to the body as possible, if hip flexion would have been created at this stage then the weight would be further away from the body, and would put unnecessary pressure on the lower back. With hip and thoracic hyperextension (possibly paired with thoracic rotation) the back is in a stronger position to reduce the pulling force.

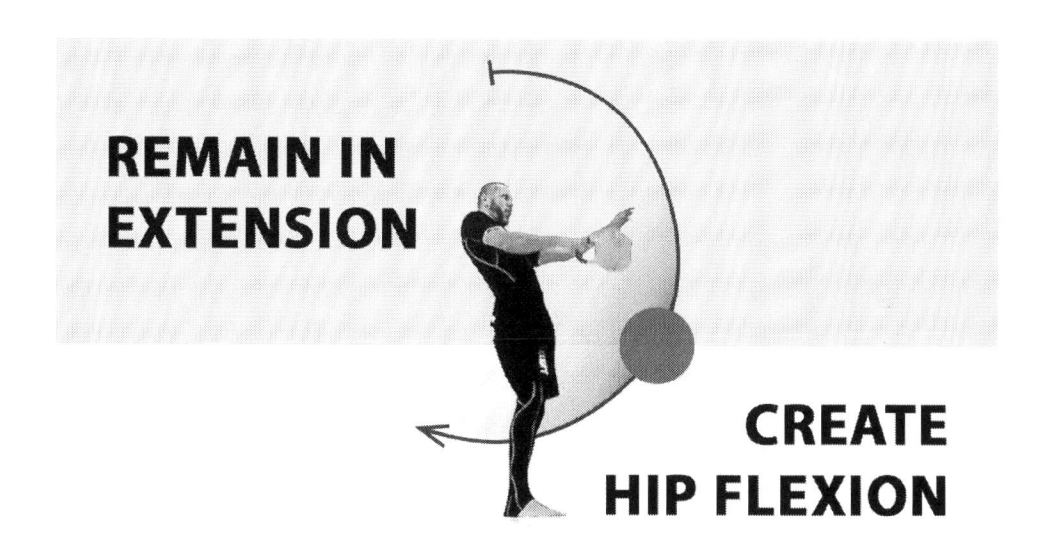

REMAIN IN EXTENSION

CREATE HIP FLEXION

Stiff back after kettlebell swings

If you're experiencing a stiff back after kettlebell swings (American, Russian, or any other swing) it can be due to pre-mature hip flexion, lack of mind-muscle connection, fatigue, too heavy, too many, not enough rest, or insufficient recovery. The pre-mature hip flexion is what I referred to above, and the same principle applies when you're swinging a kettlebell. You do not want to bring the bell further away from you after full extension (standing straight) and the weight is on its way down.

Below is a detailed video I recorded to go paired with this information.
go.cavemantraining.com/kbwc-vid6

Let's talk about the forces and moment of force (torque) taking place during the lift and why incorrect form may lead to injuries and lower back pain.

PHYSICS CONCEPTS BREAKDOWN

Center of Mass: The unique point where the weighted relative position of the distributed mass sums to zero. By moving one's body, one's changing its center of mass.

Distance (d): Horizontal distance between the weight of the kettlebell and the lifter's center of mass.

Moment of force (torque): Rotational force (product between distance and force). Just as a linear force is a push or a pull, a moment of force can be thought of as a twist to an object. The moment of the kettlebell applied on the lifter's body is equal to the distance "d" multiplied by the kettlebell's weight. So, by lowering the distance "d", one's lowering the moment of force (torque) applied. This torque is critical on the lower back.

MOVEMENT DESCRIPTION

The critical position of the exercise is the one at which the kettlebell is applying maximum torque on the lifter's body.

If at this point one does not counterbalance, then the forces on the lower back may cause injury. Buy pulling back, the center of mass moves back as well, but the distance between the weight and the center of mass becomes smaller (the kettlebell moves back even more than the center of mass when pulling), thus lowering the torque.

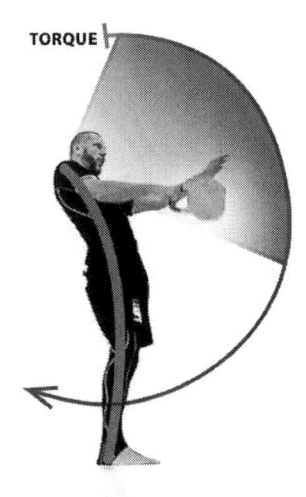

Also, the opposing arch formed by the body (when pulling) is structurally speaking better suited to stand against moment of force (torque). The torque, in this example, has a clockwise orientation (as seen in the picture), and works toward bending forward the spine with flexion. So, if you maintain incorrect posture (bending forward instead of backward) the effects of torque become critical. In this case, the incorrect posture compromises the spine, because it's harder to resist torque in this position and also a forward bend of the spine makes it easier for the torque to work towards bending it even more. The magnitude of the torque is also bigger since the distance "d" increases in this case (by not pulling back, the center of mass moves forward just a little bit while the distance traveled forward by the kettlebell is much higher, therefore the distance "d" increases).

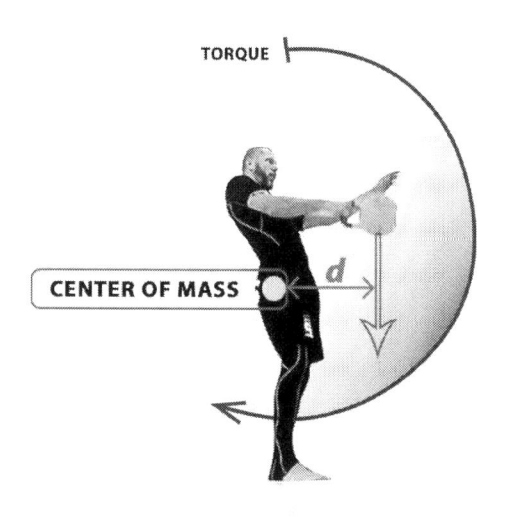

Contract the gluteus maximus

There are several exercises in which we need to create hip extension, those are (but not limited to):

- Kettlebell swing
- kettlebell snatch
- Kettlebell clean
- Deadlift
- Barbell snatch
- Barbell clean

Not contracting the right muscles is cause number two for lower back problems! I know you hear it often, squeeze the gluteals, squeeze them like you're holding on to a 100 dollar bill between your cheeks. But it's actually just your biggest gluteal that we want to concern ourselves with right now. Another reason for a stiff or painful lower back is not connecting with one of the prime movers for hip extension, the gluteus maximus. This gluteal is responsible for pulling your pelvis up, if you pull your pelvis up with this muscle then your other back muscles just need to worry about creating a rigid solid structure to protect the spine and not lifting the weight. Your hamstrings are also prime movers for hip extension, press your heels into the ground to activate them. There is much more to it which I've covered in *Master The Hip Hinge*.

Don'ts

- Don't lift with the back
- Don't break too early
- Don't lift too heavy
- Don't overtrain
- Don't neglect progression

Do's

- Contract your gluteus maximus
- Work on your MMC
- Delay the hip hinge
- Use proper progression
- Watch more of our videos and buy our books

How To Kettlebell Swing

There are a million and one kettlebell swing tutorials out there that will try and teach you how to swing a kettlebell—I know this a bold claim—but most will lack the substance to truly make you understand how and why to swing a kettlebell. This article is different.

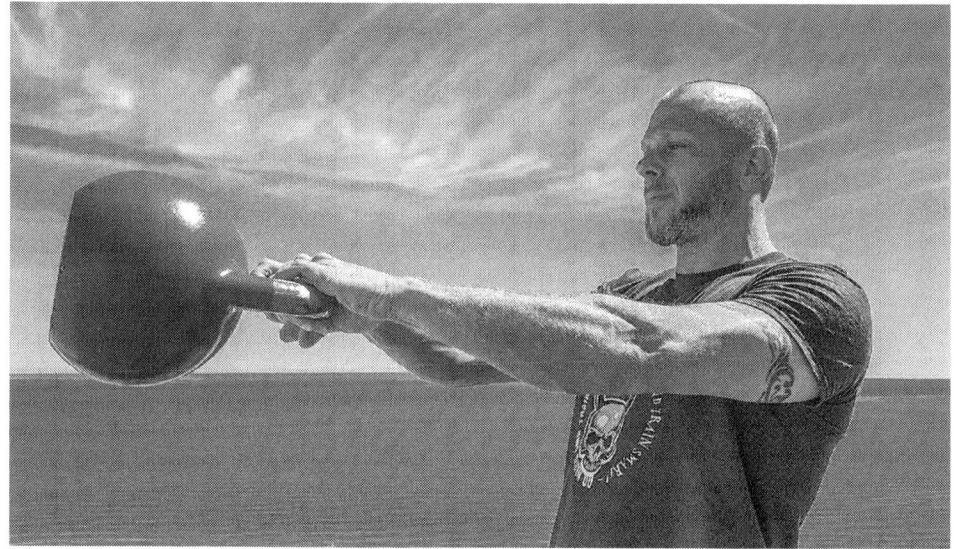

Taco Fleur from Cavemantraining demonstrates the kettlebell swing.

First, allow me to give you a quick introduction to myself, I've been swinging kettlebells for over a decade, I have plenty of kettlebell training and other qualifications, I've swung a kettlebell one third my bodyweight for 11,111 times. Enough about me, I just wanted to make it clear that I know how to swing a kettlebell efficiently and safely for multiple purposes.

A purpose is what you need to swing a kettlebell, that purpose might be to lose weight, to tone-up, to get fitter, or more flexible, whatever your reason is, you should know it, to be able to find the right kettlebell swing that is good for you.

There are plenty of kettlebell swing variations to chose from, and together with your purpose for swinging, you will be able to make an informed choice of which variation to chose. This is where this article is so different than most others, as most others will try to teach you their one way of swinging a kettlebell, without going into the reason and variations. Here are some of the variations:

- Double-arm kettlebell swing AKA Russian swing
- CrossFit swing AKA American swing
- Pendulum swing AKA Sport style swing
- Hardstyle swing

Those are some of the popular and better know variations, but there are literally hundreds of variations that exist, I won't go into those. I will say that I'll be skipping the American swing and that with the remainder of the list you can sort of break it down into:

- Double arm
- Single arm
- Hip hinge movement
- Squat movement

With the above we have enough info to create a whole arsenal of awesome kettlebell swing variations, so, let's get stuck into how and when you should use each variation.

The attributes that provide you with results are:

- How heavy you swing
- How fast you swing
- How many unbroken reps you swing
- How much rest you have in between sets

The heavier the weight, the fewer reps you'll most likely swing, but the muscles are put under more load. Muscles under more load is what you want if you want to get stronger, or bigger.

The lighter the weight, the more reps you'll most likely swing, but the muscles are put under less load. Less load is what you want if you want to go longer for a cardio purpose.

You want to pick a medium weight if you want to work on power and work with low rep ranges, with adequate rest in between. That was just a quick overview of some results you can achieve with different weights or time under load, there is much more to it than that.

What are you after? Strength, power, or endurance? Strength is what you need to move heavy stuff, power is what you need to move heavy stuff quicker, endurance is what you need to last, and that can be cardio or muscle wise. For example, you could be swinging fast and run out of breath, that's your cardio. You could be swinging long and your cardio is fine, but your muscles give up, that's your muscular endurance. With that out of the way, let's dig deeper and look at the muscles used.

What Muscles Are Used With The Kettlebell Swing?

Let's look at why you want to swing a kettlebell, what exactly can it do for your body? To figure that out we need to look at muscles involved in the swing, the muscles that action the movement, prime movers, and the muscles that keep you in place, stabilizers. I will go through them step-by-step.

First, your grip on the kettlebell, this works the muscles in your forearm. To hold on to the kettlebell handle, finger flexion is required, this is achieved through contraction of the following muscles:

- Flexor digitorum superficialis

- Flexor digitorum profundus
- Flexor digit minimi brevis
- Lumbricals

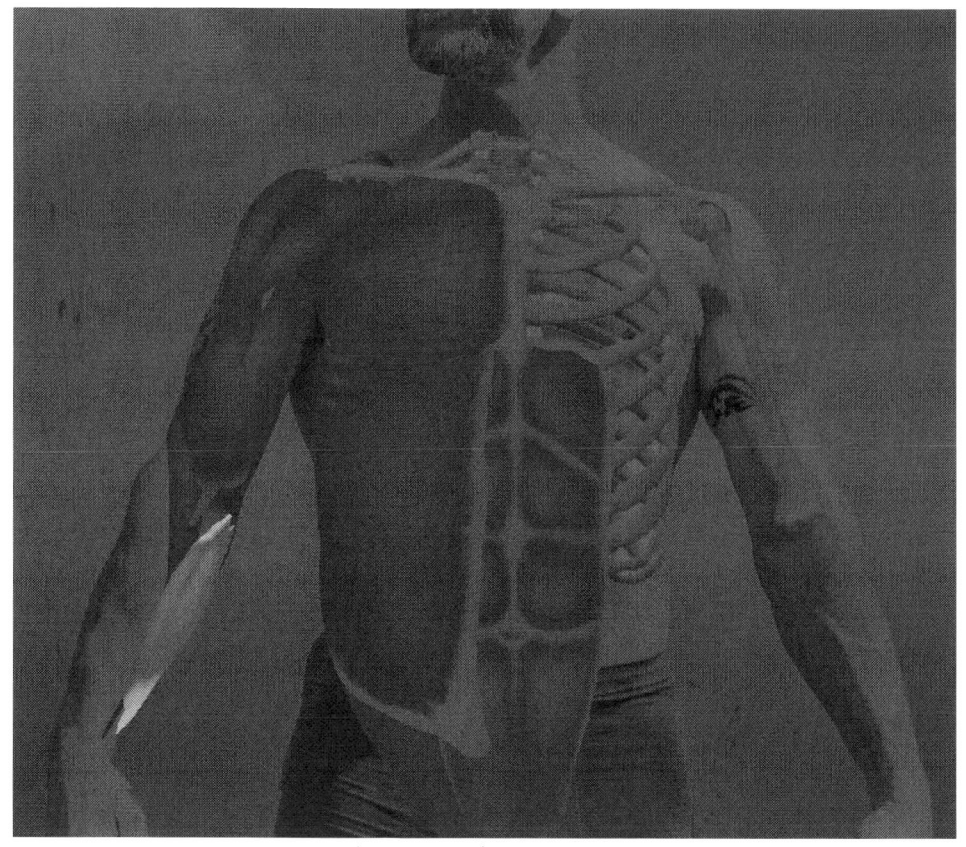

Photo courtesy of Cavemantraining.

Your arms should remain extended through the swing, so, you won't be using the elbow flexors, nor extensors (think bicep curl and arm extension). You should not be using your shoulders to raise the kettlebell, so, your deltoids should not be involved in the movement.

There is a weight pulling on you from the front, so, you should maintain good posture and keep the shoulders back and down. A good posture is achieved through slightly contracting the shoulder blades together and down. This action involves:

- Rhomboideus minor
- Rhomboideus major
- Lower trapezius

- Levator scapulae
- Latissimus dorsi.

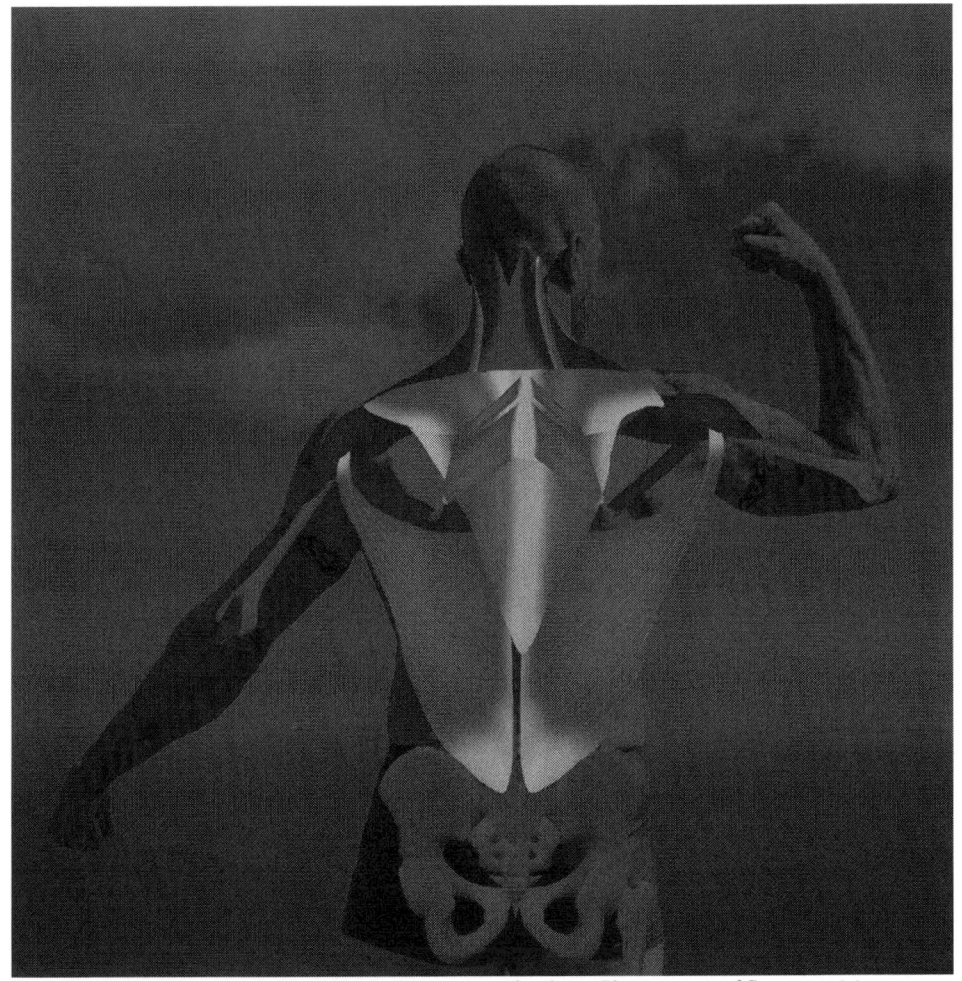

Note: Rhomboids are displayed on top of the trapezius for clarity. Photo courtesy of Cavemantraining.

Next, your spine, you'll need to work to keep it erect. This action requires you to work all spinal erectors, also known as the erector spinae muscle group, which includes the following groups:

- Iliocostalis
- Longissimus
- Spinalis

These muscle groups combined contain over 18 muscles.

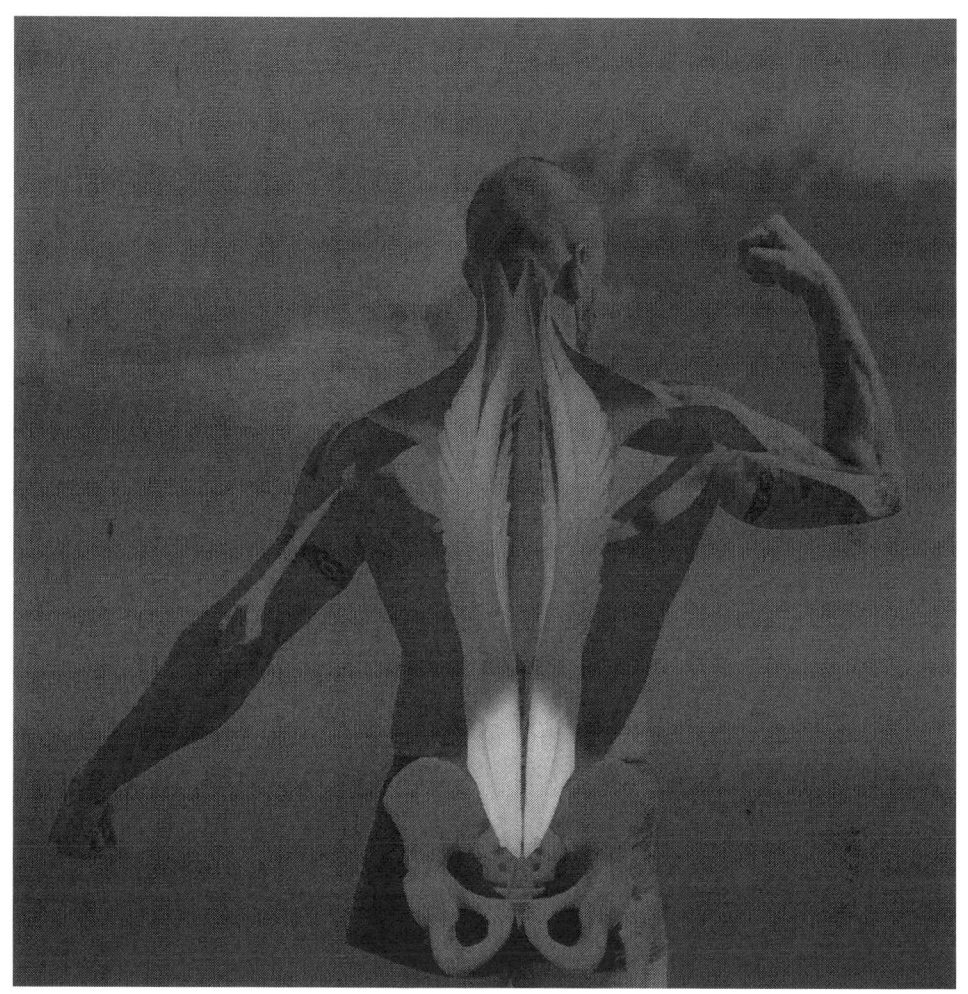

Photo courtesy of Cavemantraining.

Now we're getting to the important part of the swing, what we covered so far was great, but not the reason why you want to pick up a kettlebell and swing it. We've arrived at the prime movers, the muscles that make the movement possible, well, if you're doing the swing correctly and are not using your back or shoulders to move the weight. The gluteus maximus, also known as your buttocks or gluteals. I have to dig a bit deeper as it's important! Trainers frequently call out "squeeze your glutes", but 99.9% of the time we only want you to activate the main and biggest gluteal of them all, the gluteus maximus. You have three gluteals and they do different things, the maximus is a hip extensor, meaning it works to extend your hips, i.e. push them forward, or control the descent of the hips. The medius and minimus abduct the thigh, abduct is to take away, i.e. move the leg away from the body, or in other words, swing your foot out to the side.

We're not done yet. The other prime mover is the hamstrings, this is a group of three muscles which function to extend the hip. They are:

- Bicep femoris (long head)
- Semitendinosus
- Semimebranosus

I know that's a mouth full, hamstrings sound much better. Last but not least, the final member of the hip extensors is the adductor magnus.

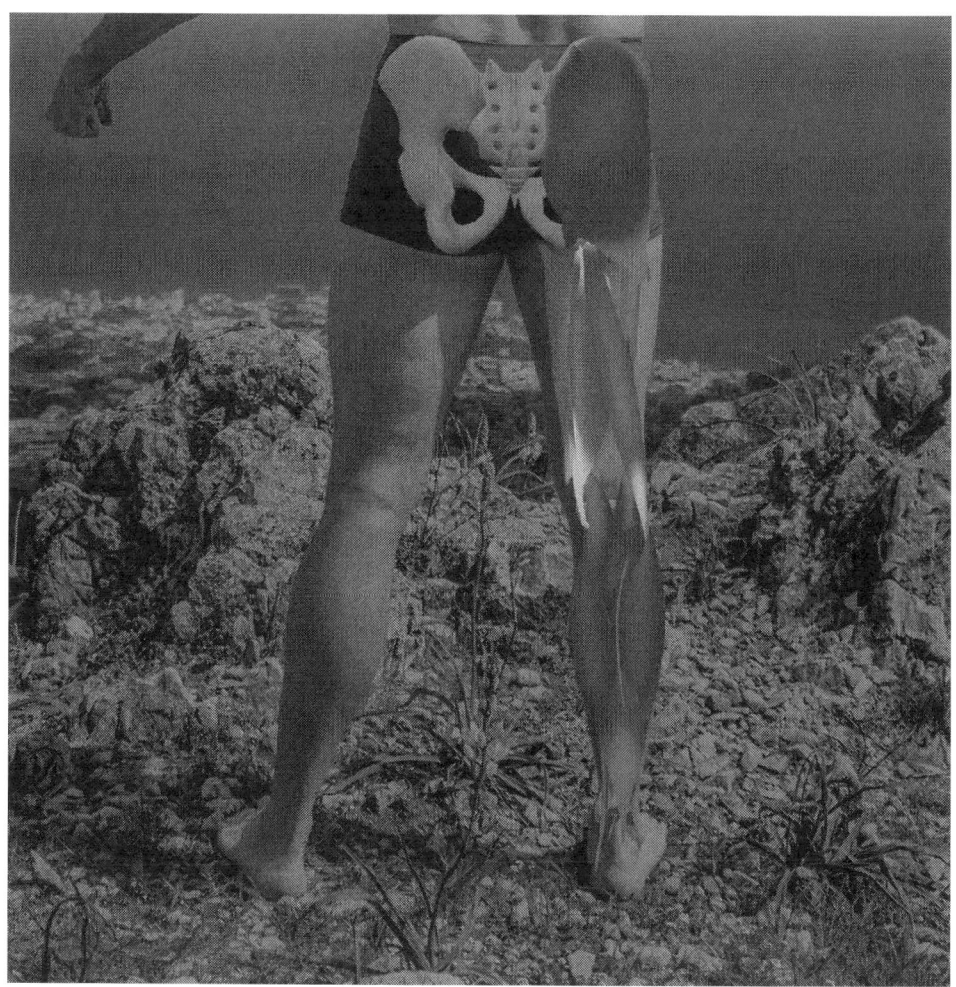

Photo courtesy of Cavemantraining.

All of the muscles function to pull the pelvis up. The first muscle I mentioned, the gluteus maximus, it is connected to the top of the pelvis and to the femur (your leg). If the muscle contracts, it pulls the top of the pelvis up. The other prime mover muscles I mentioned, they're connected to the bottom of the pelvis and to your femur. They pull from the bottom to get the pelvis upright. The pelvis sits on your femur, from there it hinges back and forth.

I know some of this can get quite complicated and might sound not useful at all, but it is, once you know all this, then you know what muscles to contract, and what muscles are doing the work. More importantly, you know how to stay safe and prevent the lower back pain that a lot of people complain about when doing kettlebell swings.

Let's go a little step further, because this is an area usually neglected, i.e. most people stop once they've covered the prime movers, not me, I'll always go that extra mile. We've basically gone from the hand, arm, shoulder, torso, hips, to the thigh. But we still have the lower leg, it does some work too. In particular, knee flexion and keeping the knee in place above the ankle. Keeping the knee above the ankle is important when hip hinging, if the knee comes excessively forward, then the movement starts to turn into a squat. This is a controversial topic, kettlebell swing and squat, so I won't go there this time. Just remember hip hinge for now. Getting back to knee flexion (bending of the knee), this is actioned by the following muscles:

- Biceps femoris
- Semitendinosus
- Semimembranosus
- Gracilis
- Sartorius
- Gastrocnemius
- Soleus
- Popliteus

Yes, those first 3 are part of the hamstrings, and we also saw these used for hip extension. Some might ring a bell with you, like the gastrocnemius and soleus, these are your calf muscles.

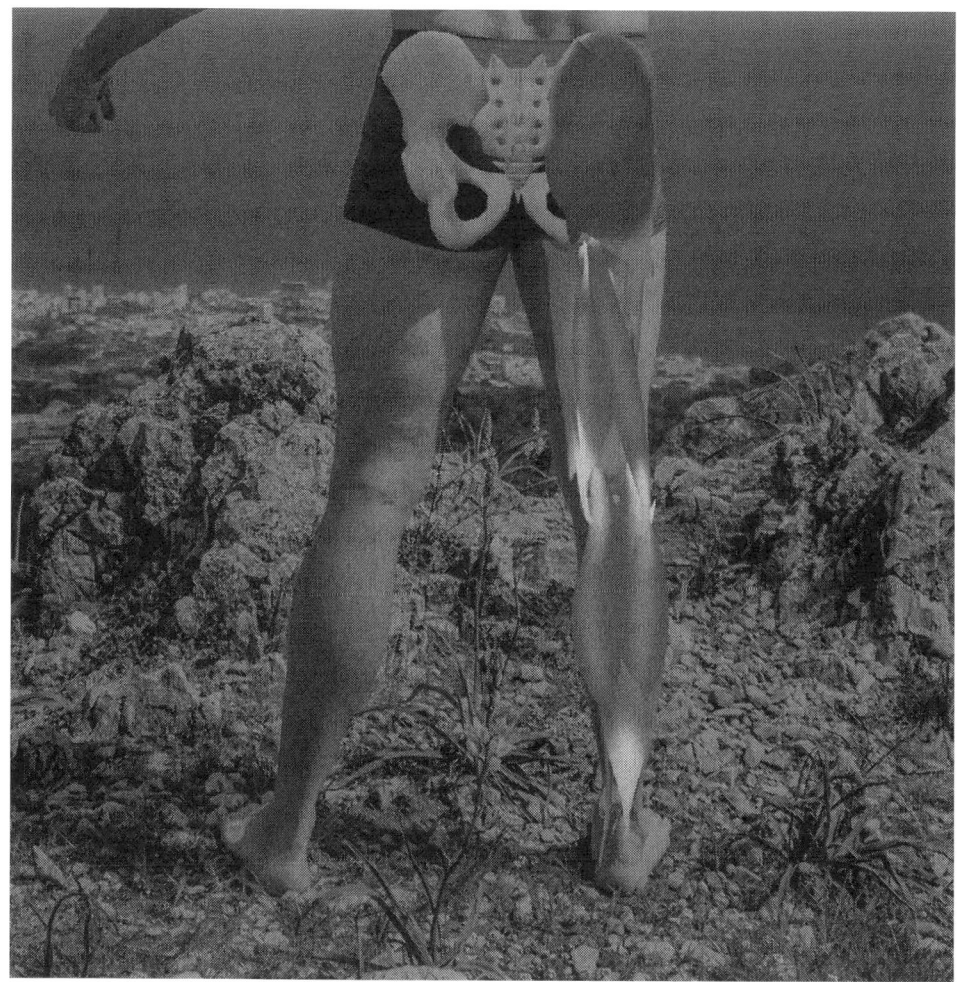

Photo courtesy of Cavemantraining.

We now have quite a big list of muscles worked and joints moved with just one exercise, which is why the kettlebell swing is called a compound exercise. A compound exercise is an exercise that includes multi-joint movements and works several muscles or muscle groups at one time. Compound exercises are great!

Hip Hinge Swing

The kettlebell swing with hip hinge movement is the most common swing. A hip hinge can be described as bringing the hips back and down while keeping the knees above the ankles, and bringing the shoulders toward the ground while keeping the back in a neutral position. The biggest difference between the hip hinge and squat is that with the squat you will be bringing your hips toward the ground and keeping your shoulders as high as possible, which is the opposite of the hip hinge. If you've deadlifted or performed bent-over rows in the gym before, then you've probably already performed the hip hinge.

Here is a clear video demonstrating the difference between the hip hinge and squat style swing in slow-motion go.cavemantraining.com/kbwc-vid9. In the vide the left side demonstrates the hip hinge, and the right the squat. You can clearly see that the hips go low on the right, while the hips remain high on the left.

How To Swing

I realize it might look like we got here in a roundabout way, but trust me, with the above information out of the way you'll catch on much quicker, and most importantly, stay safe and injury free. Here are the cues I use to teach the kettlebell swing:

1. Stand in a neutral position
2. Deadlift the kettlebell up with two hands
3. Bring the kettlebell in front of one leg
4. Bump the kettlebell out and away
5. Don't worry about the distance you bump it
6. At the same time direct the weight to the middle
7. Let it swing back through the legs
8. You're still standing straight
9. Break at the hips when the weight nears the legs
10. Push the hips back and down
11. Bend the knees but keep them above the ankles
12. Keep the spine neutral
13. Keep the head aligned with the spine
14. Let the weight come through the legs
15. Weight should never go lower than the knees
16. You should feel a good stretch in the hamstrings
17. Push the weight back a bit to get extra depth
18. The backswing is at an end when your arms hit your belly and can't go any further
19. You should be looking at the ground in-front of you

20. Next is the upswing
21. Let the weight come back out
22. Start pulling the pelvis back up by squeezing the gluteals
23. Press the heels into the ground for good hamstring activation
24. Pull the kettlebell out
25. Extend the knees
26. Extend the hips
27. Direct the weight forward and not up
28. Stand up straight
29. Pull the shoulders back and down so that your posture is nice and firm
30. Let the weight float
31. Do not pull it up with the shoulders no matter what
32. Don't worry about height
33. Generate more power on the next swing if it does not reach shoulder height
34. Let weight fall back down after the floating phase
35. Do nothing
36. Wait till the weight is near the legs
37. Break at the hips
38. Hip hinge like you did before
39. Let the weight come through the legs
40. Direct the weight to the back
41. Let the weight stop at the end of the backswing
42. You have now completed a full swing
43. Repeat the swing without putting it down

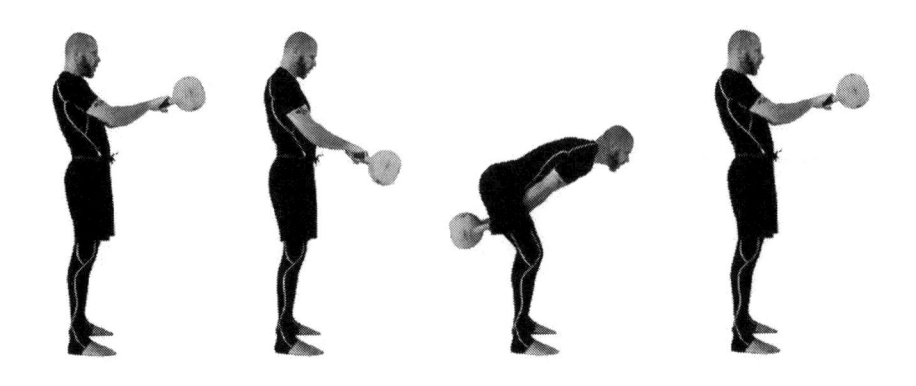

Watch a demo of the kettlebell swing described above go.cavemantraining.com/kbwc-vid10

I am swinging a heavy kettlebell, if you're just starting out, you should choose a weight that's suitable for you. Don't go too light though. Using a weight too light is a common mistake, a weight too light just doesn't provide the required resistance for a good swing. For females, I would suggest at least 12kg/26.4lbs, and for males at least 16kg/35.2lbs.

Don't worry about getting the movement perfect right away, it's not going to happen. It will take some time to perfect the swing, just pay attention to main safety and technique points:

- Use your legs and not your lower back
- Use your lower body and not your shoulders
- The weight should come through about knee height and no lower

Practice and practice until you have a good swing. The down phase of the swing is a good hip hinge with the weight pointing back, and the up phase of the swing is where you're in the same position as the static plank, but holding a weight that's swinging and now pointing forward. The plank is a good analogy for the floating phase, you need to activate pretty much the same muscles, and have the same posture at this stage as you would in the plank. Firm tight and packed chest that holds the shoulders nicely in the sockets, with the arms straight for now (bent requires more explanation).

The Single Arm Kettlebell Swing

This swing variation has the same hip hinge movement as the Russian swing. The difference is that you're using one arm to swing with. This allows you to make the swing harder, i.e. 16kg with one arm is harder than with two arms. But it also adds torque to the exercise, i.e. only one side has weight pulling, this will want to pull the swinging side of your torso forward and your other side needs to work harder to resist that torque. This is a good thing.

Watch a video of the single arm swing here go.cavemantraining.com/kbwc-vid11 another shorter demo here go.cavemantraining.com/kbwc-vid12

You might notice that I start the swing with the weight being dead. If you have mastered the hip hinge by now, you can progress to starting the swing like this, if not, stick to deadlifting and bumping it out.

Once you've mastered the single arm swing, you can start looking at switching during the swing, this allows you to last longer and keep moving while you're working on your cardio. Although the following video demonstrates a clean, it's the hand switch that you want to pay attention to go.cavemantraining.com/kbwc-vid13

You can play with the rep scheme, for example, you can do 5 swings on one side, switch, and do 5 swings the other side, repeat for 10 rounds. The great thing about single arm and switching is, you're not going to burn out your grip as easily as you would with double arm endurance swings. Eventually, you can work on your muscular endurance and stick with one arm, until you're almost fatigued, and then switch.

Kettlebell Squat Style Swing

You now know enough about the swing and are ready to learn about the kettlebell swing squat style. The squat style is where your knees come forward, and your hips are coming low while your shoulders remain high. You're looking ahead rather than the ground in front of you.

Watch a demo of the squat style swing here go.cavemantraining.com/kbwc-vid14 and I also recommend watching the side by side comparison again go.cavemantraining.com/kbwc-vid15

This is a great time to talk about whether the arms should be straight (elbows extended) or bend (elbows flexed). If you're just starting out and still have so many other things to think about and correct, then you should use fully extended arms. This is to prevent injury in the elbow flexors due to a continuous pulling force on contracted muscles. Once you understand the trajectory of the kettlebell, i.e. the path the kettlebell travels can be more outward than upward, or vice versa and more upward than outward. This is especially the case with the squat style swing, hence the reason I cover this subject here. During the squat movement the kettlebell does not go back through the legs as much as it would with the hip hinge movement, and therefore the path the kettlebell will travel is more upward than forward. When the kettlebell goes more upward than outward, it's perfectly fine to bend the elbows, as long as there is no forward pulling force. You want to feel where the kettlebell wants to go and leave the elbows bend to stay with the path of the pull upward.

The squat version of the swing is performed as following, with many of the cues from the hip hinge swing transferring to this version:

1. Stand in a neutral position
2. Deadlift the kettlebell up with two hands
3. Bring the kettlebell in front of one leg
4. Bump the kettlebell out and away
5. Don't worry about the distance you bump it
6. At the same time direct the weight to the middle
7. Let it swing back through the legs
8. You're still standing straight
9. When the weight nears the legs is when you break at the knees and hips
10. Push the hips down and knees forward
11. Keep the spine neutral
12. Keep the head aligned with the spine
13. Let the weight come through the legs
14. The backswing is at an end when your arms hit your belly and can't go any further
15. You should be looking ahead
16. Now we're going to work on the upswing
17. Let the weight come back out
18. Press the heels into the ground for good hamstring activation
19. Pull the knees back
20. Start pulling the pelvis back up by squeezing the glutes
21. Pull the kettlebell up and out
22. Extend the knees
23. Extend the hips

24. Direct the weight forward and up
25. Stand up straight
26. Pull the shoulders back and down so that your posture is nice and firm
27. Let the weight float
28. Do not pull it up with the shoulders no matter what
29. Don't worry about the height the bell comes to
30. Generate more power on the next swing if it does not reach shoulder height
31. Let the weight fall back out of the floating phase
32. Do nothing
33. Wait till the weight is near the legs
34. Break at the knees and hips
35. Squat like you did before
36. Let the weight come through the legs
37. Direct the weight to the back and down
38. Let the weight stop at the end of the backswing
39. You have now completed a full swing
40. Repeat the swing without putting it down

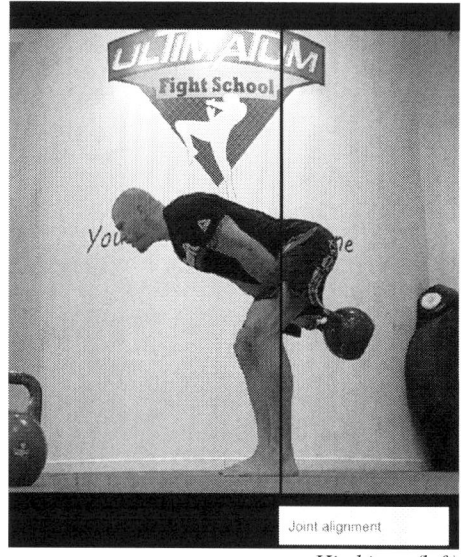

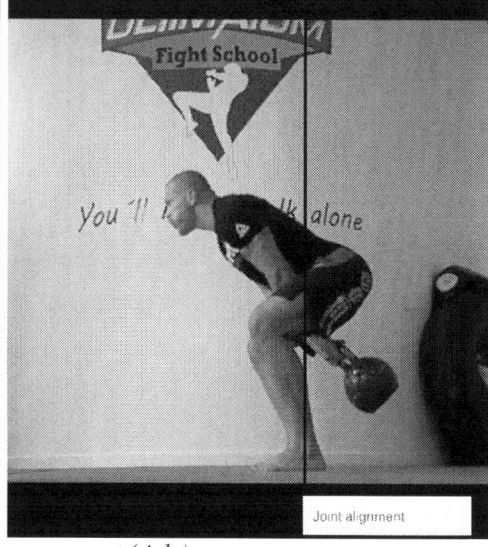

Hip hinge (left) versus squat (right)

Kettlebell Sport Style Swing AKA Fluid Style

This variation of the kettlebell swing existed before any other type of swing, this is where it all came from. Kettlebells have been a sport in Russia long before we even heard of kettlebells. This type of swing is used to improve just two things, that is, the upswing for the clean, and the upswing for the snatch. This is the reason that this type of swing does not go out, but up, and stays much closer to the body. It's designed to last longer by removing as much resistance as possible. This is in contrast to the other types of swings where you want as much resistance as possible to provide a load on the muscles, and tax the cardiovascular system. Kettlebell sport is awesome, once you get to know a bit about kettlebells, I can highly recommend looking into this. The sport is where people snatch, jerk, clean and jerk, for 10 minutes, 30 minutes, and even one hour.

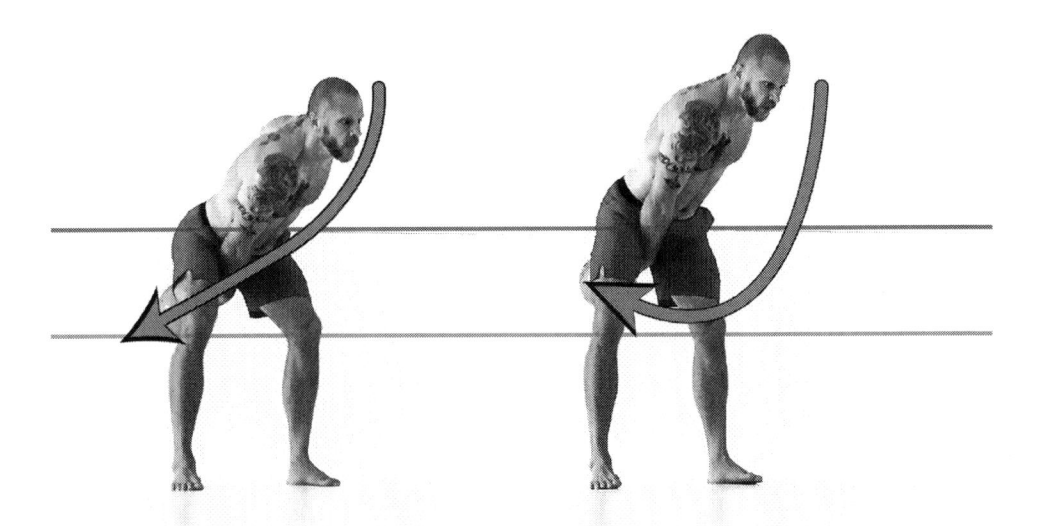

The first is that of an insert with the conventional swing and the second example demonstrates the trajectory of the kettlebell sport (pendulum) swing.

Since you're more than likely not ready to get into the sport yet, I won't delve much deeper into this swing other than, this swing movement is designed to go with the flow and push rather than pull.

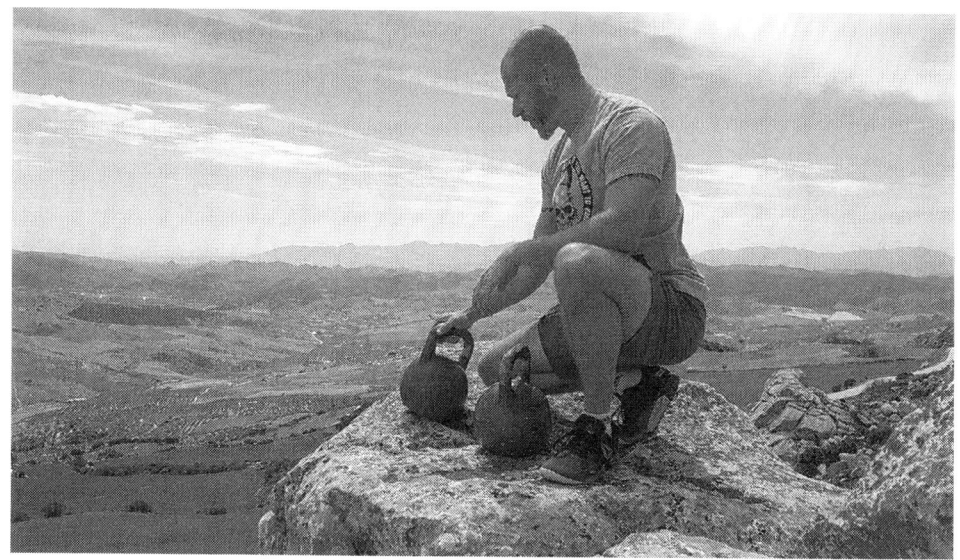

Taco Fleur. Photo courtesy of Cavemantraining.

Working Out With Swings

Now that you know more about the swing and how to perform it, you'll want to start looking at how you can incorporate this exercise into your workouts. You can mix the kettlebell swing with plenty of other exercises, for example, 10 double arm swings, 10 squats, 5 single arm swings on one side, 5 single arm swings on the other side, 10 jumping jacks, repeat for 8 rounds. If you want a serious cardio workout, then combine your kettlebell swings with jump burpees as demonstrated in this video go.cavemantraining.com/kbwc-vid16

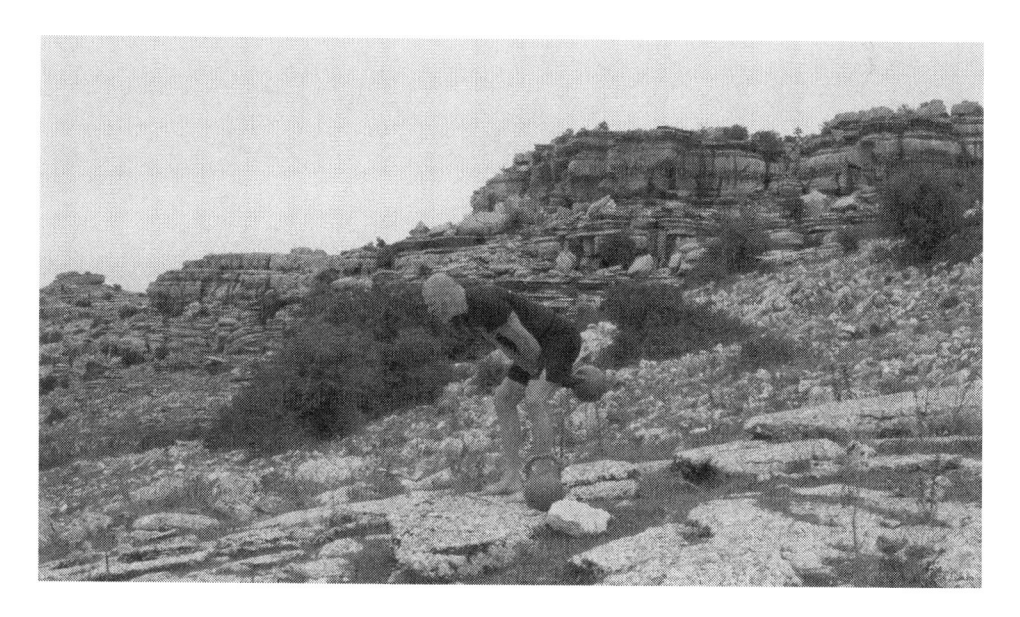

Double arm backswing end

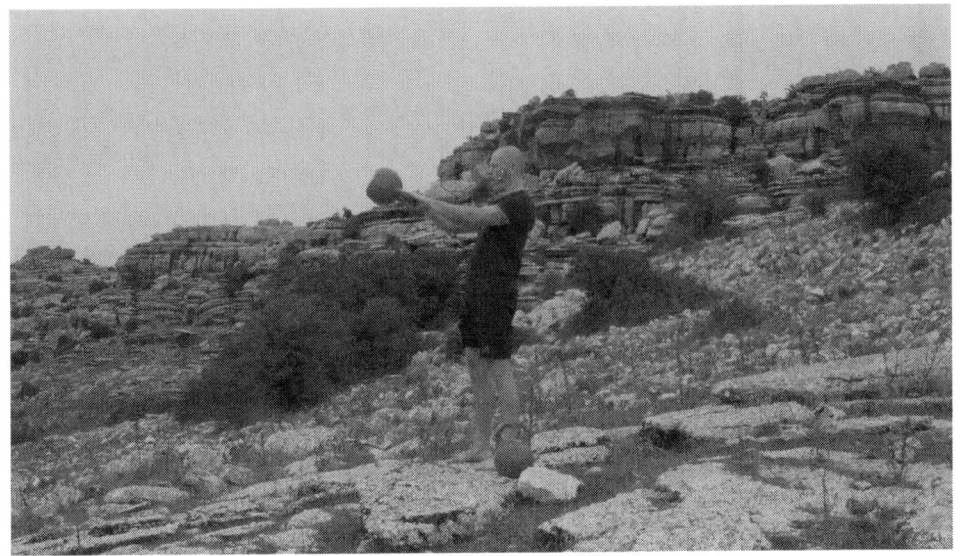

Double arm end of swing

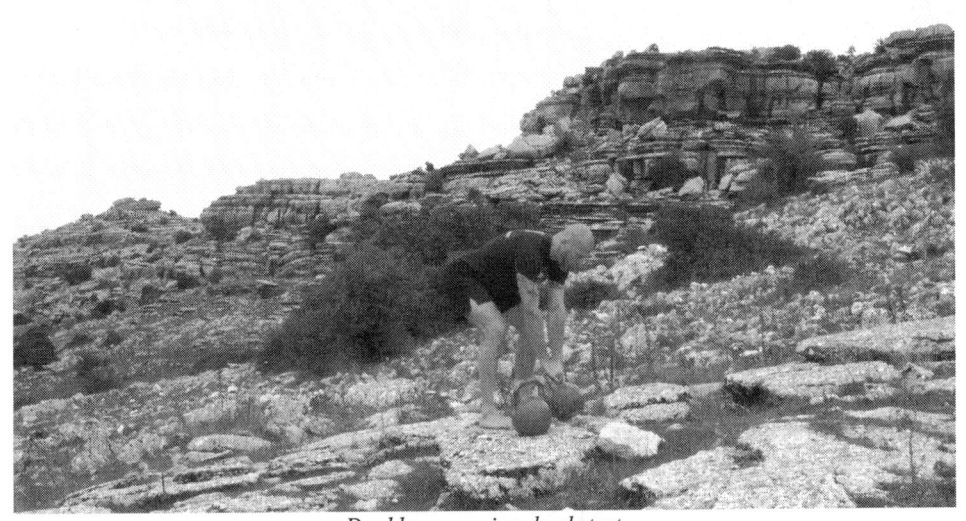

Double arm swing dead start

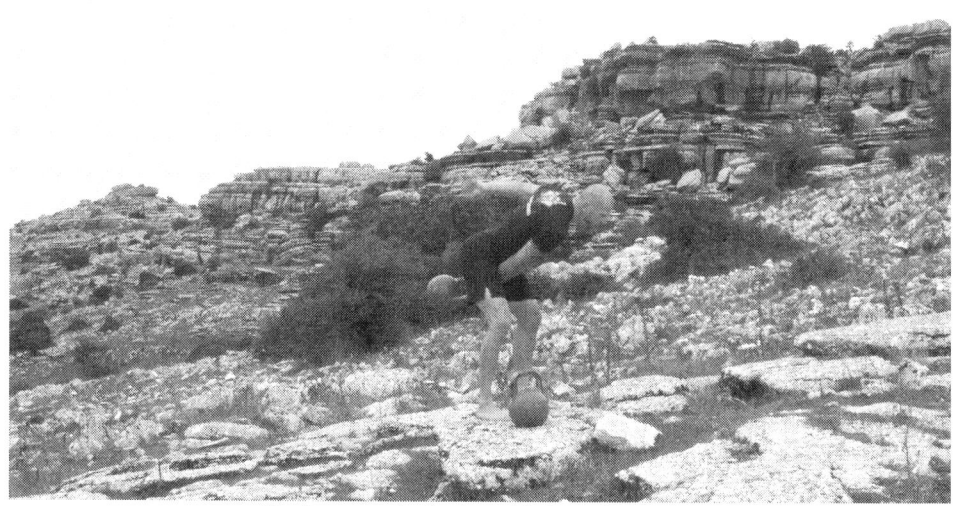

Single arm end of swing with thoracic rotation

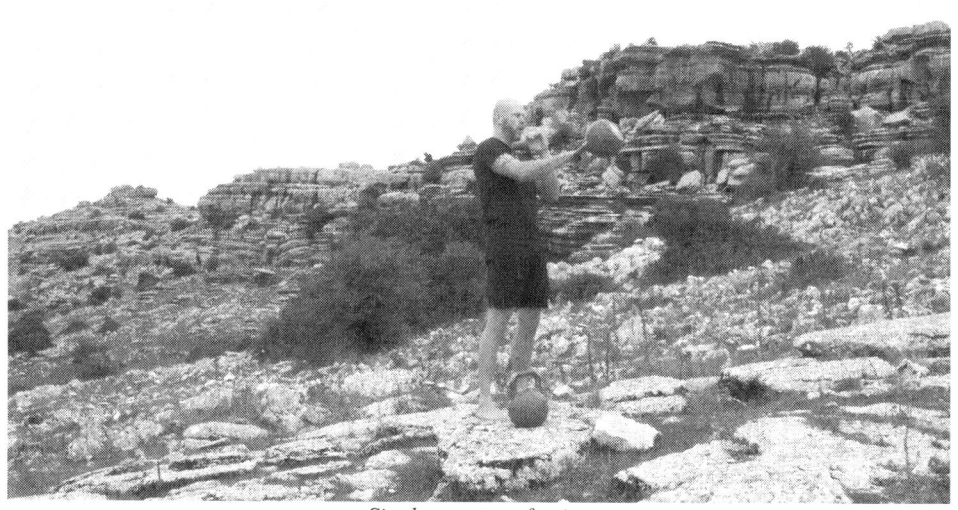

Single arm top of swing

Conclusion

The kettlebell swing is complex and there is so much more I'd like to tell you about, injury prevention, efficiency, transitioning, programming, etc. I suggest you go online and have a look for

Kettlebell Training Fundamentals, *Master The Kettlebell Swing*, and do some more research if you're interested in getting to know more about the kettlebell swing.

Kettlebell Swing Clean Fluid

There are literally 100's of clean variations, within each variation you even have slight differences and adjustments that can be made. I covered all variations in the book *Master The Kettlebell Clean* so I'm going to keep this basic and focussed on the most common clean I use.

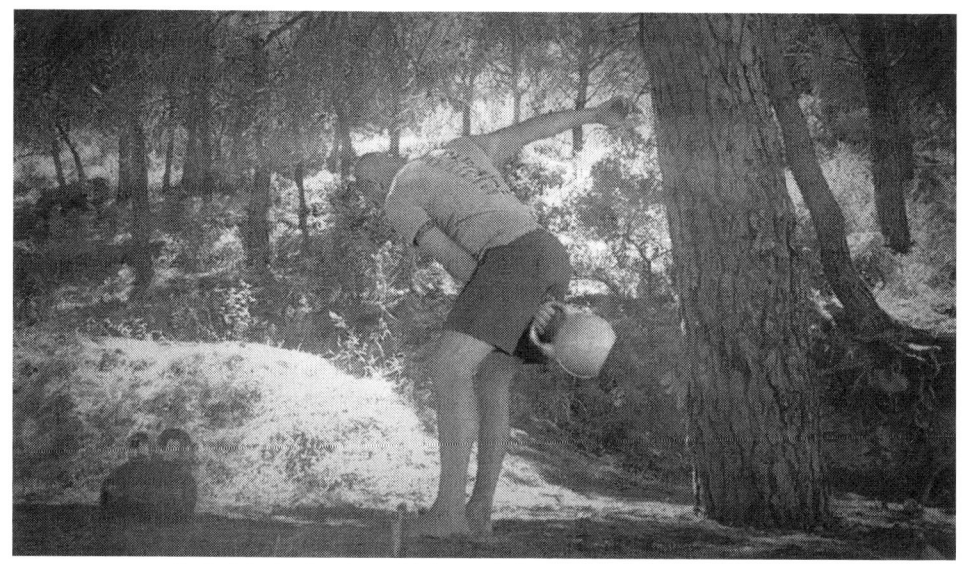

End of the backswing with internal shoulder and thoracic rotation.

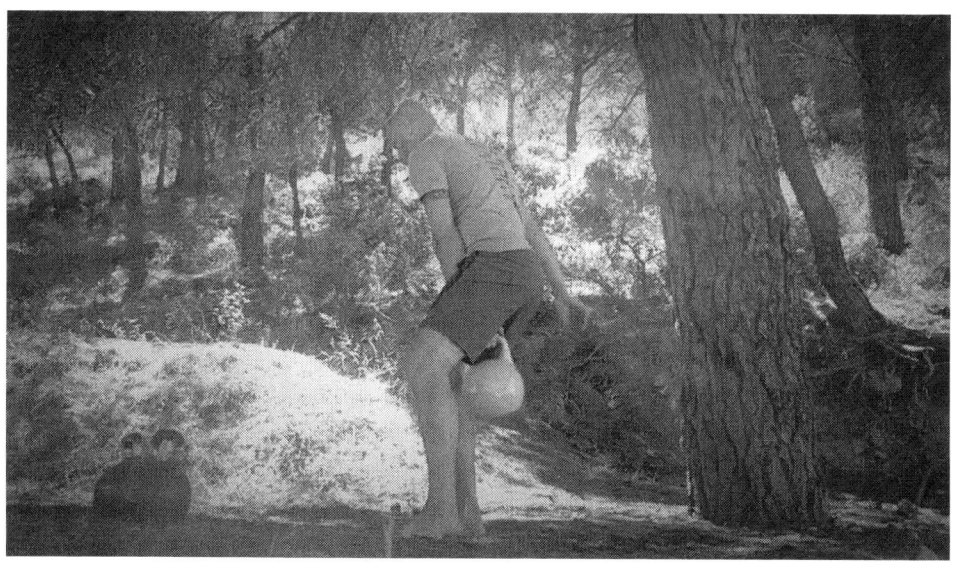

Arm stays connected while extending the hips.

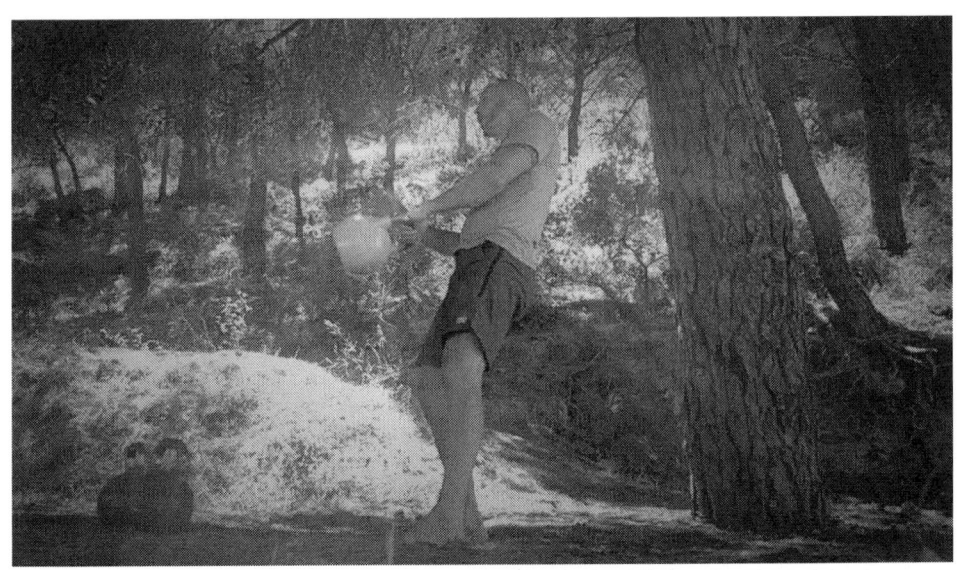

Hip and thoracic rotation paired with slightly leaning back while keeping the weight close.

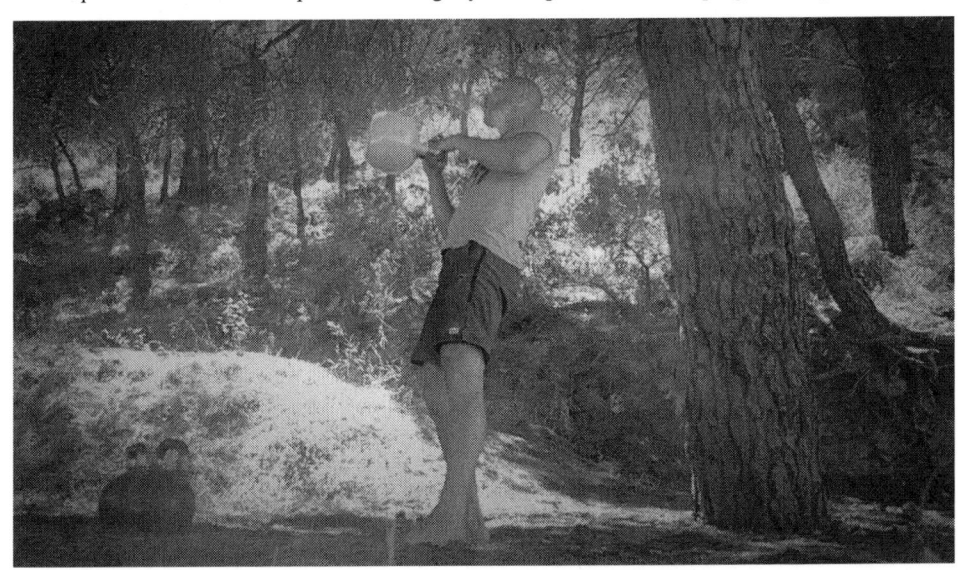

Let the weight come up to open and insert the hand.

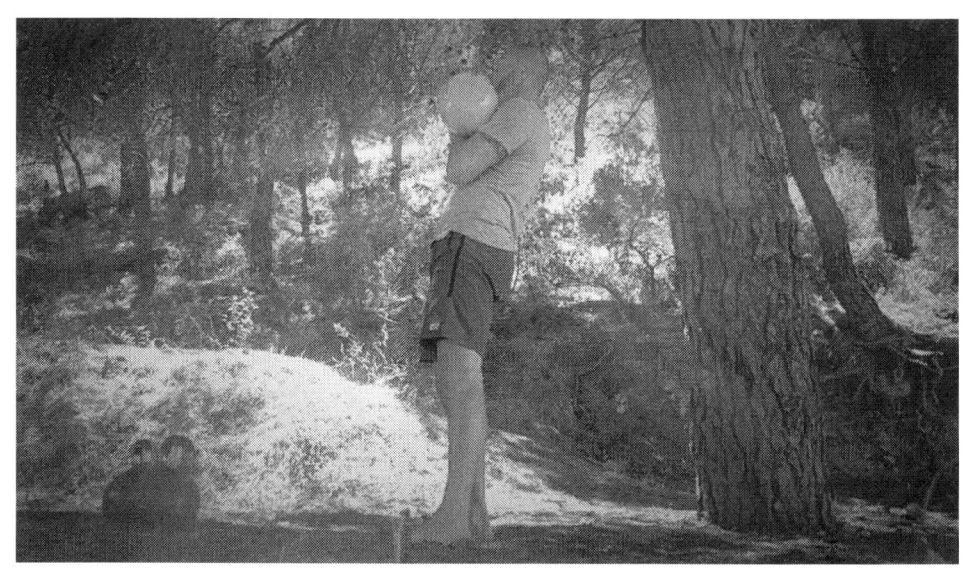

Find a good racking position.

Clean and Jerk (push press)

The clean and jerk is an advanced kettlebell combo that can be performed with double or single kettlebell. The push press is a prerequisite to the jerk and if you look at photo *8, 9, and 11*, they represent the push press apart from the heels, the heels should be driven into the ground after the push.

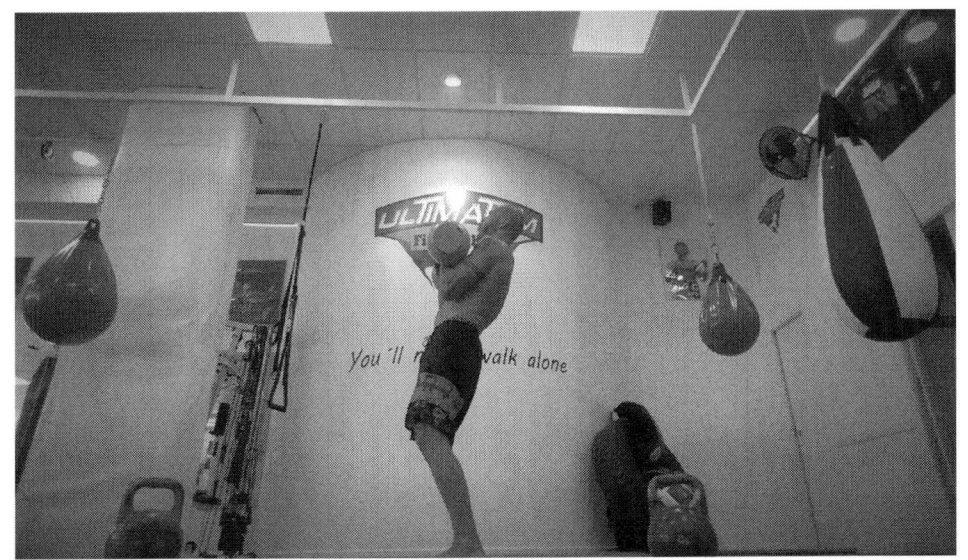

1). The weights drops from overhead into racking.

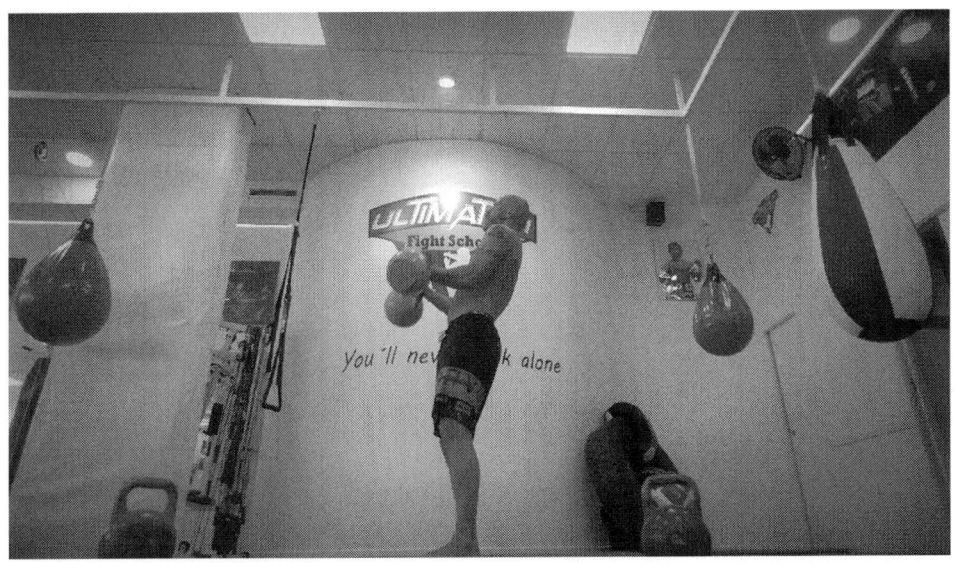

2). The weights are dropped into the backswing with the upper body coming back to create counterbalance and protect the lowerback.

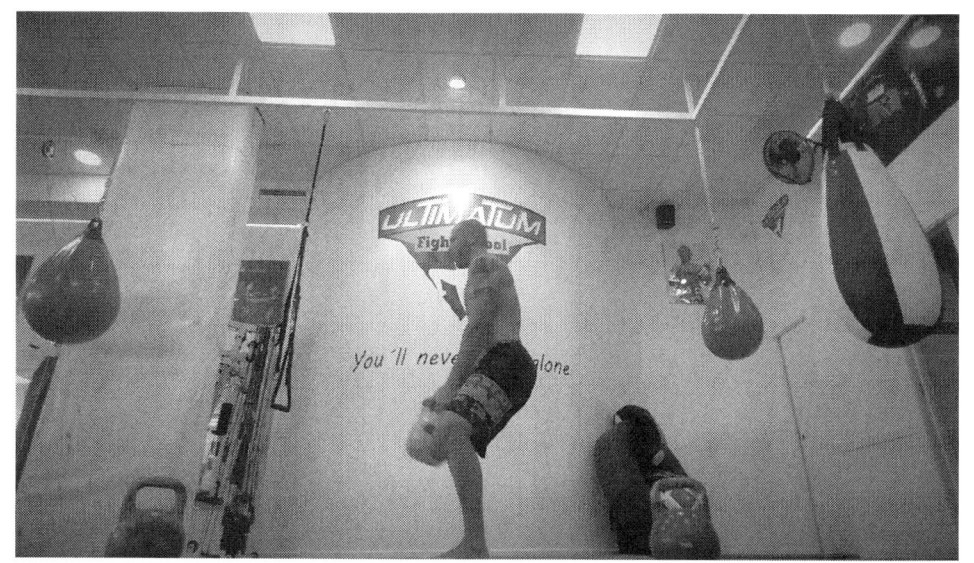

3). Pull out and let the weight come through the legs.

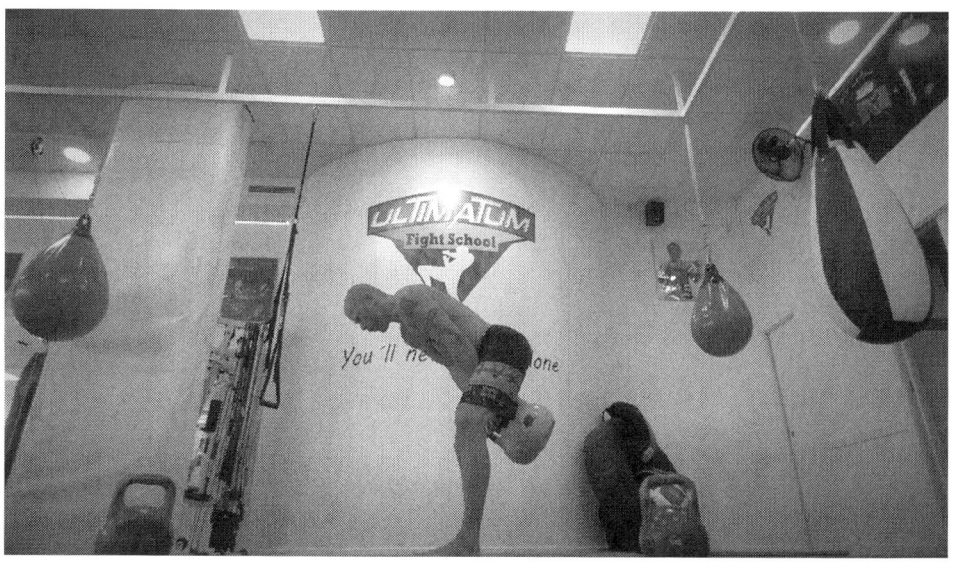

4). Hip hinge and guide the weights to the end of the swing.

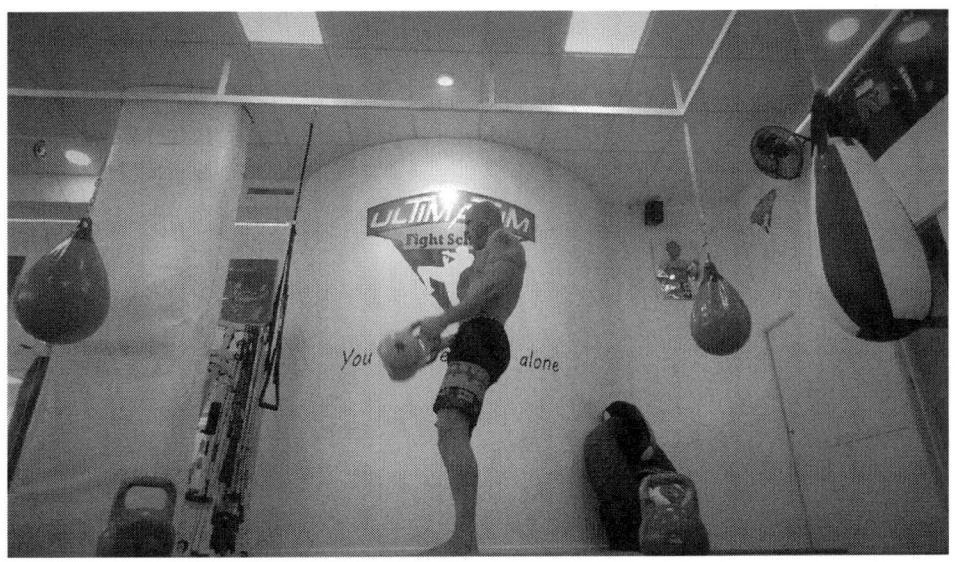

5). Let the weights come out and keep the elbows close to the body for the clean.

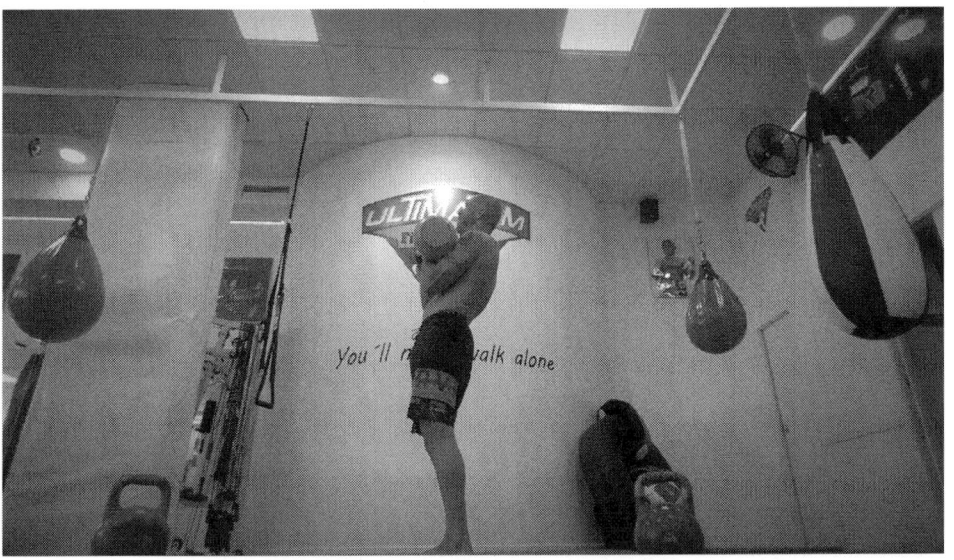

6). Clean the kettlebells and end up in a rack with safety racking grip.

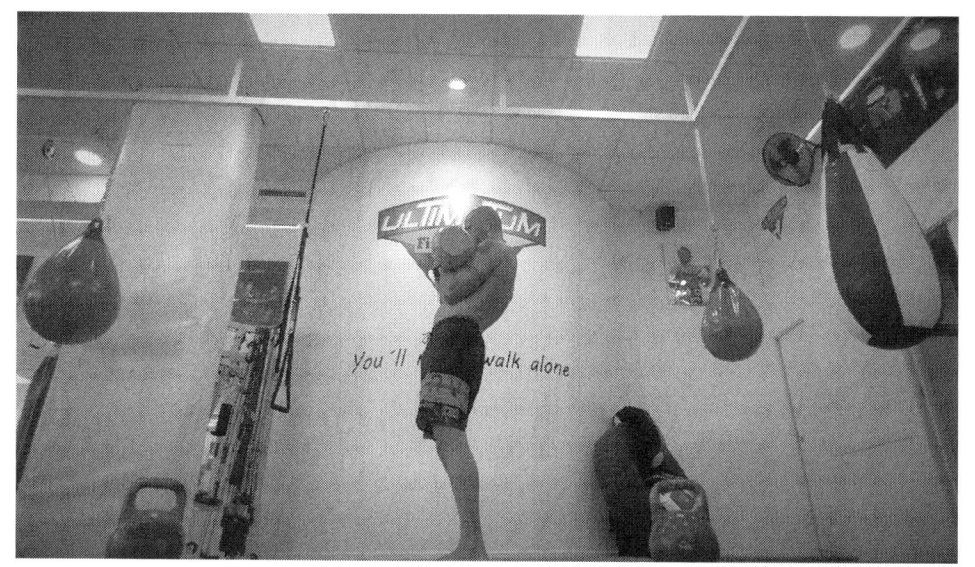

7). Create a good base for the kettlebells to be pushed off.

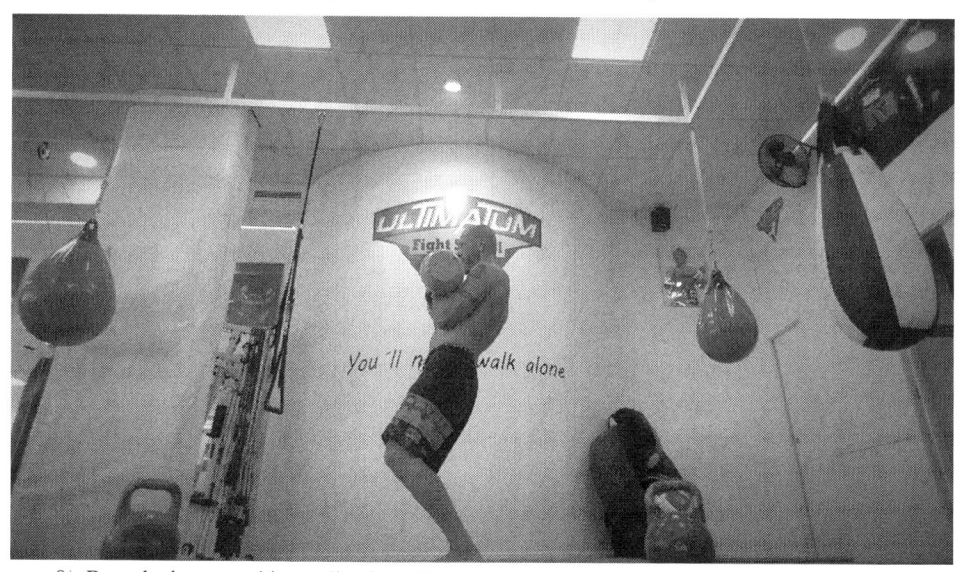

8). Bent the knees and immediately pull them back while driving the heels into the ground.

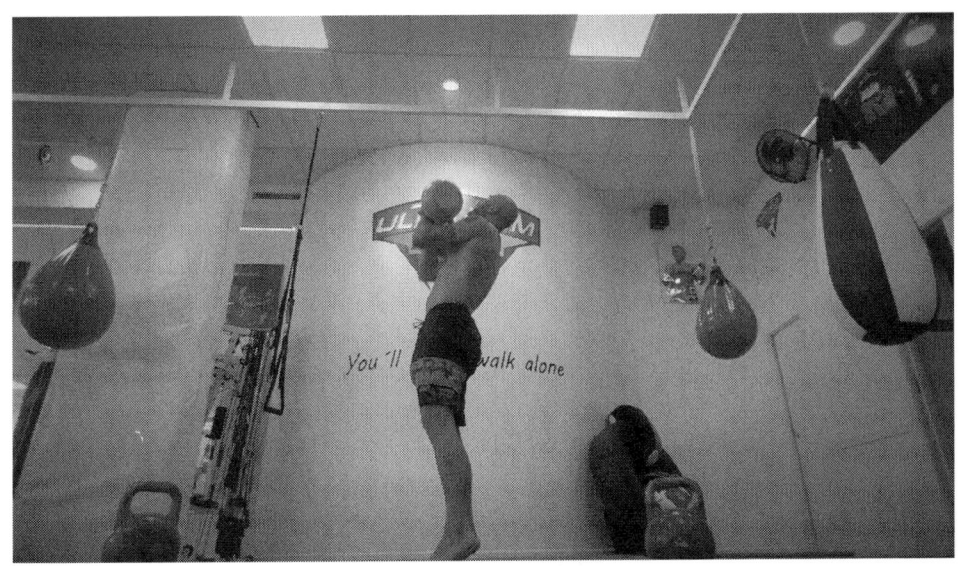

9). The force must be so great that all the work is done by the lower-body and your heels can even come off the ground if the weights was such it required it.

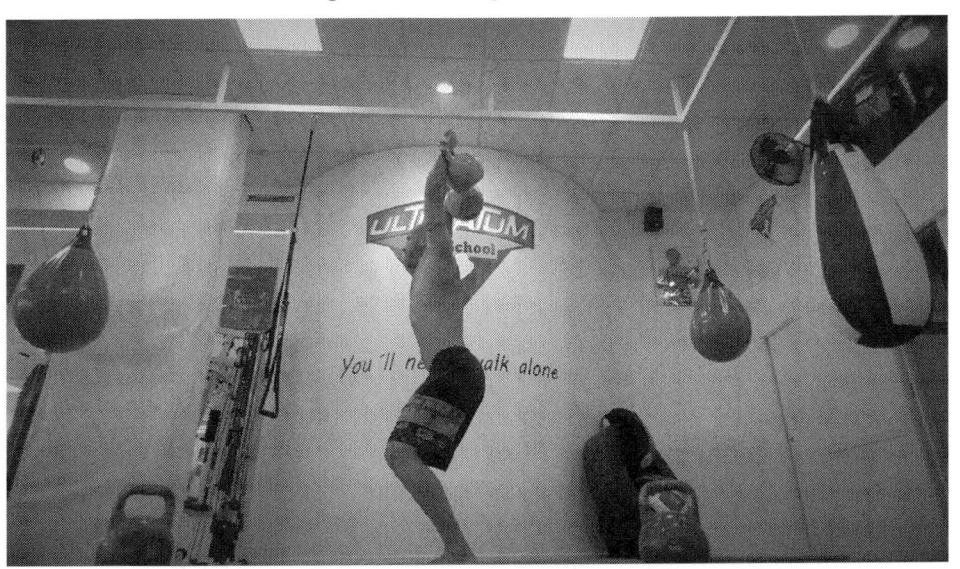

10). Dip and come under the weight with the arms fully extended.

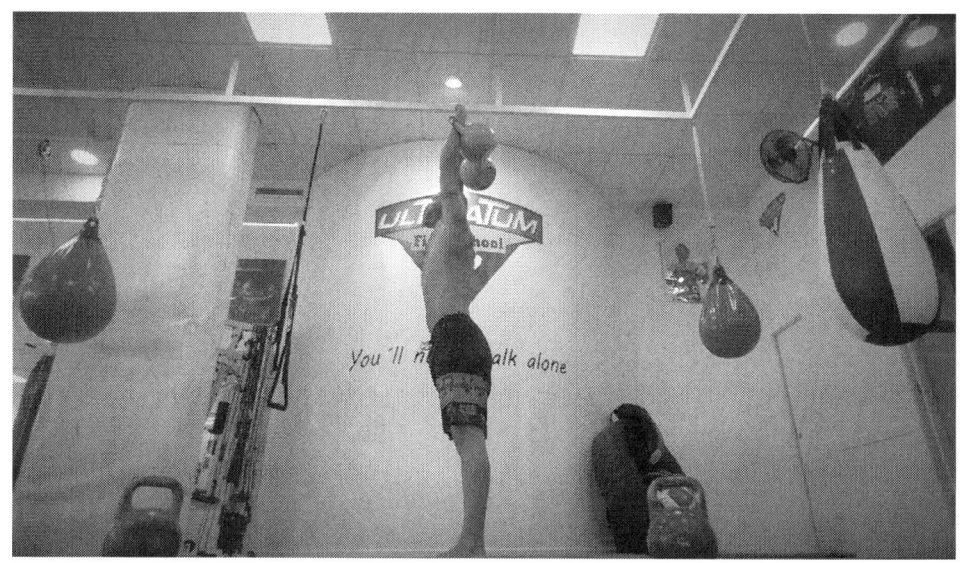

11). Brace and stand up.

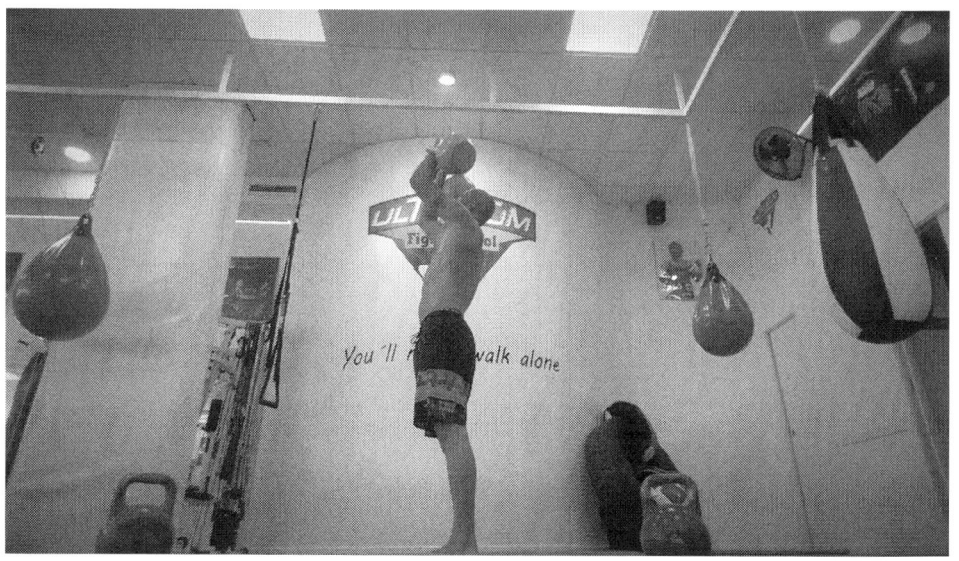

12). Drop into rack and repeat.

Gorilla Cleans AKA Alternating Hang Cleans

Gorilla cleans are a real cardio blaster and require you to get fast and explosive, one rep into another simultaneously. This exercise requires a good strong core and will put your cardio, core, and legs to the test.

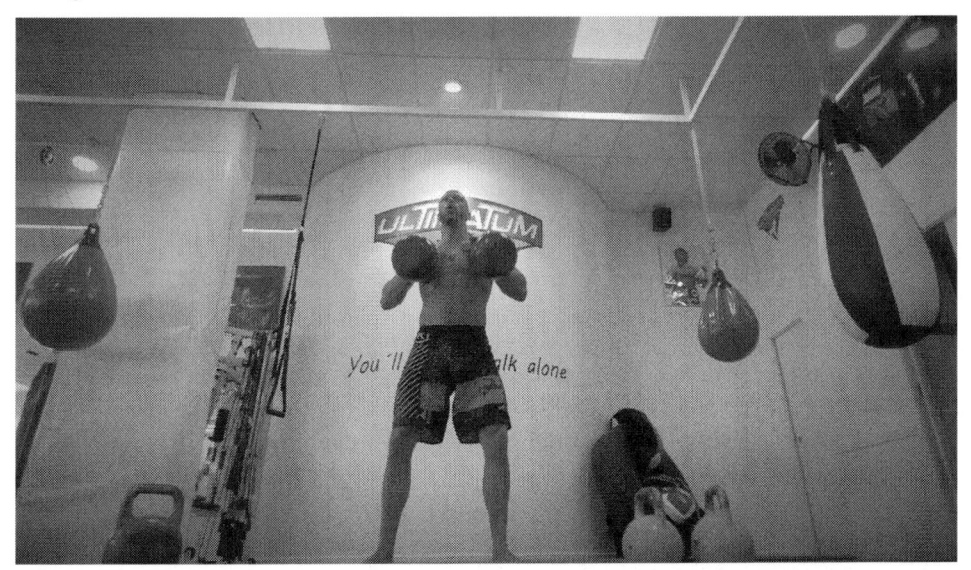

Both kettlebells are in transition with one going down while the other is going up.

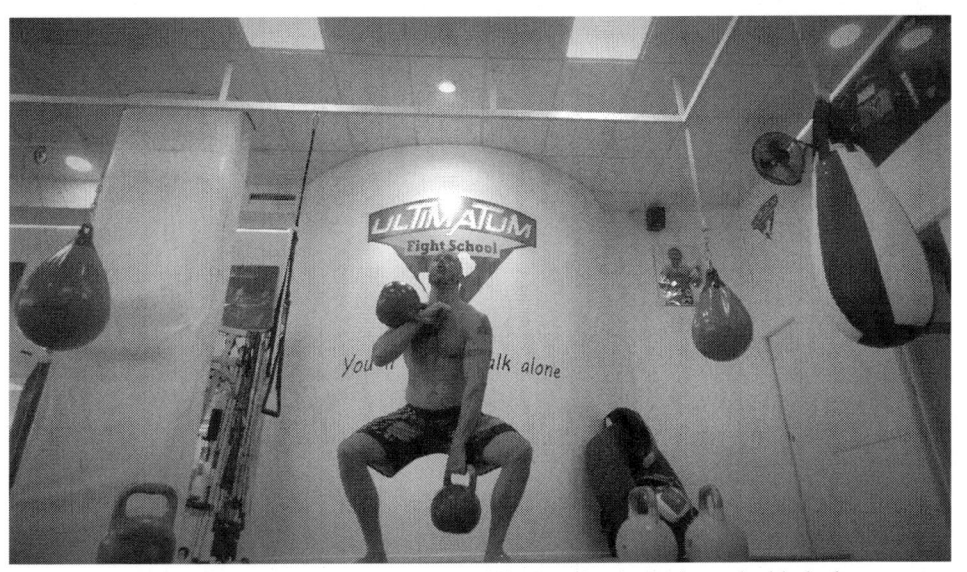

One side ends in a good racking position while the other is decelerated with the legs.

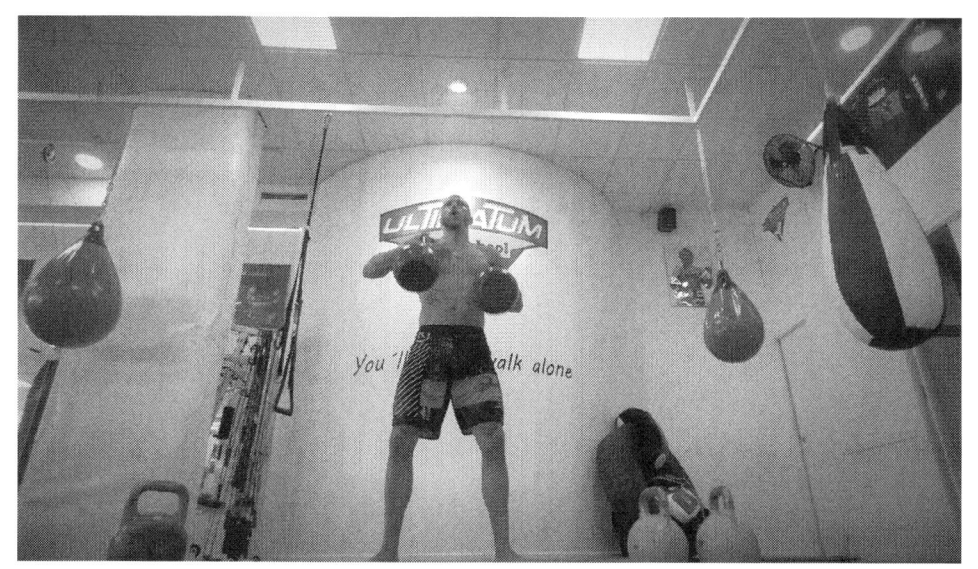

The hanging kettlebell is pulled up with the legs while the other is dropped.

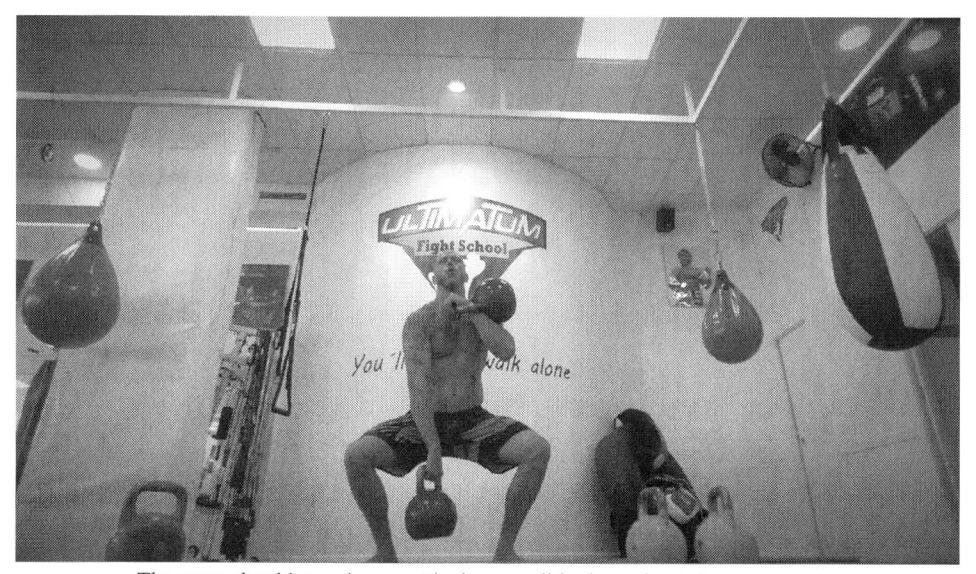

The torso should remain as vertical as possible throughout the movements.

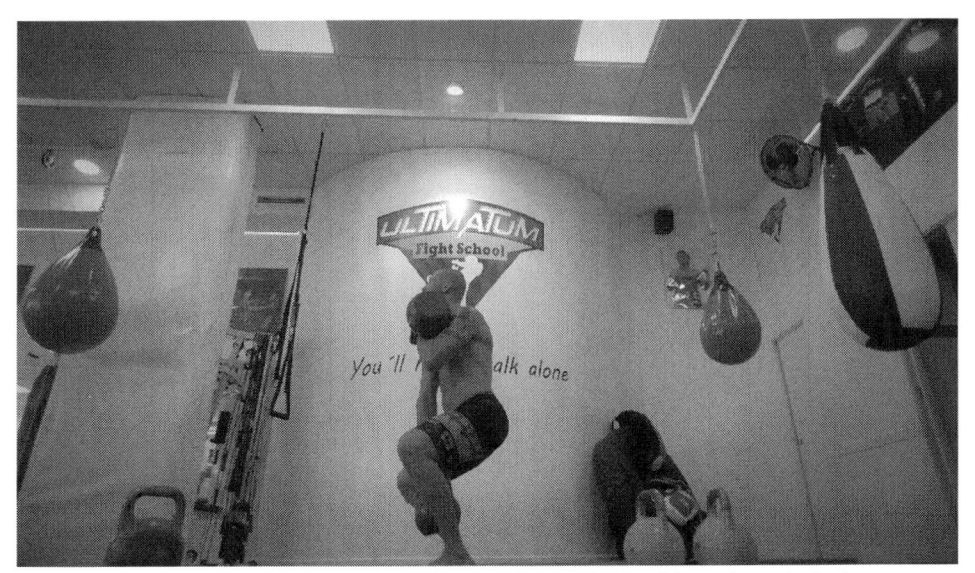

This side-on view demonstrates how close the weight should remain to the body.

Double Kettlebell Half Snatch

The half snatch is where the kettlebell return to racking position after each rep.

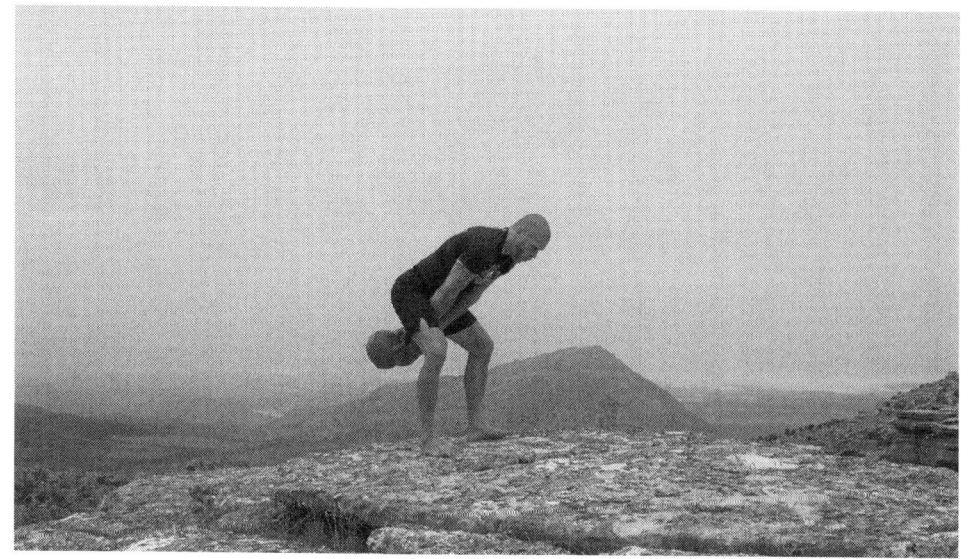

Hip hinge and deep insert.

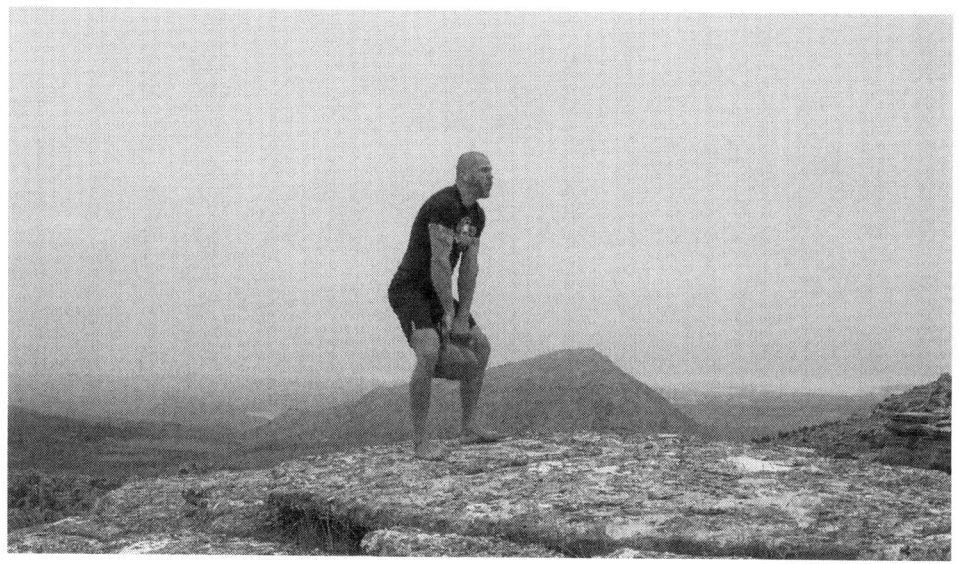

Pull out.

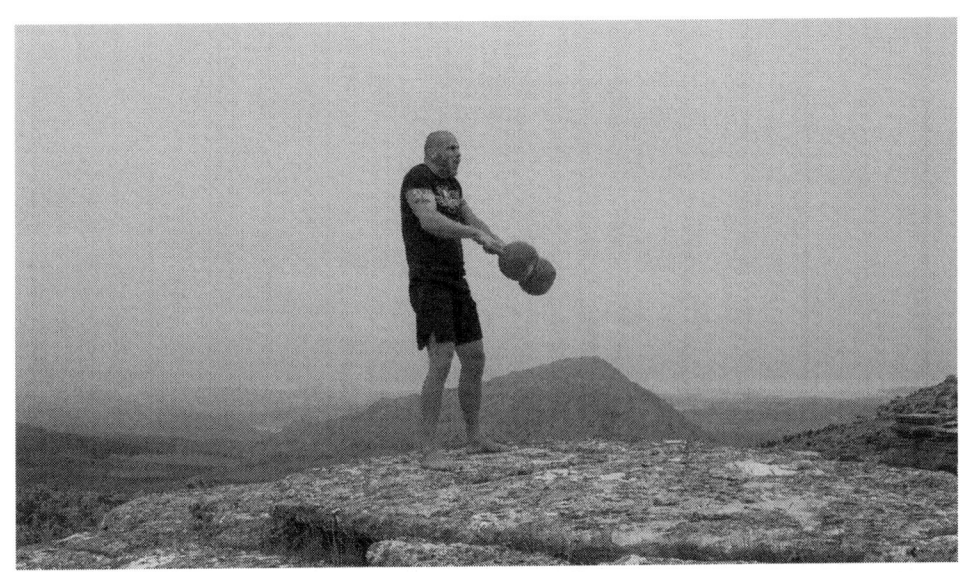

Shrug and slight pull.

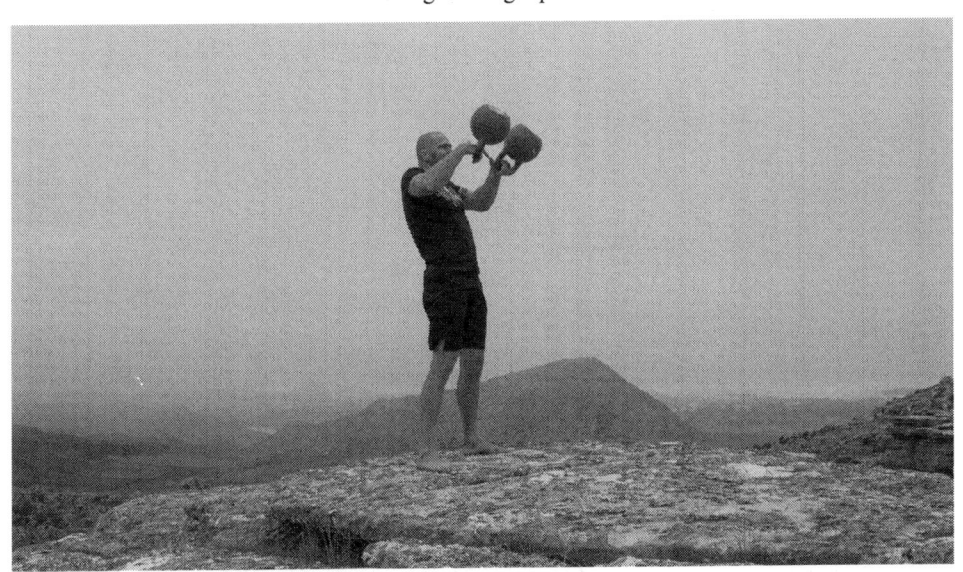

Open up to perform an insert and press out.

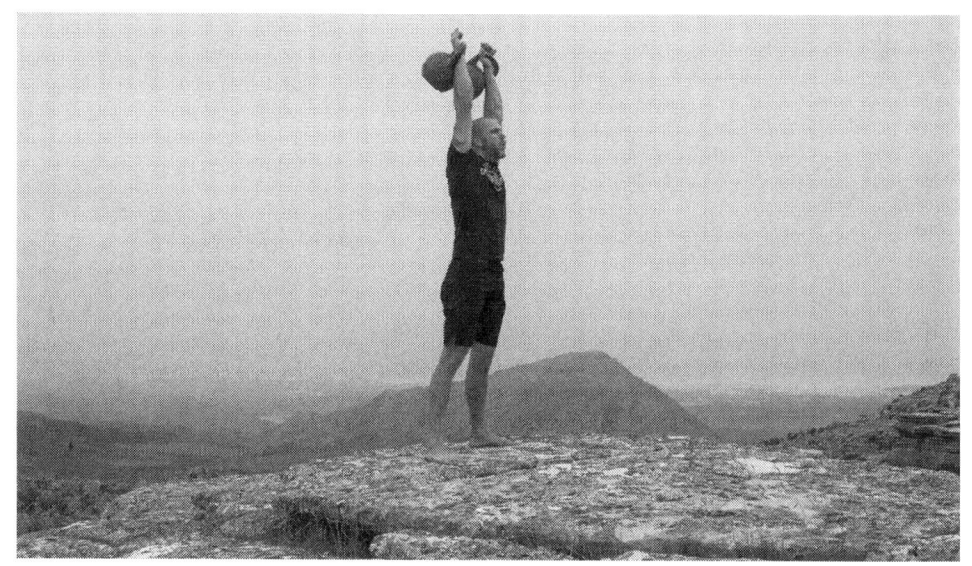

Overhead lockout.

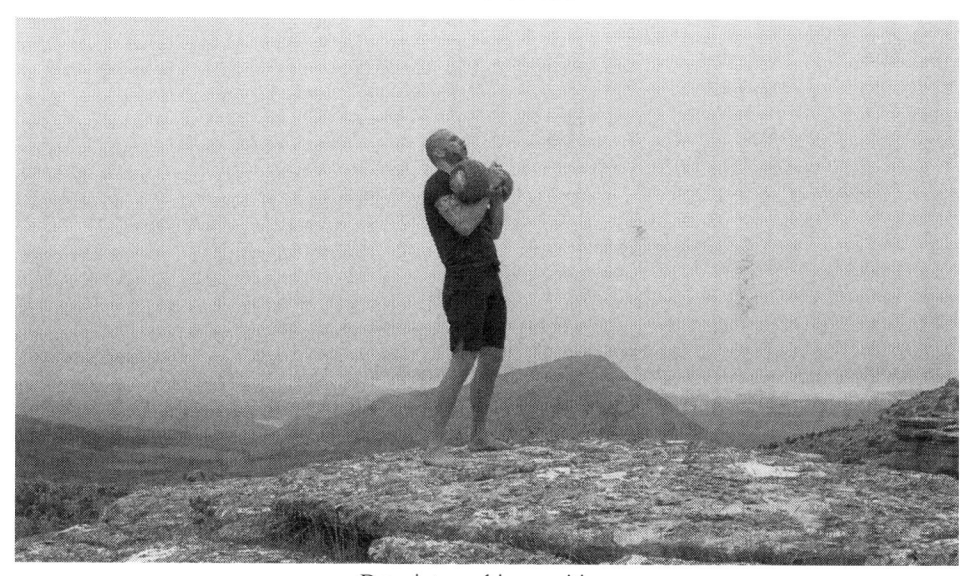

Drop into racking position.

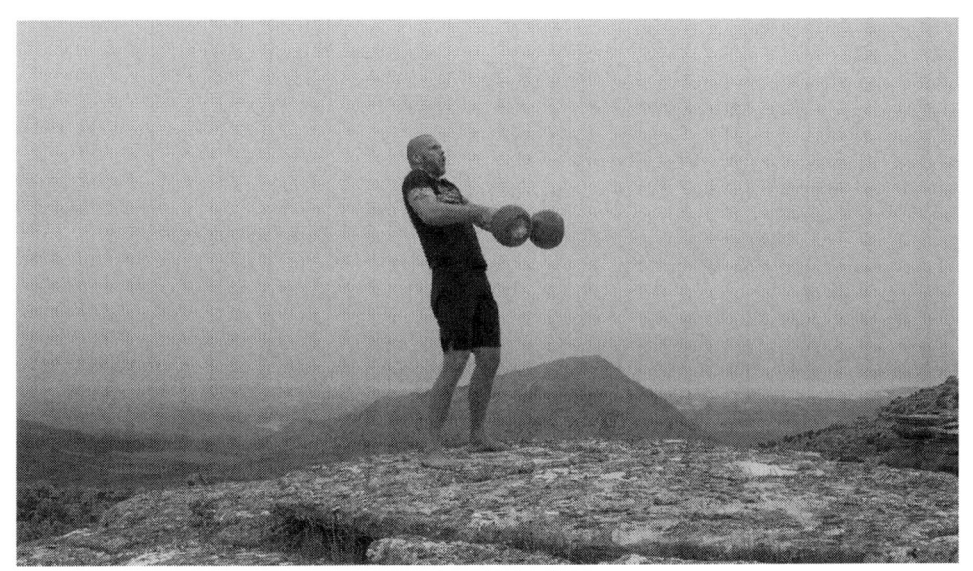

Drop into backswing.

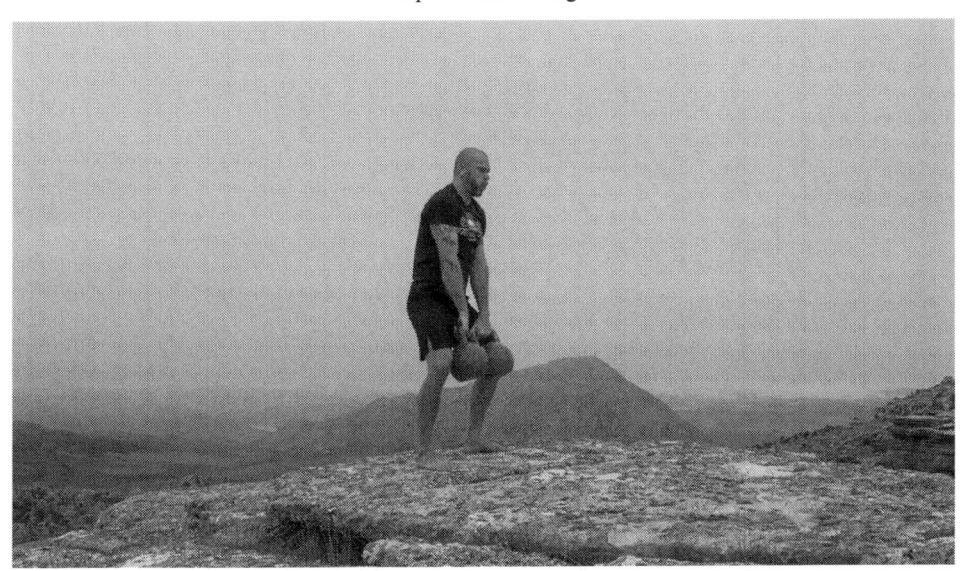

Come through the legs around knee height.

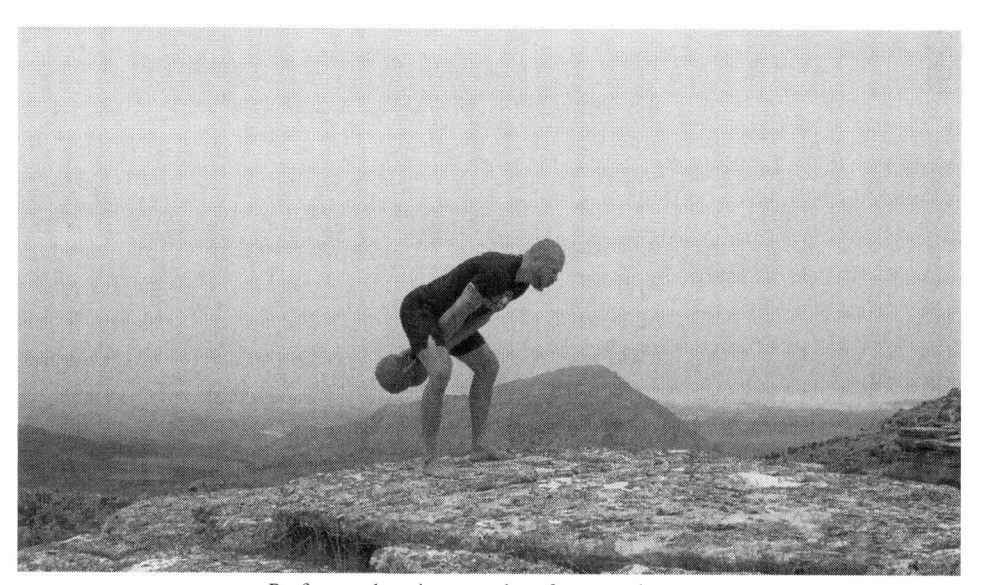

Perform a deep insert and perform another rep.

Full Snatch Fluid

The full snatch is where the kettlebell does not return to racking upon each rep. Fluid is where the movements used to create motion is such that it provides the least resistance to the body, which is great for high reps and endurance.

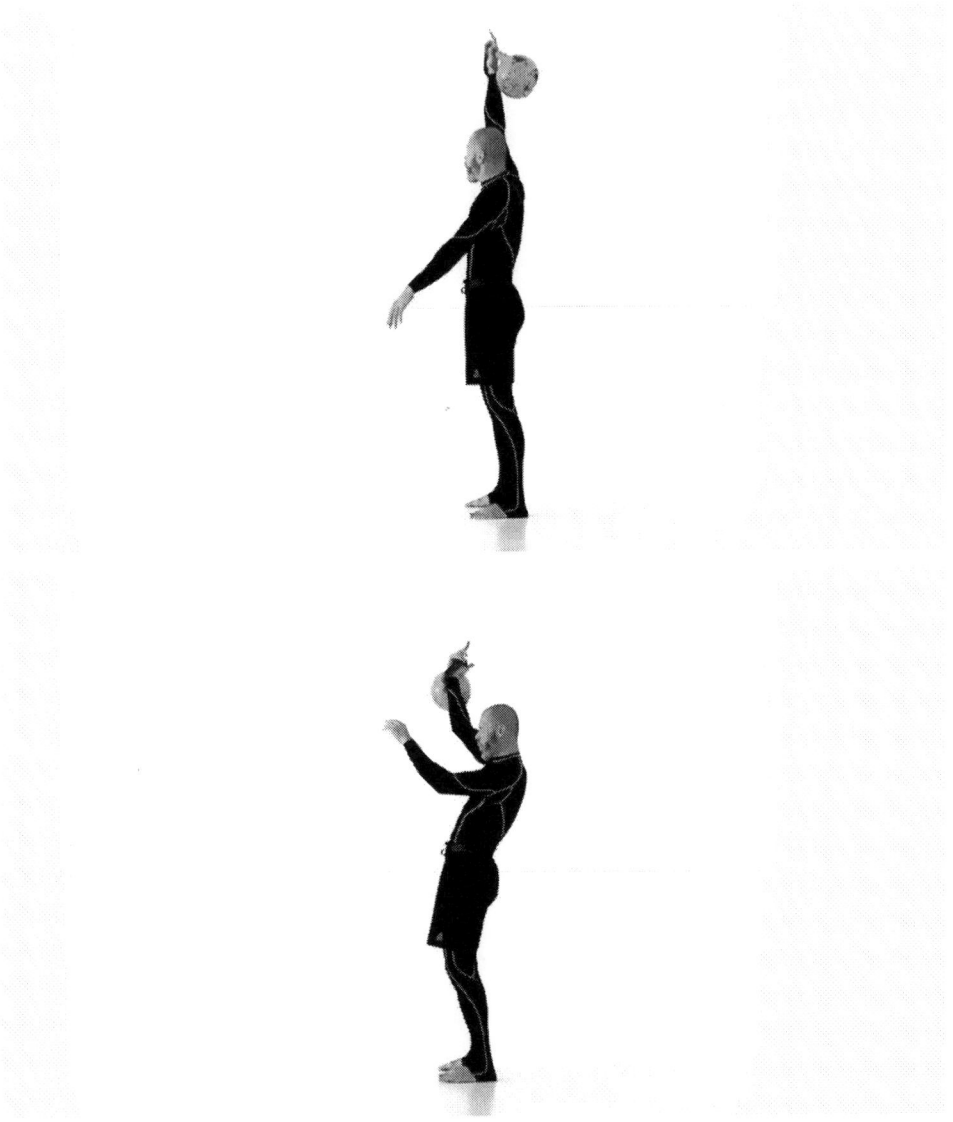

Hip hyperextension to keep the weight close to the body.

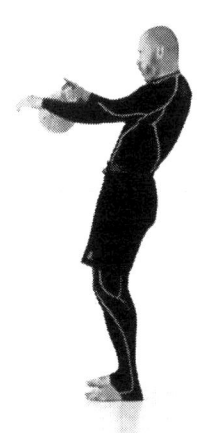

The counterbalance can be paired with thoracic hyperextension and/or knee flexion.

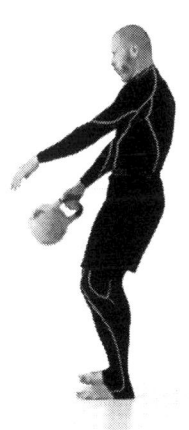

Remain as upright as possible for as long as possible.

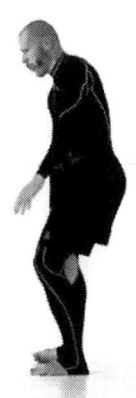

Let the weight come through around knee height so that no bending of the back takes place.

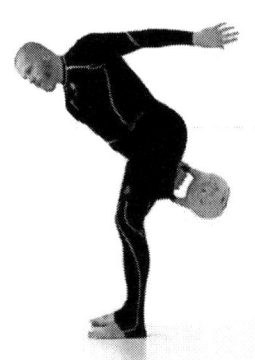

Create hip flexion to let the weight come through the legs. This can be paired with knee extension to create more space for the kettlebell.

Let the weight come back out and follow through for the snatch.

REMAIN IN EXTENSION

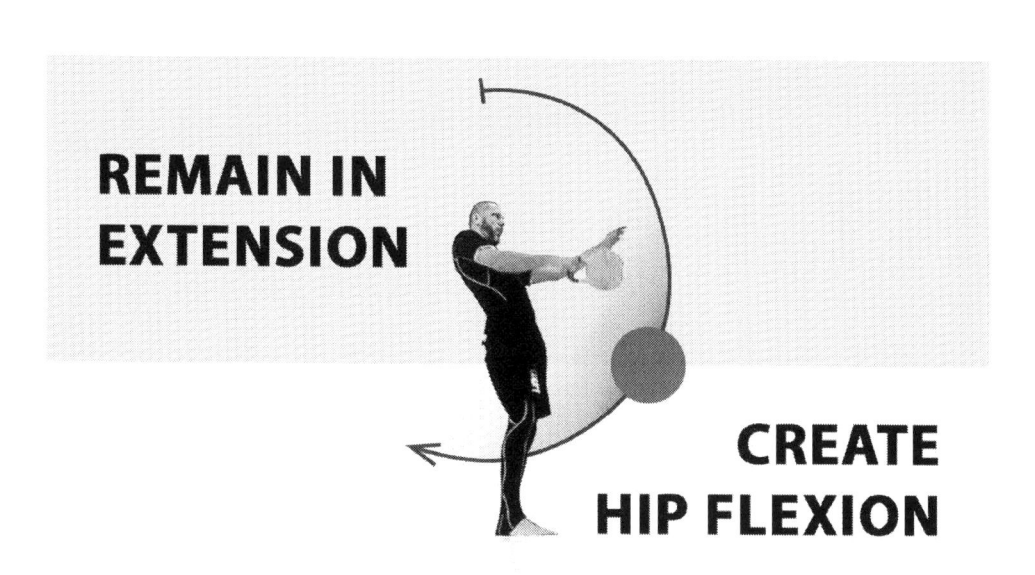

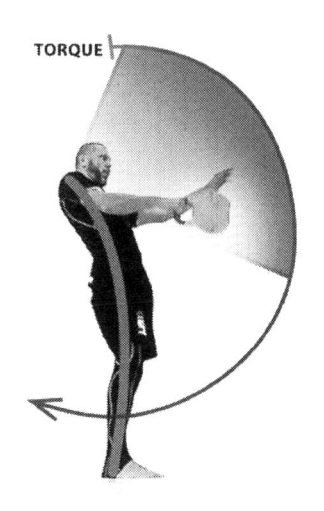

CREATE HIP FLEXION

TORQUE

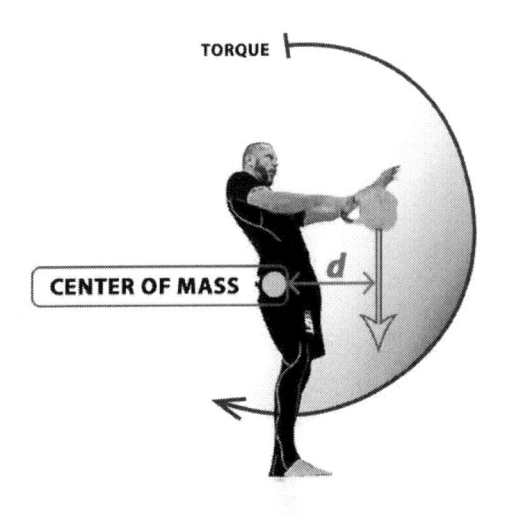

Kettlebell Snatch Hardstyle

Or as close to Hardstyle as I like it to be. The true Hardstyle snatch is where everything is rigid, in these photos I'm demonstrating some thoracic rotation (fifth photo) on the backswing which is normally not employed during the Hardstyle snatch. Everything about the Hardstyle snatch is such as to provide maximum resistance, i.e. work the most amount of muscles, resisting torque will do this (resisting rotation).

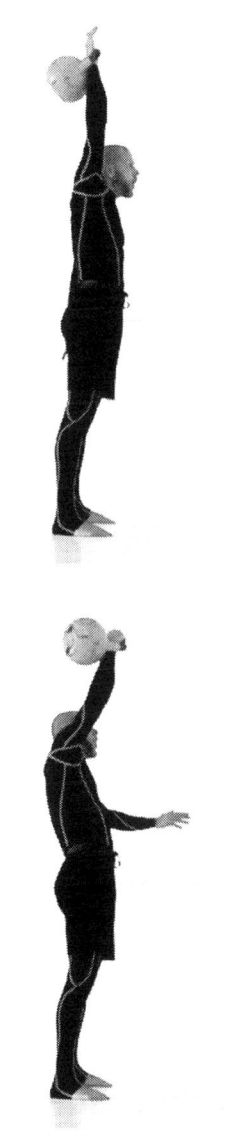

The kettlebell comes over the fist.

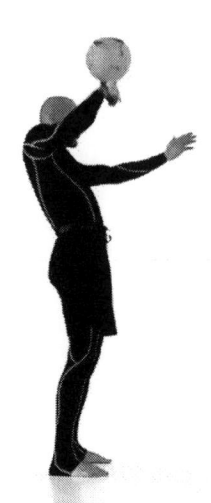

Pull out.

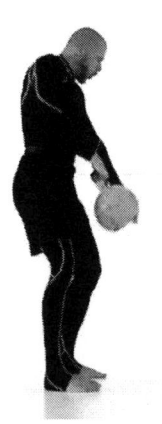

Hip hinge and insert.

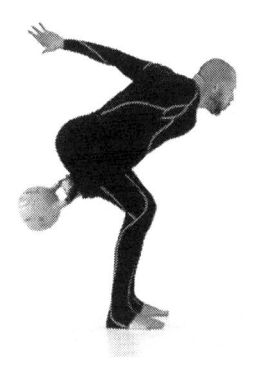

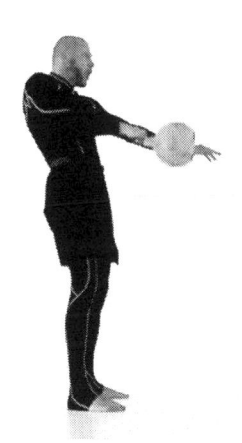

Pull the kettlebell back out.

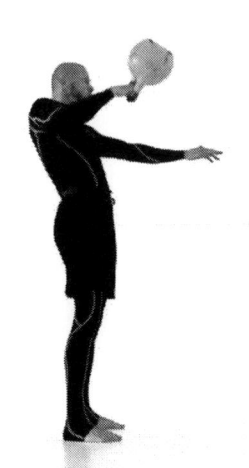

Kettlebell comes over the fist.

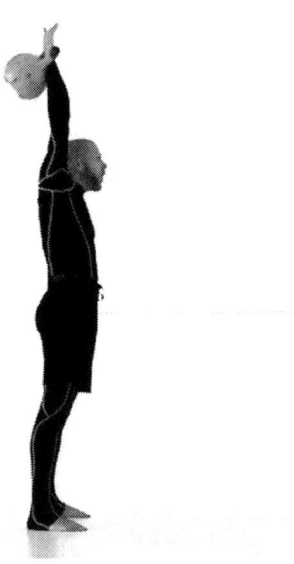

Perform an insert.

Kettlebell Halo

The kettlebell halo is great to use with a light weight for the shoulders in warm-ups. Also great to use for shoulder strength when going slower and heavier in training. The Halo is best performed with an upside down horn grip as shown in the first photo.

When you perform the Halo everything should be firm and solid with the only moving parts of your body being the shoulders. Go around the head, don't make the head go around the kettlebell. You can keep the kettlebell going in one line around eye/nose level, or you can go down to the belly button upon each rep which creates additional shoulder extension and flexion.

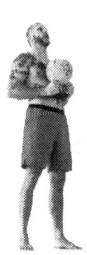

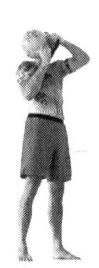

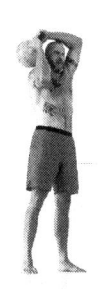

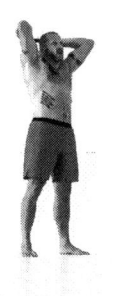

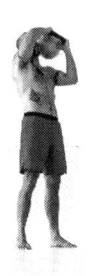

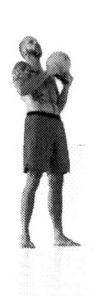

That's the end of the workouts section. I'm including some bonus content specifically aimed at trainers, explaining the basics of how to run a *Caveman Circuit* or *Caveman Boot Camp*.

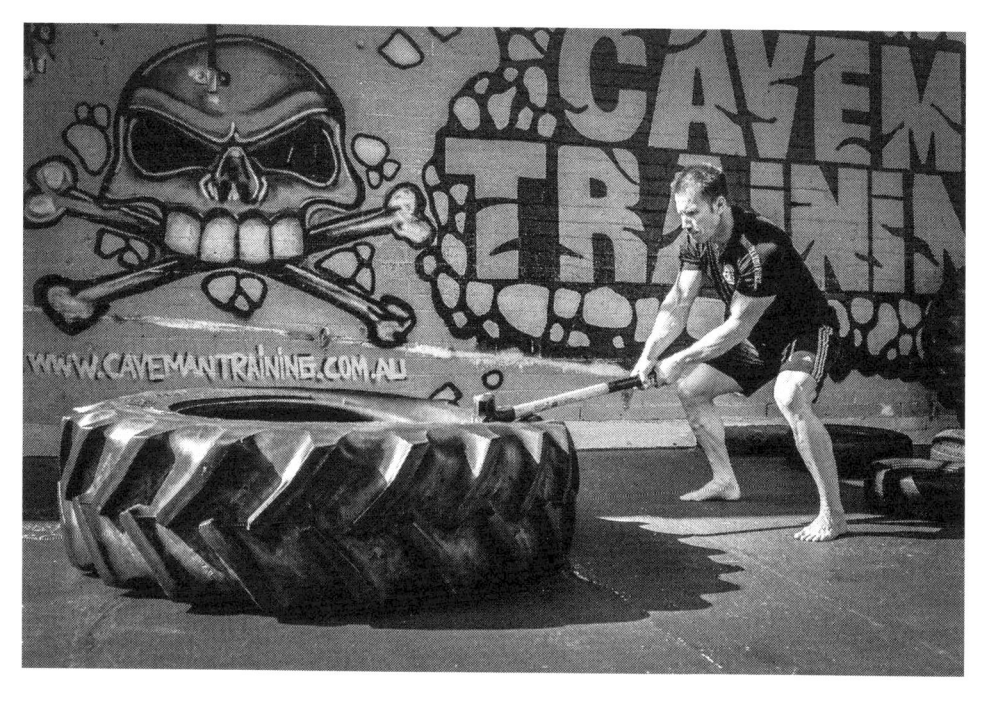

Bonus Content

Bonus: How to Design and Administer a Caveman Circuit

Provided below is information on how to incorporate the Caveman Training Circuit training principles and how to incorporate these principles in the design and administration of an effective Caveman Training Circuit.

- Designing a Caveman Training Circuit
- Training Principles
- Posture and Technique
- Verbal Instructions and Cues
- Motivation, Pushing and Encouragement
- Circuit Layout
- Stressing Nutrition

Designing a Caveman Circuit

We recommend a maximum of 10 to 12 clients per Caveman Trainer. This ensures that the trainer can effectively supervise the participants and ensure good form. The trainer would also be better able to motivate and encourage the group. If your group is larger, we suggest getting another trainer on board to help run the circuit.

There are a number of elements to analyze prior to designing any Caveman Circuit. First, check the weather conditions. If rain is forecast, you may decide to assign only exercises that can be performed inside. If you decide to incorporate outside exercises during bad weather, only include those that won't risk participants injuring themselves, for example, by slipping or dropping heavy weights. An example of a good alternative would be sandbags and slam balls. Secondly, take a look at the booking sheet and the participants scheduled to attend. If you're expecting more advanced clients, assign more difficult exercises. However, keep in mind that you should never adjust an intermediate class to suit someone you think can't do the class. Instead, advise that person to stick to the beginners' class until you feel they're ready to advance and they are invited to the intermediate sessions. If you're expecting a number of beginners, understand that the exercises you assign should reflect their abilities and that you're going to need to pay more attention to your participants. If there are exercises that you believe particular beginners will be unable to complete, be prepared to have alternate exercise ready for those people.

Set a theme for your class. Think about what workouts you assigned in prior weeks and make sure that this workout is different. Not only will you limit your clients' development by not incorporating variety, you're likely to adversely affect their motivation. You want them to show up excited to go, so don't bore them with the same exercises and same theme each week. Some examples for the theme of your workout include Cardio, Strength and Power, Agility, Progression, Full Body or Muscle Overload. Please note that because a Caveman Circuit requires mostly non-stop movement from your clients, they will always receive cardiovascular benefits due to their heart rate remaining elevated throughout the class.

If required, mix those exercises that significantly elevate heart rate with ones that hardly elevate heart rate. Stations that significantly elevate heart rate include burpees, mountain climbers, skipping and jumping. You want to ensure that each class raises the heart rate of your participants and that they end a class nearly puking, sweating and red-faced.

Always keep in mind that *Caveman Circuit* places focus on training in the red zone and features high intensity exercise (HIT). It incorporates non-conventional exercises, functional training movements and asymmetric exercises. The goal of Caveman Circuit is to develop functional strength, cardio, endurance and agility. It is not about aesthetics and building huge biceps and huge quads. *Cavemantraining* is about utilizing what's around you, using sandbags, tyres, heavy balls, slosh pipes, ropes, and one's own bodyweight. We use anything but machines.

Put together a "challenge" portion at the end of each of your circuit workouts. The challenge features a set of exercises that are to be completed within 10 minutes. This part is about seeing who finishes first. Those who finish all of the assigned challenge exercises first should be asked to encourage those still finishing, even if it's outside the assigned time. We recommend that you try to include exercises done in the circuit and/or ones that still are a part of your theme.

Following the "challenge" portion, participants will want to immediately sit down and rest and/or to hydrate. Allow them to get water, but prevent them from sitting or stopping abruptly. Instead, gather the group and take them through a structured cool down.

Training Principles

Cavemantraining develops functional strength, cardiovascular endurance, muscular endurance, core stability, agility and balance. The circuits effectively improve each of these areas because of the training principles that we focus on and implement.

Red Zone Training

Red Zone Training refers to exercising at high intensity, with your heart rate elevated to 60 to 80 percent of maximum heart rate. Red Zone Training effectively develops the cardiovascular system. Caveman Training Circuits should feature exercises that elevate clients' heart rates to this appropriate intensity and participants should move immediately from one station into the next to keep their heart rate up in the red zone.

High Intensity Training (HIT)

High Intensity Training refers to performing exercises to near muscular failure. Clients should experience near muscular failure towards the end of each assigned station.

Non-Conventional Exercises

Non-Conventional Exercises are multi-joint, multi-plane, complex movements.

Functional Training

Functional Trainings places focus on developing human movement rather than isolating muscles.

Asymmetric Exercises

Asymmetric Exercises are ones that focus on one side of the body at a time.

Posture and Technique

The main objective of a Caveman Trainer is to make sure that all participants maintain correct posture and technique, not only so that you ensure their workouts are effective, but to prevent them from injuring themselves. Circulate around the circuit floor, correcting technique and form as you walk through the various stations. Never leave the workout area. Should a trainer spot a participant with bad form or technique, the trainer should begin by correcting with verbal cues from a distance. If that does not work, the Caveman Trainer should go up to the participant and use verbal and physical cues to correct the participant. If that still fails, stop the participant from what they are doing and take them through the exercise step by step. If all else fails, the trainer will need to modify or change that exercise.

When working with beginners, place greater focus on good form. Rather than aim for exercise volume, ensure that participants are performing each exercise with the correct technique. Spend a greater amount of time going over instructions at the start of each beginner session than you would prior to intermediate classes. Feel free to increase breaks in between each round to reiterate teaching points and better explain exercises if participants are having problems with the technique at a particular station or stations.

If a participant lacks the core strength necessary to maintain a taut torso during exercises like push-ups, renegade rows and mountain climbers, do not allow them to participate in the exercise. Instead, have them get into a front static plank position and hold the position throughout the duration of that station. Once they're able to maintain proper form in the static front plank position, they can begin performing the exercises for part of the duration of the station. The participants can slowly progress to performing the exercise for the full duration.

Often we find that participants struggle with proper push-up technique. Many times they will perform repetitions too quickly without achieving the full range of motion. If assisting a male participant, place your fist on the floor directly under their chest and challenge them to touch your fist with their chest during each repetition. This will make them slow down and focus more on range of motion and technique. For females, a cup can be utilized instead of your fist.

Be sure to highlight to participants that when performing deadlifts or exercises where they are required to pick weights up, they should maintain a straight back throughout the movement. Stress to them that they should keep their eyes up and bend their knees in a half-squat when picking up the weights. This will help them keep their back straight and decrease the risk of injury.

Many of our workouts utilize a squatting movement to develop the major muscles in the legs. To decrease the stress placed on the knees, explain to participants that their knee joints should never extend forward beyond the vertical line of their toes. At the bottom of the squat, their thighs should at least be parallel to the ground. To help them understand and master the proper squat technique, have them push their hips back behind them prior to bending their knees. Tell them to imagine that they are about to sit down on a bench or even a toilet seat that's dirty.

It's a good idea to always do exercises yourself before putting the participants through them. This way you know the intensity of the exercise and how the client will feel. You'll be able to perform the exercise with the correct form and technique. A Caveman Trainer that does not perform the exercise himself first will feel guilty and won't have the full confidence required to put participants through a hardcore circuit.

Stop the circuit and re-iterate information or an exercise if required, rather than letting the circuit continue and possibly become dangerous or people become confused. Be prepared to switch or replace an exercise if you see it simply does not work. Be prepared to switch exercises if you work outside and the weather changes. Remove exercises that become potentially dangerous, even if half of your circuit needs to be removed. Replace it with burpees if you need to; there is nothing wrong with doing 300 burpees instead of what you set out to do! Safety is priority number one.

Verbal Instructions and Cues

Because Caveman Circuits move rather quickly, it's essential that a Caveman Trainer always uses a loud and clear voice to relay instructions. Cues should stay simple and remain consistent so that clients quickly and easily understand the trainer.

For example:

- Start of circuit = "GO"
- Nearing end of station = "5, 4, 3, 2, 1"
- Changing of station = "CHANGE"
- Quick drink break or rest = "DRINK BREAK"
- Nearing end of circuit = "2 STATIONS LEFT"
- Last station of circuit = "LAST STATION, GIVE IT YOUR ALL"
- End of circuit = "STOP TRAINING"

Do not change the cues as it will confuse people.

Be sure to project your voice at a loud enough volume so that each participant can clearly hear you over their heavy breathing and any moving equipment. Consider shouting "change" at a higher volume than your countdown, so that everyone understands that it's time to move to the next station. A firm and assertive tone will also galvanize participants into moving to the next station swiftly.

When participants reach the final station in the circuit, announce this clearly. Explain that you expect participants to give their all and to finish the workout strong. As a trainer, encourage your clients as necessary to ensure they use every last bit of reserve energy in their tank. Possible encouraging remarks include reminding participants that they'll be done for the day after this final station, and that they will feel a great sense of accomplishment if they push through. Remark how finishing strong in spite of their fatigue will develop their mental toughness.

Motivation, Pushing and Encouragement

Also important to a Caveman Trainer is being able to get the most out of your clients. Don't be afraid to push participants to their maximum abilities. If you find them walking to a station, tell them to run. Add on an extra station if there is too much walking. If a participant is not putting in enough repetitions on a station and resting, don't be hesitant to do what you need to do to push them. Tell them to pick up and ask them why they are here. Tell them not to be afraid to push to the puking point. If they need to puke they can do so and then get back into the circuit.

With that said, be sure that you choose your words carefully. A Caveman Trainer should motivate, not belittle. Do not curse. If the entire group is not working hard, consider picking someone out of the group that you think can handle it and use them as an example. Make it harder for them and tell the others that they can expect the same if they don't pick it up.

Understand that at times participants may get offended and mistake your encouragement for belittling or bullying. If you think someone might have been offended during the class, take them aside at the end of the class and explain your reasoning. Explain to them that this is Cavemantraining and that they pay you to push them. They pay you to correct their form and technique. They pay you to get the maximum out of them. It's likely that they will understand you after you talk to them. If not, it may be better to extinguish your training relationship as this may not be the right type of training for them. Do not adjust the training methodology for anyone.

Circuit Layout

Organize stations so that there is a logical flow to the layout. This will allow participants to quickly and easily move from one station to the next and will minimize confusion. You can use a U formation, circular, zig-zag or any other format that suits the layout of your premises. If any part of the circuit layout is not obvious, use chalk to draw arrows to the station, or make signs with clear instructions. You should also point out where all the stations are, including those that may not be immediately obvious, during the initial instructions prior to the workout.

Each station should be marked with a cone so that those working out can quickly spot and recognize the location of each station. Participants will be extremely fatigued during workouts so be sure each station is easy to find.

In addition to the cone, clearly label each station with the name of the exercise to be performed. In many cases, the equipment for the exercises will naturally mark out the exercise station. In cases where there is no equipment for the exercise, use chalk on the floor or make a sign with the name of the exercise.

Have alternate weights available at a station for those that require a lighter weight.

Once setup, test the circuit. Ensure there is enough space, so that no one gets in the way of another. Test the flow of the circuit is not confusing. Test if that ball cannot be thrown further than you think it will go. Make sure the exercises are appropriate for the type of class, i.e. beginners, intermediate, advanced or MMA Workouts.

Stressing Nutrition

Always recommend that participants eat something light before their workout. Participants should also make sure that they are well hydrated before each workout. Newcomers to the circuit sessions often make the mistake of not eating before coming for their workout only to hit the wall halfway through the workout. Having a small meal of moderate to slow-digesting carbohydrates and protein one to two hours before exercise will ensure that participants have enough fuel to complete the workout. One to two hours should also be enough time for the food to be digested. Also, recommend that participants consume approx half a litre (14 to 20 oz.) of water two to four hours before their workout. Participants will cool themselves more efficiently and be able to provide their muscles with more fuel if they're properly hydrated. Explain to them that without the fuel from food and proper hydration their body cannot perform and as a result they will not receive the full benefit of the workout.

Note: It's a good idea to share this information with participants prior to them arriving for the circuit workout.

Use the cool down period to stress the importance of post-workout nutrition. Although participants may not feel like eating immediately after the workout, remind them that taking in a meal that consists of both protein and carbohydrates within 45 minutes to an hour of exercise will help to develop muscle mass and improve recovery. Failure to eat after exercise results in the body breaking down muscle tissue for fuel. Participants who struggle to eat a full meal so soon after training can consider having a small post-workout meal within an hour of the workout to prevent catabolism, and a larger meal an hour or two after that. Remind participants to continue to hydrate themselves throughout the day to replace lost fluids, and advise beginners to keep moving and to stretch following workouts to minimize soreness.

Bonus: How To Run Caveman Boot Camp

- Group training in a Boot camp environment
- Your instructional skills—it's not just about yelling!
- Command, control and instructional techniques
- Structuring your boot camp
- Boot camp and outdoor fitness testing techniques

Do as you're told!
Our Caveman fitness boot camp is based on the military principles of training, with discipline, but without belittling people. No screaming and especially no cursing. We pride ourselves on our motivational approach!

Most Important
Check form and technique of the recruits all the time. This is the most important thing to remember and the most important part of your job as Boot Camp instructor. Incorrect form or technique can injure recruits. You are there to prevent this from happening.

We are not here to get fit ourselves! We need to be watchful, encourage and motivate all the time. If you need a workout then organize one with the business and/or other staff.

Generic Expectations
Exhaust the recruits to their maximum capabilities. We want to see them flabbergasted and sweating. This is what they are expecting from us. We push recruits to "their limits", not anybody else's.

The session always needs to keep going. No stopping or waiting for too long, for example while recruits are having drinks. Set a time limit, i.e. "You have 8 seconds to grab a drink and be back at baseline." Keep an eye out for the ones that slack off., but also keep an eye out for the ones that really do look like they need more time.

Roll Call
A roll call is to be performed at the start of every session. You need to take note of the people that did not show, as they need to receive penalties next session – the roll call also helps you to remember people's names.

Always ask if any recruits have any injuries before starting any type of exercise, and keep track of them throughout the session. Make sure you adjust the exercises to what they can do, if anything at all. Don't be scared to send a recruit home if you feel they are in no state to exercise, for example if they are sick, didn't eat enough, or are hung over etc.

Discipline and Strictness

Remember this is Boot Camp, not Chat Camp. people need to stand in line, legs apart and hands behind back, (STAND TO ATTENTION!) no hands in pockets or on hips. The same is expected from instructors. If people are talking too much or not paying attention, give them penalties. The type of penalties are up to you, but some examples are push ups, crunches, planks, burpees etc. Remember, you are in charge. Recruits will try and get away with things, or test how far they can push you, and get away with not doing what you ask.

People need to show up on time, be ready on time, and finish on time. It is very important that the sessions start and end at the same time every day. People need to get to work in the morning and count on the session finishing on time.

If someone talks back to you, give them penalties, and without a doubt, you will encounter people talking back at you, making jokes etc. This is all good, but discipline needs to be shown, and repercussions will follow. This does not have to be in a mean and negative way. You can respond to the joke but still give penalties, for example, "Yes very funny, now get down and give me 20."

If you find penalizing the offender does not work, then penalize the whole group except the offender. You'll find this will work.

Some phrases you can shout out when giving penalties.

Get down and give me 20.

Has anyone else got something to say?

Why don't we all have a laugh and get it out of our system (laugh with them); give them penalties when done.

Chatting during the session needs to be minimized; a boot camp is not a chat camp. If recruits are allowed to talk when they want, they are not paying attention to the instructions given, they are not giving it their all, and are not focusing on results.

A Boot Camp instructor always needs to wear the right attire to demand respect -- a company shirt and hat, and preferably camo shorts or pants.

Communicating with Recruits

Good voice projection is required. You need their full attention and the recruits need to know that you are in CHARGE!

There is no cursing in Boot Camp. Keep people in line through penalties and motivation. Never use obscene language.

When giving instructions, be clear with what you expect from the recruits. For example when warming-up, don't just say "Let's go!", tell them exactly what you expect from them. Say "OK we are going on a warm up. Let's slowly start running towards the houses, or the end of the road (and give direction)."

Don't give too many instructions at once. People get confused, or don't remember all of it, and they'll get annoyed. Instructions are to be given bit by bit if they entail several steps. If the drill consists of several steps, then provide the first step of the drill, and be ready at the next step to provide further details.

Blow your whistle when you require the attention of the group, however, use common sense. Keep in mind that if you are in a park where there are a lot of houses around, and it is early in the morning, keep it to a minimum and a short firm whistle. When training in areas like a sporting complex, whistles can be used with maximum force.

When demonstrating a particular exercise, do it towards recruits, not with your back to them. This can be very frustrating for everyone as some may not hear or see exactly what you are doing.

5 Steps of Instructing

- Communicate verbally
- Demonstrate
- Observe
- Correct
- Motivate

Setup of Drills and Exercises
When using markers (for eg, suicides) make sure you use ones that are clearly visible, and put them on both sides of the group. Make sure you use different colors to identify what color they are running to. Eg, 10m (red) 20m (Blue) etc, etc.

All drills, exercises and stretches need to be performed in a uniform order. Wait till everyone is present, rush the ones that you are waiting on. Make sure to keep the group busy during this time, for example, with isometric exercises like squat, push-up, plank position etc. They must hold this till everyone is present. You do not want people standing around doing nothing.

If you find a drill or exercise is not working, i.e. recruits do not understand it, it looks like they are getting bored, or not getting a work-out, change the drill immediately. If you cannot come up with another drill in time, just tell them to drop and give you 50, or send them for a lap around the oval while you think of something else.

When coming up with exercises, make sure you have alternatives in mind for recruits that cannot perform the exercise for some reason or other, i.e. injury or just not fit enough.

Make sure the obstacles are setup prior to commencing Boot Camp if there are any drills that require setup.

Creating Groups and Leaders

When splitting up groups (for example injured and non-injured, extremely fit and not so fit) always make sure you either assign a sergeant to one of the groups or make sure you give instructions to both groups.

Use your initiative. If you think you can use someone from the recruits as a leader, do so, but be clear about what you expect from that leader. Don't just say, "OK Frank, you are the leader. Let's go," instead, make it clear what you expect from them. For example, "OK Frank, you are the leader on this warm-up. Please start running to the end of the field and wait for me there, but keep active by running on the spot once you get there."

Motivate people lagging behind. Assign a leader if you are the only sergeant in the group, and get the leading people to move further with sufficient instructions. The people lagging behind need your motivation the most. Motivating from a distance is not the answer.

If there are fit people present who finish their exercises way before the rest of the team, just give them more. For example, double their amount to what everyone else is doing, tell them to keep doing exercise X,Y,Z until everyone is finished. Do not let them stand around or catch their breath.

Base

The base is where everyone meets for Boot Camp. This is where the roll call will be held and most of the drills and exercises will commence. The base line can be created with markers, talc powder or any other material that creates a clear line for people to stand behind. Put their bottles and towels behind.

Starting Time

Always arrive earlier than the recruits. Ask any new people to come a little earlier if it is their first time so you can have a little chat with them, see if they have any injuries or questions.

New Arrivals

Always make it a point to greet and meet every new member, introduce them to the rest of the recruits and make them feel welcome.

Penalties

Penalties are given to keep recruits in line, so they can see that there are repercussions for their actions. Always keep the fitness of the individual in mind when giving penalties. 10 push-ups can be a punishment for one but a breeze for another.

Penalties are given for the following, but not limited to:
- Showing up late, 25 to 50 penalties per minute late
- Talking back
- Talking during the session
- Not performing the exercise correctly

- Not giving it their all
- Not wearing the right attire

The following are some penalties to give, but not limited to:

- Tire around the neck
- Carry log or kettlebell throughout the session
- Squats
- Star jumps
- Push ups
- Burpees

Keep track of penalties. If a recruit has more than 50 penalties it's usually not possible for the recruit to perform all penalties at once. They will need to be performed throughout the session, and if need be, continued in the next session. Try not to make the rest of the group wait on someone performing penalties.

Don't be scared to give penalties. This is what people paid for, and you are in control! If you think someone has taken offense, have a little chat with them afterwards. Let them know it's nothing personal; you are here to get them fit and push them to their limits.

Make sure you give out penalties once in a while (at least once a week). Find a reason. This is part of Boot Camp. When done properly and by choosing the right person to dish out to, it can also be a bit of fun.

Fun and Games
Although the Caveman Boot Camps are very strict, they will include fun and games once in a while to break things up and work on team bonding. Whatever the game, recruits still need to work to their maximum abilities, no slacking off. Some of the games that can be played are, but not limited to:

- Bib tag
- Dodge ball
- Soccer
- Red rover
- Stuck in the mud

Difference Between 'Workout' and 'Complex'?

If you've heard the two mentioned and wondered what the difference is, read on.

To demonstrate the difference between a Workout and a Complex, let me first present to you a Kettlebell Workout and then a Kettlebell Complex.

Kettlebell Workout
- 10 x Double Kettlebell Swing
- 5 x Single Kettlebell Press Left
- 5 x Single Kettlebell Press Right
- 10 x Squat
- 10 x Kettlebell Renegade Rows

5 rounds

Kettlebell Complex
10 x Single Kettlebell Double Arm Swing
Clean
10 x Alternating Halo
Throwout
5 x Figure 8 Squat Left
Catch
5 x Figure 8 Squat Right
Catch
5 x Around The Body Left
Catch
5 x Around The Body Right
5 rounds

If you are familiar with kettlebells, perhaps you will see that with the workout you will be performing a set number of reps, put the kettlebells down, and move to another position to perform an exercise that cannot seamlessly be performed straight after.

There is absolutely nothing wrong with a well designed kettlebell workout that reaches the sett goals.

A kettlebell complex is intelligently designed in such a way that each exercise can seamlessly be performed one after the other, with no or minimal interruption to the flow. When you design a kettlebell complex it is important to explain the transitioning to your clients and write down cues for transitions. In this case the transitions are clean, throwout and catch.

In summary, the main difference between a workout and a complex is that a complex must have exercises that flow seamlessly from one into the next. A complex does not have to be done with kettlebells. It can quite easily be a complex with just bodyweight or other exercises. One such example is the following bodyweight complex I designed and call 'Corpus Construo'.

The complex consists of:

- Deck Squat
- Tricep Push-up
- Cross Mountain Climber

Perform 1 to 10 repetitions of the above complex.

- Deck Squat
- Tricep Push-up
- Cross Mountain Climber
- Jump

Perform 11 to 20 repetitions of the complex with one exercise added.

- Deck Squat
- Tricep Push-up
- Cross Mountain Climber
- Jump
- Tuck Jump

21 to 30 repetitions

- Deck Squat
- Tricep Push-up
- Cross Mountain Climber
- Jump
- Tuck Jump
- Jumping Jack

31 to 40 repetitions

- Deck Squat
- Tricep Push-up
- Cross Mountain Climber
- Jump
- Tuck Jump
- Jumping Jack
- Squat

41 to 50 repetitions

Let me know your time. I'm also looking forward to seeing videos posted on YouTube for this workout. Feel free to ask me anything about the transition or exercises.

Quick tip: If you want to upset a professional Kettlebell Trainer, ask them if you can book in for a *Kettle Ball* session. :-)

Looking for adventure? Add an experience!

All the photos you see in this book were taken during one of my outdoor adventures in the beauty of Spain. I'm available for personal training, group fitness, workshops, boot camps, seminars, hikes, challenges and other adventures.

Anything is possible:

- Mountain
- Beach
- River
- CrossFit gym
- Running
- Walking
- 1 hour
- 8 hours
- 2 days
- Filming
- Education
- Fun
- Challenges
- Training
- Working out
- Beginner to advanced
- Easy to hardcore

Watch a video where I take two people on an 11 hour hike with kettlebells: https://go.cavemantraining.com/kb-wk-vid110

To book

Me@tacofleur.com

+34 663 468 840

Inspiration

With this book, videos, and photos I also hope to inspire you to take your kettlebells outside, outside of the confinement of the gym, house, box, or other area you use to workout. I also hope to inspire you to go more barefoot, during training, but also outside of training when possible. Like the beach, nature walks, etc. I know this will help you internally as well as externally.

I hope you'll go and see parts of the world you've never seen before, I hope you'll open your mind a little to let different things in, or at least be open to them, research them, experiment with them, and don't just follow the path laid out for everyone by society. Make the best of your life, live the happiest, healthiest, and strongest life you can live. You only got one. Make it the best one.

Good or bad?

Did this book provide, as promised, 40+ awesome kettlebell workouts? If so, I would really appreciate it if you could take a few moments of your time and provide an honest review on Amazon. The more reviews it gets, the more people will see the book, and the more people we can get interested in the art of kettlebell training. Thanks in advance.

Rate it here go.cavemantraining.com/kbwc-link19

Disappointed?

It's possible. It's hard to write or create workouts that suit everyone, so I won't be offended if you're disappointed, the only thing I asked of you is that you allow me to make it up to you. I want everyone to be happy with their purchase. Email me, seriously, just let me know why and I will rectify it.

me@tacofleur.com

VOUCHER CODES

To get the course on Udemy you can directly access the following link and get 50% off.
https://www.udemy.com/kettlebell-training-for-beginners/?couponCode=CT35I1VZ09

CT35I1VZ09

Printable Copy

To get your printable copy of these workouts please use the following voucher code.

COUPON CODE: **RP8ZDSHH**

You can add the ebook to your basket and use the code at checkout here www.cavemantraining.com/shop/ebook/printable-kettlebell-workouts-and-challenges-2-0-for-amazon-purchase/ friendly URL go.cavemantraining.com/kbwc-link18

Note: You will need to use the same email address you used when purchasing this book. The print version will be imprinted and digitally signed with your personal details, hence, it should not be shared with anyone else.

To get 50% discount on the kettlebell training app that allows you to cast the videos to your TV or watch on your phone email me on me@tacofleur.com with the subject *"Voucher code for kb app from Amazon book"* and include the following verification code in the body "**291VM9OC**". I will reply to your email and send you a unique voucher code with detailed instructions to get 50% off on the app. I can't include the codes in the book due to the way Google handles the codes.

Details of the app here play.google.com/store/apps/details?id=com.cavemantraining.kb.beginners

Ready to move to the next level in your kettlebell training?
Check out the following books by Cavemantraining

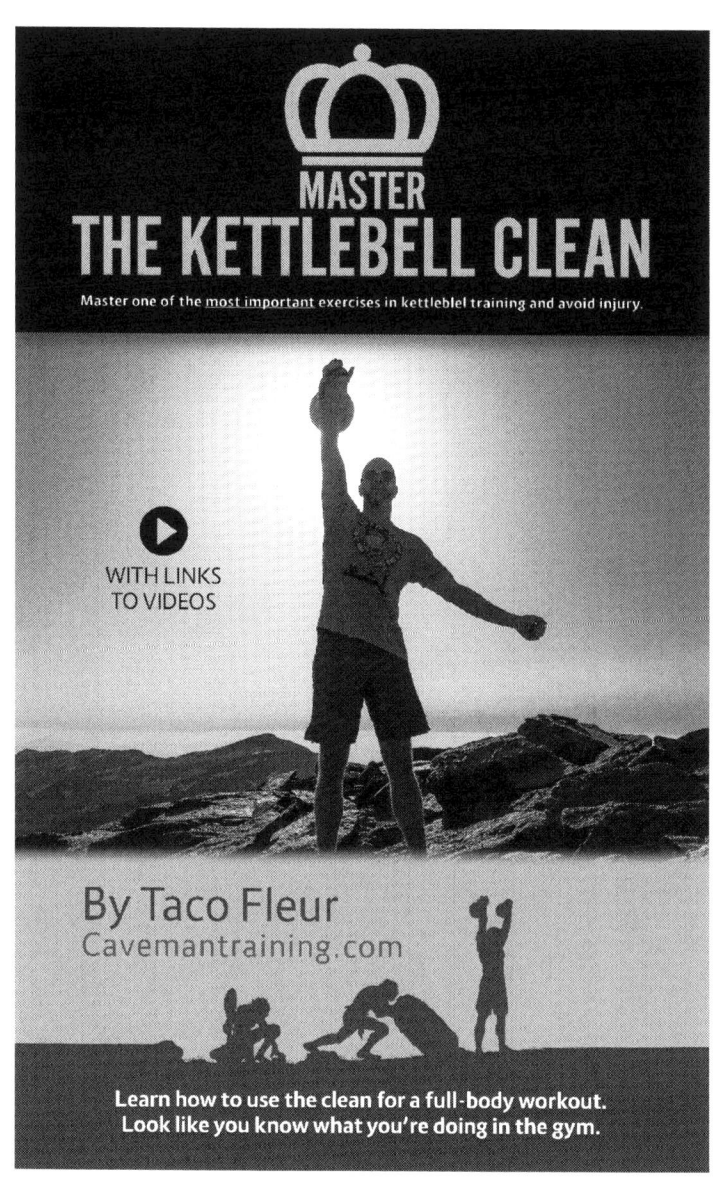

https://amzn.to/2FOJfmy

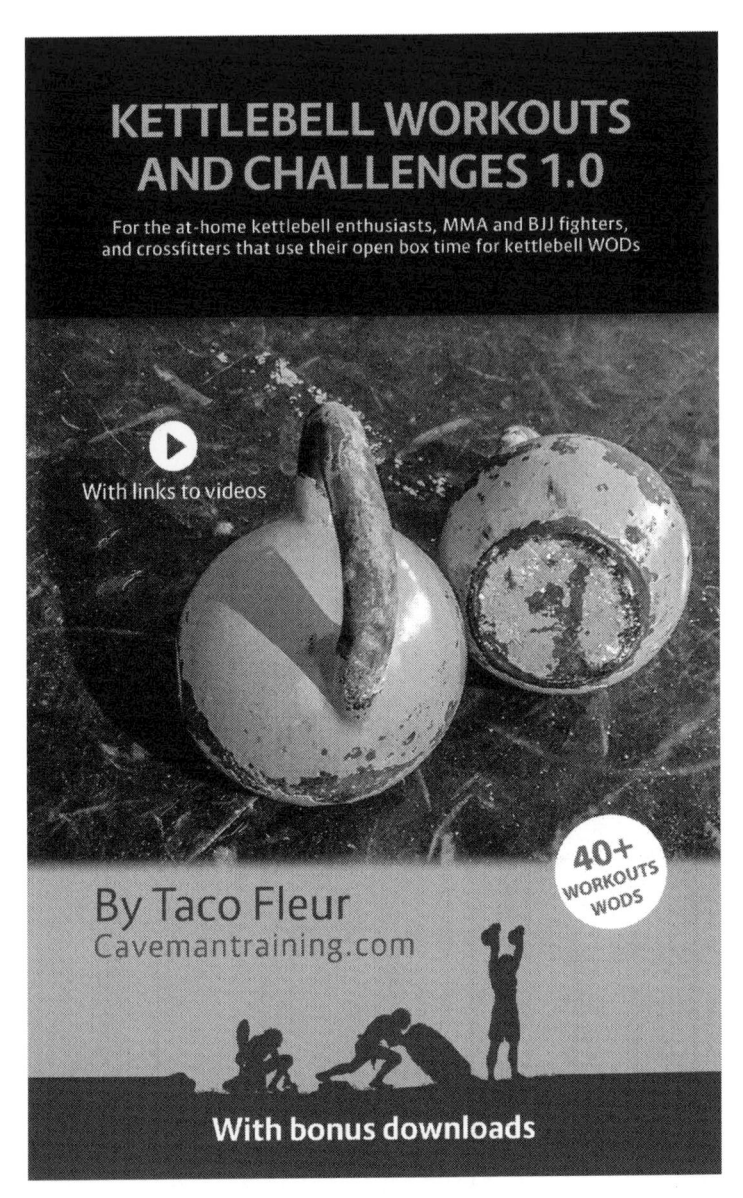

https://amzn.to/2FHgfwN

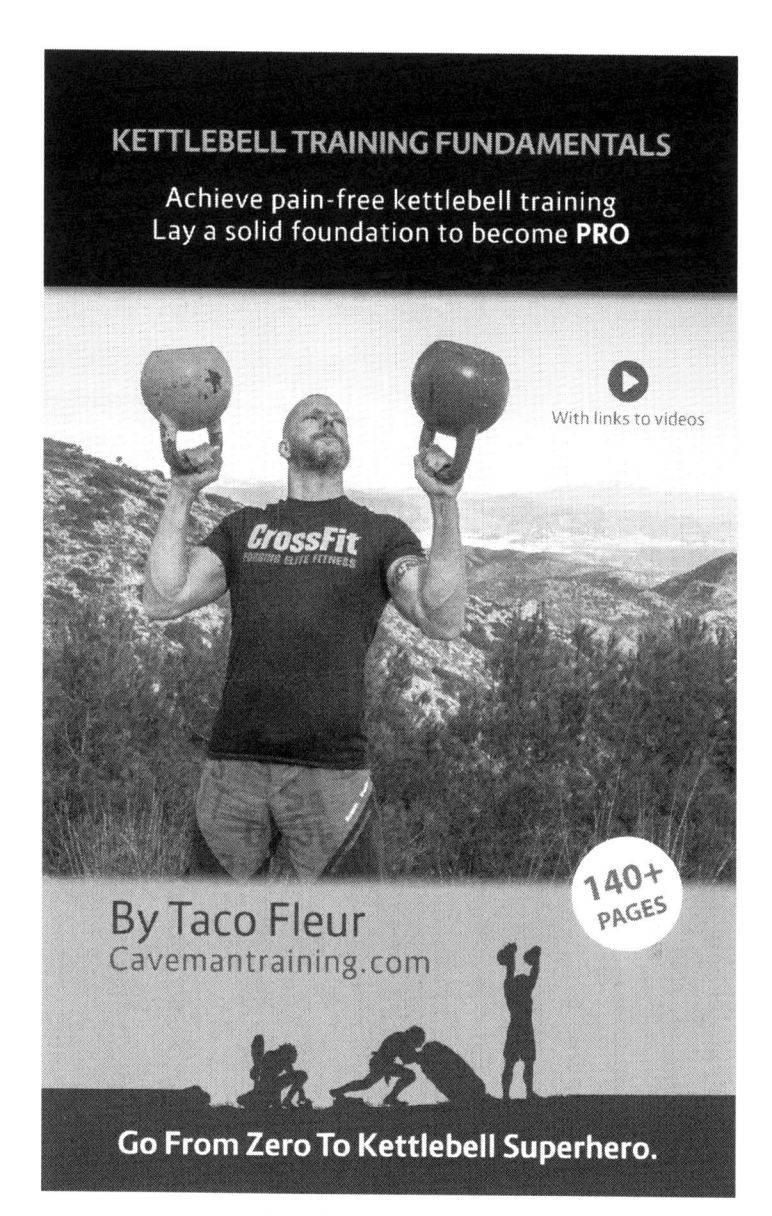

https://amzn.to/2TQYvnC

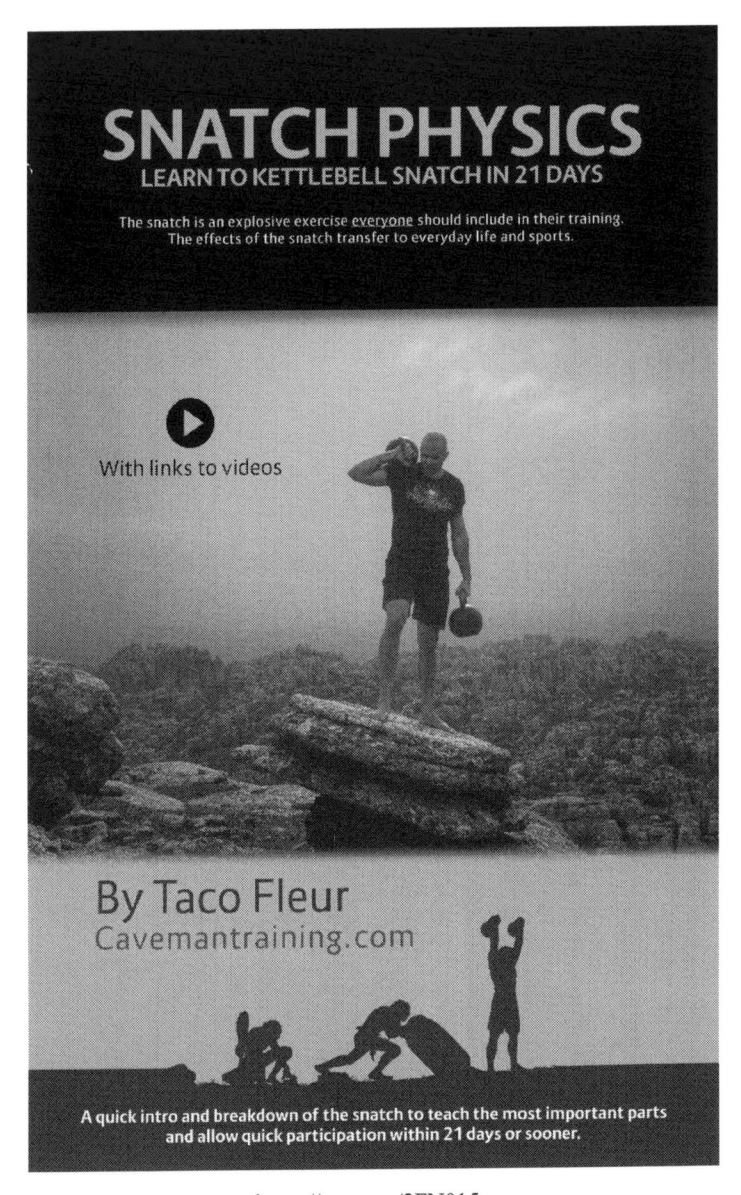

https://amzn.to/2FN015v

All books can be found here on Amazon amzn.to/2FUyaQX or on www.cavemantraining.com/shop

I hope you enjoyed this book and I hope to see more of you on your kettlebell journey, come and join me on Facebook and say hi:

The biggest kettlebell training group on Facebook www.facebook.com/groups/KettlebellTraining

Kettlebell workouts on Facebook www.facebook.com/groups/kettlebell.workout

Kettlebell training group on Reddit www.reddit.com/r/kettlebell_training

Hundreds of videos on YouTube youtube.com/Cavemantraining

Me on Instagram instagram.com/realcavemantraining/

If you can find a couple of seconds to rate the book on Amazon I would really appreciate it. go.cavemantraining.com/kbwc-link19

Thanks

Taco Fleur

Printed in Great Britain
by Amazon